Praise for *The Fall of Roe:*

'Searing and int… porting'

'*The Fall of Roe* … d outside the cabin door, … by those who lived w… ublic service . . . A … gainst legal abortion is tied inextricably to the fight for America's soul'
New York Magazine

'A rollicking read, full of complicated but passionate advocates on both sides. It's a tale of religion, power, politics and ultimately of the position of women in American society; an account of how a driven minority can triumph over a complacent majority. It's riveting'
Telegraph

'Amid it all, reporters Elizabeth Dias and Lisa Lerer were taking notes . . . The result is *The Fall of Roe* . . . A nonpartisan narrative chronicling the past decade's political chess game'
Bustle

'*The Fall of Roe* is more than an account of history. It's a warning about the future' ***HuffPost***

'A rich narrative' ***Rolling Stone***

'A fantastic narrative of the last decade that opened my eyes to how abortion rights fell apart in this country'
NPR

'The book's greatest strength is the authors' comprehensive and incisive approach to explaining that 'Roe did not just fall once, on

June 24, 2022. Roe collapsed over a transformational decade.' Devoid of rhetoric, this even-handed work exemplifies outstanding reportage' ***Kirkus*, starred review**

'The subtitle of this new book by *New York Times* reporters Dias (religion) and Lerer (politics) underscores how the conservative religious faction's far-reaching and secretive strategy of putting anti-abortion activists in the spotlight changed rights for Americans in June 2022. As the authors warn, if Democrats don't change their own strategy, we might see an entirely different nation emerge because of a single issue'
Los Angeles Times

'Great reporting by Elizabeth Dias and Lisa Lerer on how conservatives overturned Roe while everyone else slept'
Jane Mayer, *New York Times* bestselling author of *Dark Money*

'Want to read a great story with a terrible ending? Lisa Lerer and Elizabeth Dias have your back on how no one had ours'
Taffy Brodesser-Akner, *New York Times* bestselling author of *Fleishman is in Trouble*

'This book is as if the blurry portrait of abortion and womanhood that we've seen over the last several decades has finally come into view and can be captured in screaming color'
Elysse Wagner

'Brilliant. A must-read that will both chill and galvanize readers'
Michelle Bowdler, author of *Is Rape a Crime?*

'A definitive historical account of how Roe v. Wade came to be overturned' **Kirsten Powers, *New York Times* bestselling author of *The Silencing***

'Deeply reported, very needed' **Elizabeth Holmes, *New York Times* bestselling author of *HRH***

THE FALL OF ROE

Elizabeth Dias, national religion correspondent for the *New York Times*, has covered American religion, politics and culture for fifteen years. She has reported from Washington, D.C., the Vatican and across the United States. She is a Livingston Award finalist and a graduate of Wheaton College and Princeton Theological Seminary.

Lisa Lerer, national political correspondent for the *New York Times*, has written about American politics, power and elections for nearly two decades. She has covered five presidential campaigns, the White House and Congress. She was a Nieman Fellow at Harvard University and is a graduate of the University of Pennsylvania and Columbia Journalism School.

THE FALL OF ROE

ELIZABETH DIAS and LISA LERER

MANILLA
PRESS

First published in the US in 2024 by
Flatiron Books, a division of Macmillan Publishers
First published in the UK in 2024
This paperback edition published in the UK in 2025 by
MANILLA PRESS
An imprint of Bonnier Books UK
5th Floor, HYLO, 105 Bunhill Row,
London, EC1Y 8LZ

A CIP catalogue record for this book
is available from the British Library.

ISBN: 978-1-78658-412-0

Also available as an ebook

1 3 5 7 9 10 8 6 4 2

Typeset by IDSUK (Data Connection) Ltd
Printed and bound in Great Britain by Clays Ltd, Elcograf S.p.A.

MIX
Paper | Supporting
responsible forestry
FSC® C018072

The authorised representative in the EEA is
Bonnier Books UK (Ireland) Limited.
Registered office address: Floor 3, Block 3, Miesian Plaza,
Dublin 2, D02 Y754, Ireland
compliance@bonnierbooks.ie
www.bonnierbooks.co.uk

To our grandmothers, mothers, and daughters

CONTENTS

PREFACE

We set out to answer one question: How, after nearly fifty years, did Roe fall?

As journalists, we have reported on abortion in American politics and religion for most of our careers. We thought we knew the answer. It seemed simple. The decision was the result of a change in ideology at the Supreme Court ushered in by former president Donald Trump, who placed three conservative justices onto the court over the course of a single term.

But that narrative, we soon learned, kept hidden an even bigger story.

The political tale we uncovered is explosive. But the story of the fall of Roe is also a deeply human one, bound up with foundational questions of life, liberty, and the pursuit of happiness. The battle over abortion is not just about whether a woman can end a pregnancy. It is about what it means to be a woman in America at all. It is about the power of belief and the potency of denial. And it is a story of a nation fighting over what it wants to become.

This book reveals that previously unseen history. It is based on more than three hundred and fifty interviews, along with court records, academic archives, private documents, and thousands of contemporaneous news stories. We traveled to sixteen states and the District of Columbia to interview elected officials, top religious leaders, doctors, advocates, and lawyers. Our reporting took us inside the White House and statehouses, and into the back rooms of abortion clinics and the private chapel of an antiabortion pregnancy center. Our investigation discovered secret meetings, personal motivations, and a tightly networked ecosystem of lawyers, politicians, and activists who powered one of the most significant political resurgences the United States has ever seen.

History could have turned out very differently. Ever since *Roe v. Wade*, the revolutionary 1973 Supreme Court ruling that guaranteed a constitutional right to abortion, a conservative grassroots coalition had fought against the outcome. But they were losing. A majority of Americans wanted abortion to be legal, even if they disagreed on what exactly that should mean. Then, when President Barack Obama was in the White House, something began to change. A new generation of right-wing activists began to gain strength, even as the prevalence of their Christian values declined in a changing America. Methodically and secretly, an elite strike force of Christian lawyers and power brokers orchestrated a campaign to end abortion rights and remake American womanhood. The result was a strategic, top-down takeover at every level of American political and legal life.

Their opponents didn't see what was coming until it was far too late. After so many decades of taking Roe for granted, supporters of abortion rights grew dangerously complacent and disorganized in ways that made them slow to appreciate the severity of the threat. American women had more power than ever before, but the feminist movement suffered one of the biggest political defeats in American history.

These conservative Catholic and evangelical Christian operators believed they were fighting the biggest moral battle of the modern age, and forced America to debate on their terms. But despite their public appeals, they did not convince broad swaths of Americans of the righteousness of their cause. Instead, they remained a minority, and leveraged the structures of American democracy in their favor, building a framework strong enough to withstand not only the political system but also a society moving rapidly against them. They took power to remake the nation in their image. And they were far more organized than their opponents or the public ever knew.

Our book exposes legal maneuvers to craft abortion bans and game the courts, the political plan to make the Trump administration an antiabortion machine, and the infighting among abortion-rights activists that crippled their ability to fight back.

Through it all, we found that abortion is far more than simply another political clash. Again and again, as we spoke with sources across the ideological spectrum, we found that legal and political ambitions were rooted in stories of pregnancy and parenthood, and of obligations to one's self and to a future generation. The result here is two narratives: one drama that played out in courtrooms, statehouses, and voting booths, and another more intimate story inside abortion clinics and antiabortion pregnancy centers. The former is the driving story line in our book, taking place over ten years, the final decade of the Roe era in American life. We open each section of the book with the latter, a snapshot into the lives of women across the country in June 2022, the month the nation changed. All the named clients in the abortion clinic and pregnancy center gave us permission to use their full, legal names. However, given sensitivities to privacy, we chose to give every client a pseudonym.

At its core, the issue of abortion rights is about medical care and reproduction. One in four American women will have an abortion in her lifetime. But the meaning of abortion in American life encompasses so much more. It is a symbol of morality and culture, race and religion, and, of course, women and their role in the American experiment. Abortion, for better or worse, has been bound up with the story of the advancement of women for the past century. And the emerging dynamics of the new post-Roe reality will define American women—and American politics—for years to come.

The story of the fall of Roe is, quite literally, the story of the next generation of the nation. In the end, our first question led us to another, even greater one: What is America becoming?

To understand that, you have to go back to the moment Roe fell and then wind back the clock.

A • bor • tion: from the Latin *abortiō*, "abortion, miscarriage," from the verb *abortire*, meaning

to disappear

to be lost

to miscarry

PART I

THE RIGHTEOUS FIGHT

JUNE 2022

Cincinnati, Ohio

On the Catholic calendar, it was the holy day of the Sacred Heart of Jesus, and the women who led Pregnancy Center East offered up their prayers.

One prayed for their clients who were upset about untimely pregnancies. Another prayed for nonbelievers to know they were loved by God. Another for the strength to endure hardship. The center's director, Laura Curran, prayed for the nation.

"Lord, we wait anxiously for the Supreme Court decision," she said. "We pray for protection for all Supreme Court justices, all churches, all pregnancy centers, and all those who are at risk of violence after this decision comes out."

Curran and her small team were gathered in their makeshift chapel, as they were every morning before the clients arrived. Really, it was just a small conference room, with bright fluorescent lighting and dull office carpet. But at one end near the ceiling, there was a broad stained-glass panel, with white doves flanking a newborn baby Jesus, who beamed down rays of gold. Below that was a small wooden altar, carved with Christianity's timeless words, "In Remembrance of Me."

Tucked between the legs of the altar, they had added something else: A woven bassinet on a wooden rocker. Empty. Waiting.

The women joined in an ancient prayer.

"Hail Mary, full of grace, the Lord is with thee. Blessed art thou among women, and blessed is the fruit of thy womb, Jesus."

The words echoed the old Gospel story: An angel appeared to a young woman, Mary, and declared that the power of the Most High would overshadow her, and she would conceive. Mary was greatly troubled, the scripture said, but she submitted to the word of the Lord and gave birth to the Son of God.

From her chair next to the altar, Curran could see through the cracked door to the lobby. A woman had arrived and was speaking quietly with a receptionist at the front desk. Time to work.

Curran checked her phone on her way to the room where they processed the pregnancy tests—nothing fancy, just the early detection ones from the pharmacy. It was just after 10:00 a.m. When she had woken up that morning, she had had a strange feeling that the decision might come today. But so far, there was nothing. She focused on the tasks in front of her.

The sonographer passed her on her way to see their first client. Pregnancy Center East was not a doctor's office. It was one of about 2,700 similar centers across America that opposed abortion and intervened to prevent women from ending their pregnancies. They often offered free, basic ultrasounds in hopes that women would see their babies and choose to give birth.

The adoption representative was not in yet, but color-printed booklets of families wanting children lay ready on a table. That had been Curran once, before she got pregnant with "Luke the Fluke," as she lovingly called him. Still, she and her husband adopted four children with an array of health needs. Abortion, Curran believed, should be illegal at conception.

At 10:10 a.m., a phone notification popped up. Curran called out to her staff, her low heels clicking quickly back across the lobby toward her office.

"The decision is out! The decision is out!" she said, passing the women behind the front desk without stopping.

She reached her computer and tapped the keyboard. The women crowded into her office doorway as she struggled to find the opinion online. The Supreme Court's website kept crashing. The whole world was trying to load the same page. Curran kept searching.

"CBS has it on a special report . . . There's an appendix . . . This is them commenting on it," she murmured, trying to piece it together. "What's the decision? What's the decision?"

Curran had opposed abortion her whole life. She remembered when, in high school, a godfather of the antiabortion movement, Dr. John C. Willke, came to the gym and played a video of a suction abortion. The sound still echoed in her head. She and her friends bought silver cuff bracelets, stamped with the Greek letters alpha and omega and the date Roe v. Wade made abortion legal, January 22, 1973.

Suddenly she saw it. Printed on page one of the Supreme Court's 213-page ruling. The words she and the women huddled at the door had longed to hear for decades:

> *Held: The Constitution does not confer a right to abortion; Roe and Casey are overruled; and the authority to regulate abortion is returned to the people and their elected representatives.*

For seventeen seconds, silence filled the room.

Finally, Curran raised a tissue beneath her blue-rimmed glasses and straightened herself. The ruling was 6–3, someone said. Roe v. Wade *was dead. The constitutional right to have an abortion in America was gone.*

At that moment, abortion was legal for up to twenty-two weeks of pregnancy in Ohio. Within hours, a trigger law would go into effect, and nearly all abortions in the state would become illegal. By nightfall, the procedure was banned almost entirely in eight more states.

Curran could now engrave a new date on the other side of her silver cuff: June 24, 2022.

The women at the door seemed frozen, unsure whether to hug or cry or pray. It felt like the day the Berlin Wall fell, everything at once incredible and hyperreal, Curran thought. "It's going to save so many lives," she whispered. "Women are going to need us now more than ever."

No one knew what it all meant, who was safe, and who was not.

At 10:48 a.m., Curran announced a precaution to her staff. "I'm going to go lock the inside door."

At the other end of the center, a woman lay her body down on the ultrasound table. Bright lights to kill bacteria gave off a neon glow.

Her pregnancy had come as a surprise, and her sister had suggested she come here. She could see the black-and-white movement on the screen. A poster on the wall tracked pregnancy development across the first, second, and third trimesters. The sonographer said she was just about twenty weeks along.

The sticky gel dripped over her growing belly. She stared at her sonogram, unaware that beyond these walls, a new America had been born.

Curran kept a sheet of paper on her desk, to the right of her computer. It was an intake form that she'd flipped over to jot down some notes years ago, listening to a speech a professor gave the week of the annual March for Life in 2013 after President Barack Obama was reelected. "40 Years of R vs. W," she had scrawled across the top.

The 1970s were the decade when "pro-life people were blindsided" by Roe and the increasing number of abortions, she said, reading off her sheet. In the 1980s, they got "battle ready" and enlisted evangelical support. In the 1990s, they were "besieged," overwhelmed that their strategies weren't making headway, but then women started to take on leadership positions in the movement. In the 2000s, they were "bewildered," but had gotten more people to believe the fetus was a human, though "women's rights trumped the baby's rights." Then came the 2010s, the rise of social media and a "new feminism" that was conservative, she said. It was the Obama era, when everything was up for grabs.

That was a decade ago, back when all this was unimaginable.

2013–2015

1

The Autopsy

Marjorie Dannenfelser wanted to stand up and scream. She had been in this conference room so many times before, plotting the future of the conservative movement at the weekly invitation-only meeting of Republican power brokers. But today was different: her life's work was under attack.

Dannenfelser had fought for the chance to be in this room, to be part of this coalition. The attendees were a who's who of activists—from fiscal hawks to foreign policy hard-liners to National Rifle Association leaders—who came together every Wednesday at 10:00 a.m. sharp to discuss the future of the Republican Party. People in the know simply called it the "Wednesday Meeting," hosted by the quirky anti-tax guru Grover Norquist.

She wouldn't scream, of course. Dannenfelser stuck out already, a matter-of-fact mother in the largely male world of Republican politics, a Catholic in an increasingly secular Washington, who fought for her cause while shuttling around her five children. She ran on Diet Coke, an endless call list, and weekly Mass. She loved her high school friends, elaborate birthday breakfasts, and being a mom. She rarely lost her cool.

So, this Wednesday in early 2013, Dannenfelser sat and listened. But inside, she fumed. She had already read all one hundred pages of the report that the Republican strategists were presenting that day. It was all anyone in her professional world had been talking about all week. The report was called the *Growth and Opportunity Project*, a new twist on GOP. But everyone knew what it really was. An autopsy of their failures, designed to identify why their party had lost the 2012 election so badly to President Obama and how they needed to change to win.

Ever since she'd arrived in Washington as a young woman, Dannenfelser had devoted herself to a singular cause: ending abortion in America. Her organization, the Susan B. Anthony List, worked to elect like-minded politicians, in hopes that one day they would have enough power in Washington to end abortion rights. SBA was small but it had a vision to convert America to its cause, just as Dannenfelser herself had converted as a student, years ago at Duke University.

As Dannenfelser flipped through the pages, she saw a big warning. America was changing dramatically, making the Republican Party's future "precarious," the strategists said. Relying on voters who were white, male, and older would no longer work. Only 72 percent of voters were now white, down from 88 percent in 1980, they said. White people would be less than half the country by 2050. Young people were "rolling their eyes" at Republican values. Women were trending Democratic. Already, Republicans had lost the popular vote in five of the past six presidential elections.

If Republicans did not change, and change fast, they risked losing again, the strategists warned. These changing demographics seemed like political destiny to them, and this new America could condemn them to defeat for generations. To win, Republicans needed to be more "inclusive and welcoming," especially of women and voters of color, they wrote. And on the bottom of page 8, Dannenfelser saw the phrase that chilled her. Republicans needed to drop reactionary "social issues." Partially that meant opposition to gay marriage. But she knew exactly what else "social issues" meant. It was code for an issue Republican leaders found too damaging, or maybe just too futile, to even name in the report.

Abortion.

The 2012 campaign was—without question—disaster after disaster, both for her issue and for the Republican Party. Months before Election Day, a Republican congressman named Todd Akin, who was running for a Senate seat in Missouri, unexpectedly tanked his campaign in a television interview in which he claimed that women could not become pregnant after being raped.

"If it's a legitimate rape, the female body has ways to try to shut that whole thing down," Akin said, his tanned forehead shining under the studio lights.

Democrats seized the moment. Republicans, they said, were waging a toxic "war on women." Akin, a longtime antiabortion activist who had previously been arrested for protesting clinics, was labeled a Republican embarrassment. Dannenfelser's cause was guilty by association. Mitt Romney, the Republican presidential nominee, abandoned her movement altogether, going out of his way to reassure voters that he had no intention of rolling back federal abortion rights. "There's no legislation with regards to abortion that I'm familiar with that would become part of my agenda," he said in an interview with *The Des Moines Register*.

Akin lost, and Romney and a slew of Republicans lost too. Pundits, Democrats, and even establishment Republican strategists pronounced the religious right and the values it represented all but dead. Abortion was a losing issue for the party, Republican leaders decided. And those like Akin and Dannenfelser, who focused on ending it, were on the wrong side of history. The words of autopsy made it undeniable: nationally, the antiabortion movement was at its lowest point in years.

Listening to the presentation, Dannenfelser could not shake the feeling that Republicans were casting her out of the party that had been her home for her entire political life. Her allies had abandoned her. Even worse, the country had too.

The autopsy didn't say it, but 2012 was a defining year beyond politics. It marked the first time in American history that white

Christians—evangelicals, mainline Protestants, and Catholics—became a minority in America, falling to just below 50 percent of the adult population. When the Susan B. Anthony List started in 1992, white Christians were almost two-thirds of the country, a demographic supermajority. But America was growing more secular with what felt for many in the antiabortion world like alarming speed and society was changing accordingly. The values that many socially conservative Christians saw as a foundation of American life—where family was made by a husband and wife who had children and went to church on Sundays—were falling out of the mainstream. Marriage rates were dropping. States were starting to legalize same-sex marriage. And church membership was declining.

In this new America, abortion was fading as a contentious political issue for many voters, viewed as a concern from a bygone era in which women fought for basic rights, a battle fought by boomer mothers and grandmothers that had largely settled into a stalemate between liberals and conservatives. A majority of Americans accepted *Roe v. Wade* as settled law and supported legal abortion. Many Americans backed some restrictions on the procedure, although they disagreed on what those limits should be. But only 16 percent of Americans believed abortion should be illegal in all circumstances, and just another quarter believed it should be illegal in most circumstances. Dannenfelser and her allies were in this minority.

That minority had a very different vision for America's future. They largely believed that human life began at conception, when sperm and egg fused into a single cell. To them, that cell was a full human being worthy of legal rights, which meant that ending that life through an abortion was child murder and must be outlawed. A country that sanctioned the murder of babies was committing a grave moral injustice, they argued.

"The great call of our time is to reclaim the human center of the abortion debate," SBA wrote in its internal business plan in 2013.

"We do this because every human life is made in the image of God and no innocent life is ever worth sacrificing."

Ever since Roe, abortion opponents felt they were fighting a battle of biblical proportions. And in some ways, they were. The fight over abortion, over women's lives and the children they bear, touched essential questions of human existence and a fundamental one at the heart of American democracy: In the body politic, whose bodies count?

The Supreme Court answered that question for America on a warm January day in 1973, when nine justices—all men—issued one of the most consequential rulings in American history. A woman in America had the right to get an abortion until a fetus could live separately—a point the court called *viability*—which at the time was about twenty-eight weeks into pregnancy. She could make private decisions about her pregnancy with her doctor, without interference from anyone else.

The decision was instantly a symbol so enduring that it burst into American consciousness as a single word—Roe. The ruling was a watershed, hailed as the crowning achievement of liberal feminism, instantly reshaping decades of law and life to follow. The decision changed how millions of women and girls imagined their lives, offering the ability to control their reproductive futures.

Roe was a reformation. And just as quickly, it ushered in a counterreformation.

From the start, most Americans supported legalized abortion in some form, including, at first, key Christian institutions like the evangelical Southern Baptist Convention. But a small group, led by Roman Catholics and soon joined by the conservative evangelicals of the nascent religious right, never accepted the Roe decision as settled law.

For forty years, the antiabortion movement worked and prayed, grasping hope as they wandered in the wilderness of an America where Roe was the law of the land. Every town seemed to have a church with an antiabortion pregnancy ministry, or a

Catholic school that annually sent teenagers to Washington for the March for Life, or a Baptist pastor who preached against the sin of abortion.

The antiabortion movement won some critical victories and lost others. The Supreme Court opened the door to state restrictions on abortion in 1989, with its ruling in *Webster v. Reproductive Health Services*. But three years later, the court said in *Planned Parenthood of Southeastern Pennsylvania v. Casey* that those restrictions could not place an "undue burden" on a woman, a deep blow to activists' efforts to overturn Roe.

At any given moment, changes in the White House, in Congress, in the fifty state legislatures and governors' mansions invigorated one side or the other of the abortion fight. The antiabortion movement persisted, even as it was dwarfed by Planned Parenthood, EMILYs List, and other organizations that supported Democratic women who championed abortion rights. Its determination went beyond politics, driven by a higher call. Dannenfelser dreamed of changing hearts and minds about abortion, of convincing America to end—as the movement so often called it—the "culture of death" that ruled their nation. For her, and the people she represented, the political fight over abortion was at heart a spiritual battle, about the essence of being human and saving America's soul. Her movement did not think simply in electoral cycles. They planned in generations, shaped by twenty centuries of a story that stretched back to a pregnant and likely teenage girl who gave birth to a baby and laid him in a manger. The story of Christianity at the heart of their mission was one of divine birth and of resurrection from the dead.

So where the Republican consultants saw defeat, Dannenfelser saw slow progress. Like the Republican strategists, she and her movement saw Obama as a fundamental threat—an "abortion radical," as SBA called him in campaign ads. Even if Obama didn't expand abortion rights through executive actions, he put two liberal justices on the court, confirmations that ensured that the justices who most vocally opposed Roe—Clarence Thomas, Samuel Alito, and Antonin Scalia—remained a minority.

But just because Obama won a second time did not mean his vision for America would last. Since 2010, Republicans had dramatically expanded their power in the states. They now had unified Republican control of state government in twenty-three states. Democrats held only fourteen. Their party controlled thirty governors' mansions, nearing their all-time high in modern political history, in the 1920s. In Indiana, US representative Mike Pence won his race for governor. Maybe he could run for president, Dannenfelser thought. He was on her advisory board. She'd asked him to consider it before.

In this Wednesday meeting, consultants kept offering solution after solution to a problem Dannenfelser didn't believe was a problem at all. "They can't possibly mean what they say they mean," she thought.

But listening to this presentation by powerful players in her party, she realized her movement needed a new strategy if they wanted to win. For these Republicans, Todd Akin had been a scapegoat. But he could instead be a sacrificial lamb, a lesson for her cause for the future. To make the country in their image, antiabortion activists would start from within their ranks. They would consolidate their power and show Republican leaders that they would not be left behind. And then hope for a miracle.

Dannenfelser knew the zeal of her movement. She saw many people who opposed abortion, who felt that Roe ignored their voice. Official Catholic teaching opposed abortion from conception, rooted in its theology about what it means to be human. And evangelicals often shared similar beliefs, pointing to Bible verses about God knitting humans in their mothers' wombs. She did not see these Americans as a minority but as an untapped political powerhouse that just needed to be activated by the righteousness of her cause. "There's this sleeping giant, political giant," she thought. "You can't outstrip the will of the people."

Yet, abortion opponents did not need to convince a majority to change the country. People with minority positions had changed America on issues from civil rights to women's rights to gay rights, shifting public opinion through yearslong political campaigns. They could enact change beyond their size and often acted against powerful social and political norms. She did not see her cause as rooted in religion but in general human rights.

Other interest groups who came to the meeting never found their mission at risk from the party, even if most Americans disagreed with their positions. She saw the National Rifle Association as a prime example. A majority of Americans favored stricter gun control restrictions, but Republicans didn't dare cross the gun lobby even when the worst happened, like the recent horrific killings of young children at Sandy Hook Elementary School, or as the number of mass shootings increased. Through it all, the NRA held the line, mobilizing its grassroots supporters and donors and refusing to give an inch. The NRA was an unstoppable political machine, Dannenfelser thought, and that was a model for antiabortion activists.

To win there could be no compromise, Dannenfelser decided. If the Republican Party kicked the antiabortion movement out, her activists would dig in. They would do their own polling, she decided. They would find their own experts, doctors, and scientists who supported their mission to counter mainstream scientific and medical views. And they would build policy, messaging, and political institutions to compete with their enemies on their own terms.

"I am not asking anymore," she thought. "It seems impossible, but we are going to do it on our own."

Her strategy reflected the earliest lessons of her movement. John C. Willke, the Catholic doctor from Cincinnati who was a godfather of their cause, argued that to end abortion, they could not speak in religious terms. They needed people to see the fetus as a human and to see their cause as not simply a Catholic issue. "If we make it only a religious question, we lose," he explained once to a University Faculty for Life conference.

Instead, he modeled their activism after the biggest political victory of his time, the Civil Rights Act, and kept in mind something Dr. Martin Luther King Jr. had said in 1962 just before its passage. "It may be true that morality cannot be legislated, but behavior can be regulated," King said. "It may be true that the law cannot make a man love me, but it can keep him from lynching me."

Abortion opponents could not force America to embrace their belief that the first cell of a fetus deserved rights, Willke decided. But their cause could win anyhow if they could pass laws that banned abortion.

And now, in this moment of weakness, Willke's old plan found modern expression in a new cohort. The antiabortion movement was reemerging in conservative states across the country, even as it struggled nationally. The Tea Party Republicans who swept into statehouses and Congress in 2010 ran as economic conservatives, fueled by racial animosity to Obama and a backlash to the financial bailouts of the Great Recession. But they were also powered by antiabortion fervor. The next year, Republican statehouses pushed through a whopping ninety-two new restrictions on abortion, more than in any previous year—"a watershed," bragged their allies. For Dannenfelser and her movement, it was a reason for hope. "A turning point for protecting the unborn is near," she wrote in SBA's internal plan in 2013.

Dannenfelser knew they needed power at the highest levels to lock in these new laws coming from the states. SBA's first target would be to secure antiabortion control of the Senate, people who would vote for antiabortion Supreme Court justices if they got the chance. Next, they would need a president who would appoint those justices. And then they could strike at Roe.

For a brief second, as Grover Norquist's Wednesday meeting ended, Dannenfelser wondered if she was overreacting. She walked out with her longtime strategist and friend, Frank Cannon, president of the American Principles Project, a socially conservative think tank.

"Maybe we should listen more?" she asked him.

"No," he said. "It was as bad as we thought."

Dannenfelser made her decision. Unless their movement fought back, she believed they could lose everything, perhaps forever.

Dannenfelser did not see it then. No one did—not Republican leaders, and certainly not Democrats or the American public. But the autopsy heralded a birth: the final decade of the Roe era in American history had begun.

2

Joan of Arc

Cecile Richards, the head of Planned Parenthood, directed the crowd from her makeshift command station at the center of the rotunda, beneath the dome designed with a giant Texas star. In all her years of organizing, she had never seen energy like this.

It was an afternoon in June 2013, and the line to enter the Senate chamber at the state capitol in Austin snaked up flights of stairs and encircled three levels of balconies. Mothers brought young daughters. Youth organizers brandished signs. People arrived after driving three hours from Houston after work. Women milled about in burnt-orange shirts, heeding the late-breaking call from feminist activists to "come early, stay late, wear orange," the color of the Texas Longhorns and the only shirt shade available for organizers to purchase in large quantities at the last minute. They were a stark contrast to the portraits everywhere of the men who had governored Texas all the way back to the first presidents of the republic, who now stared out from gold frames.

For Richards, this moment was too critical to squander on a rookie organizing mistake. Texas was her home state. It was also where Roe started, when a pregnant waitress in Dallas named Norma McCorvey first filed a lawsuit against the state's abortion ban in 1970. Ever since McCorvey won at the Supreme Court three years later, Texas conservatives had been trying to undo the decision.

This time, their effort at a new abortion ban had reached a new—and potentially far more dangerous—level. But Richards looked around in awe. All these Texans had descended on the capitol to say no. It was a historic display of opposition in a conservative state. Even more dramatic than the women pouring into the Capitol was the scene inside the Senate chamber itself: a petite woman standing tall in salmon-pink running shoes, fighting for all of them.

Wendy Davis, a former teenage mother and current Democratic state senator, was mounting a one-woman stand against the Republican empire of Texas. To her supporters, she was "Joan of Arc," charging into battle for women across the state. "She's carrying every woman in the state of Texas, if you will, on her shoulders," Richards told *The New York Times*.

Richards was impossible to miss in the crowd. Tall and slim, with a shock of white-blond hair and a slight Texas drawl, she was a politician in her own right, even if she still saw herself as the rabble-rousing union organizer she once was. Always impeccably tailored, usually styled in a bright sheath dress, Richards was warm, while holding back just enough to reveal only what she wanted seen. The daughter of the late Texas governor Ann Richards, a legendary personality and feminist icon, Richards seemed to know just about everyone in the capitol on that day. There were friends from her mother's political campaigns, members of the state legislature, and old Texas political hands, the lawyers and troublemakers who had been part of the stagnating liberal movement in the state for years. She fielded text updates from staffers inside the chamber and calls from Democratic officials who wanted reports.

Outside the building, there were shouts and protests. Inside, Richards wanted everyone to follow the rules, shared in advance by the coalition of abortion right activists. No talking. No booing. No clapping. Nothing that could jeopardize Davis's chances, or prompt the Capitol police to throw her supporters out of the building. Public safety officers roamed the halls in their khaki uniforms and big cowboy hats, ready to bring out handcuffs at what felt like any moment. "Now might be a good time to put your ID in your bra," Richards told the women standing near her. "That way you'll have it if we get arrested later." She hadn't forgotten everything from her rough-and-tumble days as an organizer, Richards thought.

Senate Bill 5—or SB5, as it was called—would ban abortion at twenty weeks of pregnancy, directly undercutting the legal standard set in Roe. It would also impose restrictions that would likely force the closure of most of the state's forty-two abortion clinics. The bill mandated that abortion facilities meet the same standards as hospital-style surgical centers—a requirement that would involve significant and largely unaffordable renovations—and that a doctor who performed abortions have admitting privileges at a nearby hospital, a credential many facilities in the conservative state were unwilling to grant. If enacted, it would be the most radical new law in the country. But about 60 percent of Texans supported banning abortion at 20 weeks, split largely on partisan lines.

Texas wasn't the only state embracing these new restrictions. Even though the national Republican Party was wary of the push to end abortion, local Republicans in conservative states were embracing laws that went further than ever before—as Marjorie Dannenfelser had noticed. Nearly a dozen other states had already passed laws banning abortion at twenty weeks, the result of flagship model legislation pushed by the National Right to Life Committee. Other states were pushing even further, with twelve-week and six-week bans. After abortion-rights organizations sued, those earlier bans were enjoined by courts, making them unenforceable as the litigation moved forward. But some of the twenty-week bans stood.

A twenty-week federal ban would not stop many abortions. Only about 8,600 procedures in the country happened after that point in pregnancy in 2013, just 1.3 percent of the total that year, according to the Centers for Disease Control and Prevention. Generally, abortions that late happened in tragic circumstances—situations like pregnancies resulting from child sexual abuse and life-threatening maternal and fetal conditions. But curbing abortion wasn't the only point of the laws: the idea was to strike at the legal precedent set in Roe, which said abortion was legal until viability. That marker was now at about twenty-four weeks of pregnancy, about a month earlier than when Roe was decided in 1973, because of medical advances.

Democrats in Texas knew they had little hope of stopping the twenty-week ban. Republicans controlled the legislature and the governor's mansion. They had called a special thirty-day legislative session and were trying to ram through the abortion bill at the very end. But Democrats came up with one last-ditch idea, and a woman to lead it: a filibuster. If their side could run out the clock, Democratic leaders knew, the special session would end before the Republicans could pass their bill. For everything to work, Davis had to get the microphone on the senate floor and keep talking until midnight, when the session ended. She could not sit, eat, drink, use the bathroom or even lean on her desk, or her filibuster would be declared dead, and the Republicans would call the vote. Davis would stand alone.

Richards had flown in from her offices in New York City to help manage the strategy. She was the most powerful symbol of abortion rights in the country, a Goliath commanding a force nearly unmatched in American politics. Planned Parenthood had about seven hundred health care centers, three primary national offices, and a political action arm backed by separate political action committees operating regionally and nationally. The legal office was essentially an in-house law firm. Its doctors participated in dozens of research studies and, in 2013, its lobbyists spent more than $1.5 million advocating for abortion rights and women's health care. Internationally, they worked with more than one thousand partners in countries across the globe. The antiabortion movement had no such organization.

During her seven years at the helm, Richards had transformed Planned Parenthood from a women's health organization struggling for influence into a feminist power symbol dripping in hot pink—the signature color of its brand. By the time Obama won reelection in 2012, Richards commanded seven million supporters and a budget of more than a billion dollars. She was a political superstar, twice named to *Time* magazine's list of most influential people, with celebrity endorsers and an open door at the White House.

She also represented the prevailing view in America: that abortion should largely remain legal and that Roe, the law of the land for two generations, should stand.

In liberal America, the new Republican abortion bans felt outrageous and backward. The message Democrats had taken from Obama's win was that America was shifting in their favor. They believed that a diversifying electorate of immigrants, young people, women, Black and Hispanic voters would be more liberal and overpower the white conservative Christians who had dominated Republican politics for decades. The arc of history was long, as Obama was fond of saying, but it was certainly bending toward their sense of liberal progress.

But the national promise of Roe had always been bigger than the reality, especially in Texas. For years, opponents had chipped away at abortion rights, with laws creating extensive rules for doctors, patients, and clinics that made it more difficult to get an abortion in the state. Texas required women seeking abortions to have transvaginal ultrasounds and waiting periods, and doctors to convey claims about the dangers of abortion. Many of those laws passed with little public outcry.

Now, abortion-rights activists were pushing back, with Davis as their champion. Early that morning, Richards had stopped by Davis's office to wish her good luck. A sign hung on her door: STAND WITH PLANNED PARENTHOOD.

"I want to make sure every senator has to walk by this sign on their way to the floor," she told Richards.

In the Senate chamber at 11:18 a.m., after a doctor threaded a catheter into Davis's bladder so she could avoid ending her thirteen-hour stand by leaving the floor to use the bathroom, Davis opened her thick binder of research, legal arguments, and some thirteen thousand testimonials from Texans speaking out in opposition to the bill. She read aloud a story from a seventeen-year-old girl named Ellen, who said she wanted to kill herself after a man raped her, until her mother took her to an abortion clinic to end the pregnancy. Patricia from Baylor said she felt the real sin was not abortion but carrying a child into the world and not being able to care for it. A man named Paul said that in Judaism, the health of the mother is paramount, the fetus considered to be a part of her body, not a person with preferential rights, and worried that the bill would impose Catholic or Baptist views that life begins at conception.

Davis wanted Republicans to listen to science. The Texas Medical Association, on behalf of its forty-seven thousand members, argued that the medical community should determine care, not legislators. The Texas district of the American College of Obstetricians and Gynecologists said the bill flouted scientific practice by defining a two-week embryo as a "child"—a "child," the doctors said, was a person from birth until eighteen. Davis dictated these statements into the record, her voice steady and strong.

After two hours and forty-six minutes, Davis flipped the page to the testimony of a woman named Carol from Austin. Her voice wavered, ever so slightly. At her twenty-week pregnancy appointment, Carol got the news that her baby girl had hydrops fetalis, a condition in which an abnormal amount of fluid had built up inside her, and that it would be terminal in her case. Carol had to make an impossible choice—go through with the birth and watch her child die, induce labor now, or have a dilation and extraction procedure. "When you are given the news that there is nothing that can be done to save your baby's life, it feels like your soul has been ripped apart," Davis read aloud from Carol's letter, her voice slowing.

Until now, she had been able to stay strong. But she struggled to get through what came next. "I held her, kissed her, watched her get baptized, told her that I loved her, and I said goodbye," Davis read, unable to stop her tears.

Her thoughts traveled to a memory. She had been elated when she got the news in the fall of 1996. It was her fourth pregnancy. Her first happened right after high school, when she was still a teenager living in a trailer park with her boyfriend, and it was followed by a shotgun marriage, a rapid divorce, and a series of low-end jobs. Her second happened much later, when she was remarried to Jeff Davis, a Princeton-educated lawyer, and taking the LSAT with dreams of getting into law school. Her third, an ectopic pregnancy, happened after she had worked her way through Harvard Law School and was practicing law back home in Texas. It ended with the removal of one of her fallopian tubes.

Davis prayed that if God willed it, she would get pregnant one more time. And at thirty-three, when she was mounting her first political campaign, running for city council of Fort Worth, it happened. Davis was determined that everything would go right this time. She read all the books. Ordered skim milk instead of wine. She even chose a name, Tate Elise.

The maternal fetal medicine doctor cried when he told Davis the diagnosis: Dandy-Walker syndrome. Tate's brain had developed incorrectly, with parts that might never grow at all. Davis and her husband saw a specialist in obstetric neurological diagnoses, got a third and a fourth opinion. "Likely incompatible with life," the doctors all said.

Davis remembered feeling Tate's little body tremble inside her and sensed she was suffering. Weeping, she promised Tate that she would not experience further pain. In the medical office, with tears flowing down their faces, she and her husband watched her doctor still Tate's beating heart.

After a delivery by C-section, Tate was brought to her in a tiny pink dress and knit cap. Davis held her, cried over her. They took photographs and had her baptized by an associate minister from their church. And as Davis lay in the hospital sobbing, her hand over her womb, Tate's body was taken away and cremated. Davis would never forget the blackness that followed. The deep despair that came in crushing waves. When she emerged, after nearly a year, she was forever changed.

All these years later, it was still too personal, too painful, to share aloud. Davis kept reading.

Richards listened to the stories unfolding in the chamber. She had heard so many like them over the years. And she understood how personal they were. After having her daughter, followed by a set of twins, Richards had felt her family was complete. Then, she got pregnant again. The abortion wasn't a particularly emotional decision. She did not feel guilty or anguished. Instead, she felt lucky. Having an abortion in Texas back in the 1990s wasn't "the nightmare that it is now," she reflected. But, like Davis, her experience also wasn't something she went around sharing publicly.

The private nature of both of their stories underscored an inescapable reality of abortion. The issue wasn't just political; it was deeply personal. Women understood intuitively how choices about pregnancy affected their lives. But the stigma and shame that surrounded the procedure kept the stories of women who had an abortion largely cloaked in silence. For abortion-rights supporters, the public debate was most often conducted not in intimate terms but in the more bloodless language of medicine, law, and politics.

Younger abortion-rights activists were trying to grow those stories into a movement. It's easier to deny someone rights when they are simply invisible, they reasoned. They encouraged women to, in a phrase coined by one activist online, "shout their abortion." Social media helped spread their effort. That spring, a twenty-five-year-old woman who worked at an abortion clinic filmed and posted her own procedure. The video was viewed one million times, sparking a tsunami of responses, including some so threatening that YouTube disabled comments. But it inspired other young women, who began talking about their procedures online and at events on college campuses. Abortion-rights activists had used the internet to their advantage. And as Davis spoke in Texas, they were doing it again.

In the rotunda, women paced in slow circles around Richards, chanting, "Won't go back." Above them, women lined the balconies live streaming their protest to the world. With help from organizers at Planned Parenthood and their allies in the movement, the word spread on Twitter, then a relatively new social media platform with untold capacity for disruption. Outcry reached the highest levels of Democratic power. At 5:53 p.m., House Speaker Nancy Pelosi posted her support. Obama soon followed, with a tweet read out loud by a protester in the rotunda: "Something special is happening in Austin tonight." Richards and Davis suddenly understood: people were following along with their fight—and not just in Texas. "The whole world is watching," Richards realized.

By 10:30 p.m., #standwithwendy was being posted on Twitter 1,500 times per minute, huge numbers for the young social media platform. By the end of Davis's filibuster, it was tweeted nearly 730,000 times. The online moment was so notable that Twitter's founder would later tout it as illustrative of his technology's ability to foster grassroots democracy.

Richards was amazed by how the wave of resistance in her home state inspired people across the nation. Generally speaking, abortion rights didn't energize supporters as much as opponents of the issue. In the run-up to the 2012 election, only about four in ten Democratic voters and 29 percent of independent voters said abortion would be very important to their vote—far less than the 51 percent of Republicans who said the same. That dynamic made sense: it was a basic rule of politics that those pushing for change—like the Republicans who wanted to roll back Roe and abortion rights—tended to be more motivated than the voters who were comfortable with the status quo.

That enthusiasm gap between the two parties meant that in election after election, Democratic voters dismissed risks to abortion rights as little more than political posturing, the same-old, decades-long battle. Even after Republican statehouses began passing a deluge of abortion restrictions in 2011, research found that voters who supported abortion rights remained largely unaware of the new laws or how the landscape was starting to shift. Over the course of 2013, Tresa Undem, a pollster who studied issues related to gender, conducted 150 focus groups with independent and Democratic women. When she'd flash a list of abortion restrictions on a screen, the women would be shocked and outraged—*Who is passing these*, they would ask, *and why didn't I know about this?*

Now, activists in Texas put abortion rights front and center across America, including in liberal states that hadn't really understood those rights were at risk. An issue that a majority of the country believed to be settled law suddenly drove the political narrative. To Richards, it felt like a national awakening to the new threats abortion rights faced in conservative states, and it was thrilling.

Richards and many of her liberal allies believed that this was how progress happened. With the right organizing efforts, personal beliefs could grow into mass actions, which could change laws. If her side could convince enough of their supporters to speak out in protest, they could show Republican legislators in Texas that they would pay a political price for restricting abortion and convince them to abandon this law. The abortion-rights movement had drawn its own lessons from Martin Luther King Jr. and the civil rights era. In the years before Roe, King spoke of the intertwined relationship between his movement and Planned Parenthood's. He praised the group's founder, Margaret Sanger, for her nonviolent actions promoting birth control, which he said made his own movement more resolute. For King, mass demonstrations were necessary to shift the country. By organizing, and marching, they could force the government to act. "We had confidence that when we awakened the nation to the immorality and evil of inequality, there would be an upsurge of conscience followed by remedial action," he wrote in a letter to Planned Parenthood in 1966. "We had to organize, not only arguments, but people in the millions for action."

That's exactly what Richards hoped was happening over all those hours in the Texas Capitol, as Davis spoke and Republicans tried to find ways to end her filibuster. They gave Davis one procedural strike when she discussed the state budget and Planned Parenthood funding, a reference that Republicans said was outside the scope of the current bill. When she put on a back brace with the help of a colleague, she received a second strike for accepting outside support. On the third, a simple majority of Republicans could vote to end debate, and she would have to yield the floor. That came two hours before midnight when she mentioned a previous law mandating a sonogram before getting an abortion. A gavel sounded, and the objection was upheld. "Let her speak! Let her speak!" opponents of the bill chanted from the upstairs gallery.

Davis could feel the floor vibrating from the stomping. Her Democratic colleagues tried to eat up time at the microphone, speaking in their slowest Southern drawls. With fifteen minutes to go, state senator Leticia Van de Putte attempted to address the floor. She kept getting overlooked, and at one point, her mic was cut off. When she finally got her moment, her emotion—not just about abortion rights but equal pay, women's power, and how the issues that impact women the most are simply overlooked—exploded.

"At what point must a female senator raise her hand or her voice to be recognized over the male colleagues in the room?" she asked.

The crowd in the Senate gallery erupted. The clock ticked. Davis raised her fingers in a V—a sign for victory—and the crowd above grew so loud that it became impossible for Republicans to move forward with the legislation. The shouts grew like a wave, reverberating to the larger crowd outside the Senate chamber's doors and then to Richards in the rotunda. Richards threw her arms in the air, signaling to raise the volume even more. The protesters started counting down the minutes. Davis pointed to the clock—"Midnight! It's midnight!" she said.

At 12:03 a.m., three minutes past the deadline, the senate passed the bill, voting 19–10. The vote did not count, though Republicans spent hours arguing the legislation went through three minutes earlier. A screenshot on Twitter finally proved them wrong. Still, Davis couldn't imagine that her Republican colleagues would flout the public outrage and bring the bill up again the next term. Around 3:00 a.m., she sent a text to Richards.

In the rotunda, surrounded by iPhones recording and streaming the moment, Richards read the message to the crowd: "First, I love you guys. The lieutenant governor has agreed that SB 5 is dead." The deafening applause became a chorus of "The Eyes of Texas," the fight song of the University of Texas Longhorns. Richards broke into a grateful smile, swelling with pride for what they had accomplished. "We love you too, Wendy," she shouted. In deep-red Texas, she felt possibility, and hope. This night in Texas, a fuse had been lit, Richards thought, one she hadn't seen since her mother won the state back in 1990.

Richards glanced up at the portrait of her late mother, the first woman to be governor of Texas elected in her own right, staring boldly out of her own gold frame in her royal-blue blazer, alongside the portraits of all the men. Richards had been eight months pregnant with twins, her toddler, Lily, in tow, when she watched her fifty-seven-year-old divorced, progressive, and recovering alcoholic mother, Ann Richards, become the state's forty-fifth governor and hold up a T-shirt in victory: A WOMAN'S PLACE IS IN THE DOME! it said.

Oh, thought Richards, how Mom would have loved this.

3

A Conversion Story

Marjorie Jones Dannenfelser was older than Roe, but not by much. Her mother was barely pregnant with her in 1965, when *Life* magazine published the first photographs of a human developing in utero—a glowing eighteen-week fetus, floating in an amniotic sac against what looked like a starlit sky. An astonishing eight million copies sold in days. The images of the fetus were both a revelation and a fairy tale. They showed it developing over time, but not the woman growing the fetus with her body and blood. America met the fetus on its own, a pioneering cosmonaut exploring the womb, without the literal ties of motherhood.

But the bond between mother and child shaped Dannenfelser from the start. Not long after she was born, her parents moved back to her mother's hometown of Greenville, North Carolina, to live near her mother's mother. Dannenfelser would listen to her and two great-aunts tell stories of their lives growing up on the Perquimans River, where their father ran a hardware store and two of them got married on the same day. She learned from their strength and loss. Their fourth sister, the baby of the family, had died suddenly at age thirty back in 1939. The death certificate said she had an infection following a surgery that removed a dead fetus, and died of cardiac failure. She left behind her husband and two small children.

The Episcopal Church tied together generations of Dannenfelser's family. The church was becoming more progressive, and it supported Roe. Before the ruling, Americans across party lines backed some form of abortion rights, including 68 percent of Republicans—more than the 59 percent of Democrats who agreed that "the decision to have an abortion should be made solely by a woman and her physician," in a poll released by Gallup in August 1972. Abortion opponents, often Catholic, were largely a nascent collection of regional groups and had no significant national organization.

Like many Republicans of their day, Dannenfelser's parents were conservative on matters of economics and foreign policy, but liberal on social issues. They believed abortion was a "necessary evil," Dannenfelser later wrote, so she did too. When she followed her mother's footsteps to Duke University, she was eager to study medicine, like her father had. They were close, and when she worried she might be pregnant the week of her freshman orientation, her father helped her see a doctor to get a pregnancy test.

Dannenfelser knew she would get an abortion if it came back positive. She holed up in her room, anxious, and did not want to talk about it. It was 1984, about a decade after Roe. That year, more than 1.3 million American women had abortions. The Duke paper carried a regular ad, tucked between classifieds for a $6-per-hour housecleaning position and a typist job that paid $1.25 per page: "Abortion to 20 weeks. Private and confidential GYN facility with Saturday and weekday appointments available. Free pregnancy test." Dannenfelser had her family, and she would have their love and support no matter what. She vowed she would not withdraw from college on the first day, that she would not be both a freshman and a mother. But it was a decision she never had to act on. The test was negative. She did not recount the story for years, until she was one of the most prominent antiabortion activists in the country.

The incident, and how it shaped the rest of Dannenfelser's life—as Davis's loss of Tate Elise affected hers—was another illustration of how the intimacy of abortion made the issue unlike nearly any other in American life. Pregnancies—intended and unintended, joyful and tragic and routine—shaped the lives of the women and men on all sides of the political fight over the procedure. And it is the inescapable closeness of the issue that has made it as formative for the nation as it has been for its major political players.

With the pregnancy scare behind her, Dannenfelser jumped into college life, and for her, that meant the College Republicans club. Its campaign to reelect President Ronald Reagan was in full steam, and she was fascinated with politics. Decades before Donald Trump made it his motto, Reagan had promised to "Make America Great Again," and like most voters, Dannenfelser didn't take his antiabortion views seriously. Two-thirds of Americans opposed the constitutional amendment he supported that would outlaw all abortions. Plus, it was hard to believe he would really do what he said, because before Roe, when he was the Republican governor of California, he signed a law that legalized abortion in cases of rape, incest, or the life or health of the mother.

But unlike in the world Dannenfelser knew back home in Greenville, where it was not uncommon to be a Republican and support abortion rights, the Republicans she met at Duke were so divided on the issue that the club had two different factions, one that was "pro-choice," one that was "pro-life," the political shorthand for supporters of abortion rights and their opponents. The split mirrored the division growing in the Republican Party across the country in the 1980s. A new movement, the "religious right," as it was called, was gaining power and had been making abortion a significant, politically divisive issue.

Paul Weyrich, one of the fathers of the religious right, and his allies saw abortion as a way to mobilize Christian voters against Democrats like President Jimmy Carter, whom they blamed for forcing evangelicals to desegregate their Christian schools to keep their tax-exempt status. They organized Christian conservatives into a significant political coalition for Reagan—and he won, twice. Though Catholics often led antiabortion groups, evangelicals quickly became a more consistently reliable antiabortion cohort. And Reagan became the most high-profile champion of their cause.

After Reagan won reelection, Dannenfelser refused to go to an event at Duke where antiabortion activists screened a film that the president himself had shown at the White House. *The Silent Scream* was a twenty-eight-minute film depicting a suction abortion at twelve weeks of pregnancy in graphic detail, made to look as if the fetus were crying out during the procedure. Medical experts disputed that a fetus could feel pain at that stage, but Reagan declared that fetuses felt "long and agonizing pain" during the procedure. The footage was edited, with the speed altered for dramatic impact. It gave the impression that a twelve-week fetus, in reality less than two inches long, was like a full-term baby thrashing about in alarm before an abortion. The White House showing was a high-profile win for the new antiabortion movement, which aimed to get the film in front of as many elected officials and Supreme Court justices as possible. The effort made Dannenfelser angry. She remembered how she felt when she thought she might be pregnant.

"When you become a woman, come back and talk to me," she told men who questioned her views.

But the shifting Republican politics were a powerful force as she came of age. Her interest in medicine was rapidly being replaced by a growing ardor for politics. She wrote to the Heritage Foundation, Weyrich's conservative think tank in Washington. The group was part of an effort to build a new generation of conservative leaders in public policy, working alongside other new groups like the Federalist Society, which aimed to shape the future of conservative law. In the summer of 1986, Dannenfelser got a spot in a group house for ten young Republicans on O Street in Georgetown, called the Right House, part of an experimental project to network top young Republicans from around the country.

Warm summer evenings at the Right House became a time for Dannenfelser and her new friends to sort out their place in the shifting Republican order, with boozy ramblings about philosophy.

Members of the Right House fell generally in two camps, the libertarians, who, like Dannenfelser, supported abortion rights, and the social conservatives, who were often Catholic and opposed Roe as "a tragic betrayal of our nation's founding principles," she later recalled. Most of the house focused simply on politics, but she grew smitten as one recent Catholic philosophy graduate, Chris Currie, made impassioned political arguments from a place of moral conviction. They would argue over Catholic dogma, and she pressed the case for why the church should allow birth control and divorce. He was "the best apologist" for Christian faith she had ever met, she said.

As the summer went on, they dated, and she started doubting her past beliefs on abortion and on faith. His Catholic worldview seemed so big, with philosophy and history stretching all the way back to the first century, and her Episcopal faith started to feel inadequate. She encountered the book that catechized antiabortion activists, John C. Willke's 1971 *Handbook on Abortion*, filled with images of mangled fetuses and arguments to defend their cause. She admired the way the Catholics lived their lives. When one of the Catholic guys in the house found a pornographic video in the VCR, he destroyed it. The house manager, a libertarian, demanded he pay for lost property damages, citing principles about freedom of speech. But the Catholics, including Currie, replied that they ultimately answered to a moral call higher than law: pornography, the church taught, violated human dignity and harmed the community. The libertarians kicked them out of the house, and Dannenfelser chose to leave with them.

The death of a childhood friend that summer also pushed her toward faith. "How to handle loss for the Christian is all tied up in the whole story of salvation and humanity," she reflected later.

Religion and politics were blending in a new way for Dannenfelser. Back at Duke, she decided to major in philosophy, with a second in political science. And when Pope John Paul II came to the United States in September of her senior year, she and Currie traveled to see him in Detroit, the final stop of the pope's whirlwind ten-day trip. Before leaving to return to Rome, the pope urged action against abortion.

America's majestic mountains and fertile plains were indeed beautiful, John Paul II told a crowd gathered at the airport to send him off. But America's greatest beauty and richest blessing was instead found in the human person.

"Every human person—no matter how vulnerable or helpless, no matter how young or how old, no matter how healthy, handicapped or sick, no matter how useful or productive for society—is a being of inestimable worth created in the image and likeness of God," he said. "If you want equal justice for all, and true freedom and lasting peace, then, America, defend life!"

Dannenfelser soon felt a tug she could not ignore. As she got to know the Catholic Church through her boyfriend and the pope's teaching, she fell in love with the faith. And like falling in love, religious conversions are often hard for those on the outside to truly understand. Her mother absolutely disagreed with Catholic opposition to birth control, abortion, and divorce. The conversion to Catholicism meant saying goodbye to her old self, her whole identity, and in many ways to the women who had shaped her for generations. Yet spiritually, Dannenfelser felt drawn to what Pope John Paul II often called the "feminine genius" of Mary, the mother of Jesus. History had long excluded women and limited their economic, political, and social participation because it penalized motherhood instead of rewarding it, he argued. Mary was a model for full human dignity and female service to society, grounded in being a mother.

It was this vision of womanhood that Dannenfelser grew to love, even as her religious conversion to Catholicism and her political conversion to the antiabortion cause blended into one. Her personal transformation mirrored the shift of conservatives of her time. Over the fourteen years from Roe to the time of the pope's visit, the Republican Party had gone from mostly supporting abortion to being defined by opposing it. The story of her conversion was also the story of a new Republican Party, driven by a conservative Christian flank.

Not long before Dannenfelser graduated, after she saw the pope in Detroit, she went to see Reagan when he came to speak at Duke's Cameron Indoor Stadium. The editorial board of *The Duke Chronicle*, the student newspaper, criticized the president, "this most moral of leaders," for forcing his morals on the public by opposing abortion rights. A fight broke out in its pages as students fired off opinion letters to the editor about abortion—for weeks.

Men can never understand "the desperation, the anguish, the physical and emotional suffering" of a pregnant woman considering abortion, a junior named Stacy Pollina wrote. What about the forty-year-old mother of five who jeopardizes her own life with another pregnancy? Or of a thirteen-year-old raped by her father, a child carrying a child? Biologically, women have no choice—no freedom. "To make abortion illegal is only to rape women of what freedom they do have—the freedom to choose to have an abortion or not, in accordance with their own moral values," Pollina wrote. "To make it illegal is to impose certain moral values upon every woman in the form of control over her body through legislation."

Reading Pollina's letter, Dannenfelser decided it was time. Unlike when she was a freshman, she was now with Reagan all the way.

Dannenfelser replied with a five-paragraph letter of her own, her first real public declaration of her new opposition to abortion. LIFE DESERVES A CHANCE, the headline announced.

She used to agree with Pollina, she wrote, and she understood "the desperation, the anguish, the physical and emotional suffering" that Pollina described, alluding to her own pregnancy scare. "I can testify to the fact that concern for oneself—one's body and reputation—is natural and understandable," she wrote. "But the difficult and crucial challenge in life is to come to the point where one can reach beyond the self and feel concern for the life of another."

The right to life is the most fundamental of all rights, she went on. No one knows for sure at what point we can be called human, "given the elusive physical and spiritual nature of the human being," she reasoned. "This means we must not assume that an unborn life is not human; even the smallest chance that it is, that is, is enough. Life is too precious a gift to gamble with."

Dannenfelser settled in Washington a converted woman in the late 1980s, eager to follow the political principle of her first boss on Capitol Hill, an antiabortion Democrat, Representative Alan Mollohan, cochair of the House Pro-Life Caucus: "If you shoot a bear, you have to kill it." It felt strange to her, working for a Democrat, but helping him advance the antiabortion cause came first. She married a cradle Catholic, a colleague and mentor working on antiabortion issues, Martin "Marty" Dannenfelser, and temporarily retired to start a family.

But she remained devoted to the antiabortion cause, determined to bring her own conversion to America. It was not long before she helped to start a new group, the Susan B. Anthony List, to shoot down the bear of Roe. And now, after four years of losing in Obama's America, she refused to let her own party prevent her from killing it.

4

Her Mother's Texas

Cecile Richards was, according to her mother, a beautiful but fussy baby. To get her to nap on weekends, her parents would drive from their home in Dallas to Austin, where they would meet up with their political buddies at Scholz Garten, a beer hall that was a gathering place for the lawyers, politicians, journalists, and gadflies who comprised the state capital's progressive scene.

Her father, David, was a rising star in liberal legal circles, defending civil rights leaders, unions like the International Brotherhood of Teamsters, and people who were accused of being communists amid the tumultuous cultural changes of the 1960s. The family never quite fit in in Dallas, a place her father described as "a pinched-up, buttoned-down wasteland for the soul." When Richards's sixth-grade teacher questioned her on why she refused to say the Lord's Prayer with her class after they recited the Pledge of Allegiance, she replied: "We don't read the Bible in our house." Her parents, who attended the progressive Unitarian Church, "weren't particularly religious folks," Richards later recalled.

The family soon moved to Austin, an island of liberalism in conservative Texas, where her parents embraced the hippie ethos of the era. Ann ordered hundreds of ladybugs to grow a pesticide-free garden. Richards, her siblings, and their friends stuffed envelopes for political candidates at the dining room table and watched as liberal stalwarts like the columnist Molly Ivins acted out the Watergate hearings by the pool with their parents. David was, as Richards would later remember, always "the smartest guy in the room and the center of attention."

But as David fought to create a more liberal Texas, it was Ann who was home taking care of Richards and her siblings. Her brilliant, hilarious mother carried baby Cecile to early NAACP meetings in Dallas and pushed her around in her stroller, canvassing Black and Latino neighborhoods for Democratic candidates.

It was Ann who took Richards to swimming class and Girl Scouts. Who sewed her baby clothes and her Halloween costumes and made dinner. Who created massive Easter egg hunts and made chocolate meringue pie to celebrate special days. Who took Richards to Scarborough's to buy new wool, midcalf A-line skirts for college and organized raucous group campouts across Texas so she could experience the beauty and diversity of her home state.

It was Ann who Richards told when she was disciplined by the principal after wearing a black armband—made of felt scavenged from her mother's sewing kit—to school as part of a day of national protest of the Vietnam War. How dare that principal "intimidate you just for standing up for what you believe?" Ann fumed that evening. The feeling, Richards later recalled, was "exhilarating," like they were fighting for justice, mother and daughter together.

And in 1972, it was Ann who started campaigning for Sarah Weddington, the twenty-seven-year-old lawyer who had just argued Roe at the Supreme Court, cluttering the dining room table with canvassing plans to get her elected to the state legislature. The position on her campaign was the first professional action of Ann's adult life she'd taken without David—but not without Richards, a teenager just about a dozen years younger than Weddington herself, who helped to phone bank and door-knock. Richards watched as Weddington's primary opponent called her "that sweet little girl" instead of using her name and complained that she was trying to confuse the voters; one day she would wear her hair up, the next day she would wear her hair down.

Weddington won anyway. Roe was decided thirteen days after she was sworn in. Female political power, and the whole project of women's equality, seemed bound up with abortion rights. Ann took a job as Weddington's legislative office manager at the state capitol, working outside the house for the first time in nearly two decades. After years of watching her mother run their family, Richards saw her run something bigger. Suddenly, it seemed like Ann could do anything.

Ann was, in many ways, a woman of her era, coming into her own professionally at the same time as Gloria Steinem and Shirley Chisholm and Billie Jean King. These women represented a second wave of feminism, one that expanded the work of their foremothers, who fought for women to have the right to vote. Abortion rights became a central part of their fight for equality. Equal rights for women were not the legal rationale of the Roe decision, which was based in a right to privacy and personal liberty rooted in the Fourteenth Amendment. But Americans understood the decision in terms of equality and new freedoms for women.

Women's lives were changing, and Richards was watching her mother ride that wave. In 1975, Ann was recruited to run for the Democratic nomination for county commissioner, after David turned down the chance to run. She feared that if she ran and won, it would end her marriage. She did it anyway.

When Richards left for Brown University, seeking a chance to see beyond Texas, her parents were married and her mom was home. By the time she graduated in 1980, her mother was an elected official and a rising feminist star. Her parents were divorcing, and her mother would soon enter rehab in Minnesota for alcoholism. The new feminism hadn't just roiled the country, it had transformed Richards's family. Women's liberation had remade her mother's destiny, put her on track to become something more influential. And the way such big political changes could reshape women's lives became a foundational story not just for Ann but for her daughter as well.

After college, Richards became an itinerant union organizer, camping out in her car and traveling from New Orleans to Los Angeles to the Rio Grande Valley, organizing campaigns for garment workers, nursing-home workers, and janitors. In 1981, her mother called her home to help with her next campaign, a run for state treasurer, where she was battling criticism that a woman could not handle the state's money. Richards traveled the state in her car and was so good, Ann boasted, that her campaign got an editorial endorsement in a town she had never visited.

By 1988, Ann had become so admired for her political instincts and quick wit that she was chosen to deliver the keynote address at the Democratic National Convention in Atlanta—the second woman to be selected for that slot. Her speech—in which she famously described Vice President George H. W. Bush, the Republican presidential nominee, as "born with a silver foot in his mouth"—turned her into a political icon. As Ann basked in the applause that night, she wrapped an arm behind a beaming Richards, standing onstage by her side smiling in a bright yellow dress.

When her mom ran for governor in 1990, Richards was married to Kirk Adams, another union organizer, and raising their toddler, Lily, in Los Angeles, where the couple were hired to organize the most important union campaign of their lives. But Ann called and Richards packed her life in Venice Beach into a U-Haul and drove home to help her mom once more.

The gubernatorial race was a match between two larger-than-life Texas characters. Ann Richards was a big-haired, wisecracking grandmother who defied the expectations for stay-at-home mothers. Clayton Williams was a conservative cowboy businessman rich from oil, banking, and cattle, who promised to return the state to its traditional ways—"to make Texas great again," he said. It was a clash of values between the ol' boys' Texas and the "new Texas" that Ann described on the campaign trail, a place that empowered women and Black and Hispanic voters. A choice not only of politics and policies, but over changing roles for American women.

Like Todd Akin in 2012, Williams roiled his campaign with a comment about rape. Sitting around a fire with reporters he had invited to his cattle ranch, he compared the heavy fog enveloping the campsite to the violent sex crime. "If it's inevitable, just relax and enjoy it," said Williams, taking a bite of beans from a blue tin cup. It was "just a joke," he said later, when questioned later about the remark by the reporters, adding, "that's not a Republican women's club that we were at this morning."

Ann cast him as a pig from the past. "Rape is not a joke. It is a crime of violence," she told a gathering of Democratic women. "It is time we had a governor in the state of Texas who recognized that women are not cattle, that they are not there for servicing."

At the time, the joke was considered uncouth but not that uncommon. The comment barely dented his chances, and Williams still led Ann by fifteen points almost six months after the remark. His real trouble started after he refused to release his taxes, telling a reporter that he paid nothing in 1986, the year of the oil bust that cost hundreds of thousands of Texans their jobs. "The guy's a Donald Trump in a cowboy hat, selling one failing business to shore up another," Ann's campaign manager Mary Beth Rogers said, a reference to the high-profile financial collapse of the then New York real estate developer. On Election Night, Texans agreed: They backed Ann by 49 to 47 percent.

Suddenly, Ann became the most powerful elected woman in America. Richards saw firsthand how women's equality, and the inherent right to abortion she believed it included, could conquer even in Texas. "My name is Ann Richards, and I am pro-choice and I vote," her mother declared at the party's national convention in 1992.

Her victory was a harbinger of new power for Democratic women. During Ann's first year in office, Americans were riveted to their television screens, watching the fourteen white men of the

Senate Judiciary Committee interrogate Anita Hill, a Black law professor who alleged that Clarence Thomas, President George H. W. Bush's nominee to the Supreme Court, had sexually harassed her. Only two women served in the US Senate then—one Republican, one Democrat—and neither was on the committee.

Women responded by running for office in droves in 1992, determined to transform Washington, and they won. The number of women in the Senate tripled to six. Forty-seven women won House seats, a new record for female representation in the chamber. Media outlets declared "the Year of the Woman." Nearly all these new women were Democrats and supported abortion rights. Any antiabortion agenda seemed gutted after the election, especially after the Supreme Court's ruling that year in Casey.

A new president, Bill Clinton, nominated Ruth Bader Ginsburg to be the second woman and sixth Jewish justice of the Supreme Court. Abortion restrictions, Ginsburg told the Senate during her confirmation hearings, treated women "as less than a fully adult human responsible for her own choices." In her new Supreme Court chambers, she put a silver mezuzah on the doorframe, the first ever affixed by a justice.

Hillary Rodham Clinton, the lawyer and powerhouse who helped drive her husband's successful campaign to the White House, predicted the moment was the start of lasting change. "We'll have a woman president by 2010," she told an audience in Los Angeles. She may not have been elected herself, but she was the most visible embodiment of the spirit of the moment: a Yale-educated, liberal feminist, who graduated from law school the year Roe was decided. She rode into Washington from Arkansas making no excuses for her staunch support of abortion rights.

But something shifted by the time Ann Richards ran for reelection just two years later in 1994. She lost to George W. Bush. He wasn't the only Republican who won: in Washington that same election, a "Republican revolution" delivered unified control of Congress to the GOP for the first time in more than four decades. A different political force had risen, one Richards had not seen coming.

There had been a clue. A few weeks before the end of her mother's reelection campaign in 1994, Richards traveled to a plant gate in Beaumont to hand campaign flyers out to factory workers. What she heard startled her: union guys attacked her mother as a "baby-killer" who plotted to take away their guns. These were the same kinds of guys Richards once organized. But now, they were mobilized by a new movement—the Christian Coalition. These right-wing religious conservatives were determined to remake the country with cultural appeals aimed squarely at undercutting the secular, liberal version of Texas that Ann and her family had spent decades trying to build. The New Texas, it turned out, was something else entirely. More conservative. More Christian. And it wasn't just Texas.

Richards saw a national threat: the conservative Christian backlash to the Democratic female victories had become a force feminists could not ignore. She started her own organization, the Texas Freedom Network, to push back on conservative Christian pastors who sought to influence public school curriculums by banning books, teaching Bible stories about Earth's creation alongside the scientific theory of evolution, and promoting abstinence-only sex education. When George W. Bush ran for president in 2000, Richards warned that feminists and abortion-rights advocates would be foolhardy to ignore the Christian right. "We think their ideas are goofy, so we think no one's going to listen to them," she said that year, addressing a conference on the future of the women's movement in Baltimore. "But look at the Christian Coalition. They showed what a well-organized minority can do when they put their mind to it." If the feminist movement could be as politically involved as the conservative Christians were, she said, "we will win."

Richards moved to Washington, becoming a top aide to Nancy Pelosi charged with rallying liberal forces behind the lawmaker who, as House minority whip, occupied the highest leadership position ever held by a woman in Congress. After that, she founded America Votes, a coalition that coordinated the political activities of the richest, most influential unions and liberal advocacy groups for the 2004 elections. Her work was getting noticed: "She could be the president," Pelosi would later tell *The New Yorker*.

Richards chose a different path. When she took over Planned Parenthood in 2006, Richards saw an opportunity to give the feminist movement the political power to push back against the religious right. They had a lot of work to do. The antiabortion forces had made significant gains after Bush won and now championed their cause from the White House. Yet their problems weren't limited to Republicans. When Bush signed legislation banning so-called partial-birth abortion, he had support from seventeen Democratic senators who defied the opposition from Planned Parenthood to vote for the bill. Democratic leaders openly recruited Democratic candidates who opposed abortion rights, arguing they would be better positioned to win in more conservative states. "We're the very best at what we do, providing reproductive health care for women," Jill June, the head of Planned Parenthood in Iowa, told Richards when she interviewed before the hiring committee that year. "But we keep losing ground in the political arena." The board wanted someone to transform the ninety-year-old women's health care provider into, as Richards would later say, "the largest kick-butt political organization."

Building stronger political support wouldn't be easy. But Richards—the sixth leader in the organization's history and the only one without a background in women's health—saw an opportunity. Planned Parenthood's hundreds of clinics served nearly three million people annually. One in five women had visited one of its offices. The majority came not for an abortion but for birth control pills, HIV tests, or breast cancer screenings. Richards would convert those patients into political activists who would help build popular support for their cause. "The most important thing that we had to do as an organization was match up our incredible health care footprint in all 50 states with an engaged movement in these states," she said.

To start, she would organize voters to block abortion restrictions at state legislatures. "No one gets up every morning and thinks about the Supreme Court," Richards told *The Dallas Morning News* shortly after Bush elevated Samuel Alito to become the newest member of the highest court. "But everybody has a legislature, and everybody knows that legislature has an enormous impact on every aspect of our lives." Her first major test came just three weeks after she started, when South Dakota's Republican governor signed the nation's most sweeping abortion ban since Roe, criminalizing the procedure unless a woman's life was jeopardized. She launched a petition campaign so voters could directly overturn it at the ballot box through a referendum, and won, by a margin of twelve points.

When Ann died, less than a year after Richards took the position, the loss was devastating to Richards and symbolic for the country. "She ultimately was my mentor, I suppose, in addition to being my mom," Richards would later say. If her mother's life was the story of women winning abortion rights in America, Richards's would become the story of the fight to protect them.

When the Obama administration swept into Washington in 2009, Richards saw an opportunity to advance her mission. She lobbied for the president's new health care bill, beating back the sixty-four antiabortion Democrats in Congress—nearly one-quarter of the Democratic majority—who wanted it to include a ban on abortion coverage. When the bill passed, Richards believed they had made history. The legislation prevented insurance companies from considering pregnancies preexisting conditions, added birth control to the list of mandatory services insurers had to offer, and covered a fleet of preventive services like mammograms. It wasn't everything they wanted; shortly after entering the White House, Obama said pushing for a law protecting abortion rights by codifying Roe into federal law—a promise he made to Planned Parenthood during his campaign—wasn't his "highest legislative priority." But the health care law was the kind of political victory that occurs only once in a generation. "A big fucking deal," as Joe Biden infamously put it as he leaned a little too close to the microphone at the signing ceremony.

Two years later, Richards notched a second high-profile victory, one that exposed the creeping guerrilla tactics of her adversaries. After Republicans won control of the House in 2010, they launched an investigation into whether Planned Parenthood was using federal funds for abortion services, a practice banned by the Hyde Amendment. Soon after, the prominent breast cancer charity Susan G. Komen for the Cure announced that it would no longer give money to any group under federal, state, or local investigation. The only grantee that fit that description was Planned Parenthood, which received annual funding for breast cancer screenings. It was a coup for the antiabortion movement, which had targeted Komen for underwriting breast cancer screenings at Planned Parenthood clinics for years.

Nancy Brinker, Komen's founder and chief executive, insisted the decision had nothing to do with abortion. She asked Richards to keep the policy change quiet to avoid controversy, Richards later recounted in her memoir. "We don't want to make a big deal of this," Richards recalled Brinker saying. "It would be better if it were just understood between us." Instead, Richards blasted the news to her million-strong email list, asking their backers to help make up the funds. Planned Parenthood's supporters took to the internet to express their anger, firing off 1.3 million posts on Twitter mentioning the issue. Within four days, Planned Parenthood raised four times as much for its breast cancer program as it would have received from Komen's annual grant that year—nearly $3 million in total. Komen, meanwhile, saw a drop of $77 million—about 22 percent of the foundation's income—in contributions and sponsorships.

Richards used the victory to cement an image of Planned Parenthood that defied the caricature drawn by its opponents. Over and over, she pounded a message that most services offered by Planned Parenthood are universally supported procedures like cancer screenings—exactly the kind of work championed by Komen. Planned Parenthood was about women's health care, she stressed, not just abortion. She skillfully refocused the ire on her real enemies. "My issue was not with Komen," she told *The Dallas Morning News*. "The same people yelling at women outside our health centers were the same folks urging boycotts of their walks and turning the screws on them, finally pushing them over the edge."

Just weeks after the Komen uproar, Richards faced off with her adversaries directly. Catholic bishops were objecting to a part of Obama's health care law that required religious charities, hospitals, and universities to pay for contraception for their employees. Richards argued against an exemption to the rule to White House aides. After a fierce lobbying campaign, Richards won for a third time. Contraception would be free in the new health care law. "No matter how much birth control Planned Parenthood provided, and we were probably the biggest in terms of a health care provider, it meant anyone could get it," said Richards. It was, she thought, "a radical change." Richards was thrilled when Obama called her himself to announce the news. "I'm making three phone calls today: the Catholic bishops, the Catholic Hospital Association, and you," Richards said Obama told her. "Suffice it to say, I think yours is going to be the happiest phone call I'm going to make." It was the proudest moment of Richards's career.

Even as the Catholic groups took their case to the courts, the victory showed the influence Planned Parenthood held in Obama's Washington. Planned Parenthood was no longer a liability, the Obama campaign realized. It could be a political weapon. Internal polling commissioned by White House political aides found the organization to be more trusted than the Democrats, Congress, and the White House. Richards was the campaign's most important surrogate for the 2012 presidential race, outside of the vice president and First Lady, David Plouffe, Obama's political strategist, told aides. Obama's political operation asked her to take a leave of absence to campaign full-time for his reelection bid.

Weeks before Election Day, Richards stood in the wings at the second presidential debate and was thrilled to hear Obama mention Planned Parenthood from the stage for the first time in history. Not once. Not twice. But five times. Obama didn't use the word *abortion*, and he offered no clear promises to expand abortion access, even as the wave of restrictive laws swept statehouses. But Planned Parenthood, the president implied, was a trusted health care provider, not the corrupt abortion peddler that its opponents on Capitol Hill and in churches across the country described. To Richards, it felt like power. In just six years, they had "cracked the code" in the Democratic Party, she thought.

On Inauguration Day, Richards stood on the inaugural platform with the most important Democratic officials, looking out over the crowds stretching to the Washington Monument, to witness Obama's second swearing in. It was, she believed, a moment for celebration. The antiabortion movement was losing ground. The Republicans had imploded over Akin's "legitimate rape" language, and party officials were running away from the religious right. In Mississippi, one of the most antiabortion states in the country, a ballot measure to grant constitutional rights to a fetus from conception failed.

Planned Parenthood could claim some measure of responsibility for these wins: the Supreme Court's 2010 ruling in *Citizens United v. FEC* opened the door to unlimited political spending from advocacy groups, and Richards had taken advantage. Planned Parenthood's political operation poured nearly $12 million into campaigns for Democratic candidates—more than fourteen times what it had spent just four years earlier and four times more than the Susan B. Anthony List, which spent less than $3 million. Shortly after his second term began, Obama became the first sitting president to address Planned Parenthood's national conference—a thank-you gift delivered after winning reelection. The antiabortion activists had state laws, but Richards had the president and the Supreme Court.

Still, Richards hadn't fully seen the possibilities in her deep-red home state. Not until that night under the rotunda with Wendy Davis.

Hours after Davis and Richards celebrated in the capitol, Republicans called another special session to try one more time to pass the twenty-week abortion ban. And once again, Richards and Davis were ready. They rallied outside the Capitol and crisscrossed the state to energize supporters in orange buses nicknamed "Ann" after Richards's mother and "Maggie" after Margaret Sanger, the founder of Planned Parenthood.

Feminist writers heralded a "Wendy Davis nation," where abortion rights would motivate Democratic voters. An internet meme circulated showing Davis as Daenerys Targaryen from *Game of Thrones* with a dragon on her shoulder: "In the game of Texas Senate, you either filibuster or Republicans own your uterus," it read. Progressives in Texas saw the start of a rebirth, a wave of activism that could lift them back into power.

Days before the second vote, Richards hosted a rowdy party in Washington called Sex, Politics, and Cocktails. Hundreds of young supporters, joined by several dozen members of Congress, sipped their drinks in the airy atrium of the Newseum. They chuckled about the party favors: hundreds of condoms with wrappers that read PROPER ATTIRE: REQUIRED FOR ENTRY.

Liberal women believed they were watching democracy at work. They believed Davis would win. A new Texas and a new America were here.

BUT THEY LOST.

The second vote on the Texas abortion ban happened less than three weeks after the first. This time, Davis could not run out the clock, because Republicans introduced it early in the session. Democrats tried to add exceptions for rape and incest into the legislation. They failed. After all the yelling, the organizing, and the protesting, the final vote—19–11—remained nearly unchanged from the first. On the day that the governor signed the law, Planned Parenthood announced that three of its Texas clinics would close. Republican lawmakers cast Richards's protesters as unruly renegades trying to take over the capitol and overpower an elected majority doing the work of the people. In Texas, the law was popular, particularly with Republicans. Concern about the threat to abortion rights faded away as liberal America moved on to the next outrage.

Still, Richards believed in the power of what she witnessed in her home state. Her people would keep fighting. Organizing, protesting, and shifting public opinion: that was how they would strengthen abortion rights and roll back these laws, she believed. "It's not enough, in this area, to just be great at what you do. You have to back it up with people," she said. And in Texas, they had. Along with Davis, her movement had shown the nation what was at stake with all these new abortion bans and restrictions. And as far as Richards could tell, the country had been riveted by their fight. In deeply conservative Texas, she thought, they'd "woken up a sleeping giant."

5

Teaching the Men

Not long after Obama's reelection, Marjorie Dannenfelser sought the help of one of her oldest and most trusted allies: Kellyanne Conway. Antiabortion activism was in Conway's DNA, Dannenfelser would say, encoded from her childhood at a Catholic school in New Jersey. Like Dannenfelser, Conway believed the problem for Republicans wasn't opposition to abortion but how they sold that view to voters. Their men—Republican candidates—avoided the issue or said the wrong thing entirely, like Todd Akin did. The dynamic was an immediate, and significant, problem: of the 233 House Republicans who would soon be serving in the new Congress in 2013, only 20 were women.

They needed to teach the men.

On a cold day in early 2013, Conway headed to a golf resort in Williamsburg, Virginia, to start their reeducation effort. She was scheduled to appear with two of the party's prominent male consultants on the first evening of a private retreat of House Republicans to talk about what had gone so very wrong for the party during the 2012 race.

As gigs went, it was hardly inviting. The mood was somber, with none of the giddy optimism of when many of the Tea Party members were still new to Congress two years earlier. The overwhelming focus of the lawmakers were the looming fiscal fights.

But Conway came to deliver a different message: abortion could win elections for Republicans—so long as their candidates followed her and Dannenfelser's advice.

Looking out at the overwhelmingly male audience, Conway didn't mince words. Akin's views that rape couldn't result in a pregnancy weren't that unusual among socially conservative activists. They were deeply rooted in the antiabortion movement, going back to a book published by John C. Willke in 1985. But to the general public, they were unscientific and immediately cast Akin as a misogynistic dinosaur. In her comments, Conway offered some clear advice to avoid making the same mistake. She spoke from experience. Akin had briefly been a polling client, though Conway resigned after his comment. "Rape is a four-letter word," she told the crowd. "If your mommy told you not to say four-letter words, remember rape is one of them."

By this point in her career, Conway was used to lecturing men. Over her two decades working as a conservative pollster, she had learned that delivering these kinds of presentations at Republican gatherings could feel, as she joked, like entering a bachelor party in the locker room of the Elks Club. She had also become what antiabortion activists called the "gold standard" of polling for their movement, arming them with data to craft their messaging and legislation. Conway worked for socially conservative Republicans like Dan Quayle, Newt Gingrich, and Mike Pence, who needed help reaching female voters, and for advocacy groups, including the Susan B. Anthony List.

As a girl, Kellyanne Fitzpatrick had been raised in their movement, growing up in a matriarchy with her single mother, grandmother, and aunts in a house adorned with crucifixes and saint statues. Her childhood was cards, church choir, and boisterous Sunday dinners after Mass. Starting at twelve, she worked summers packing blueberries for sixteen cents a crate in the shed of Indian Brand Farm, an operation owned by her parish youth group leader. She didn't like to lose, eventually winning the New Jersey Blueberry

Princess pageant and the World Champion Blueberry Packing competition. That contest was initially called a tie, until she asked for a recount. "The faster you went, the more money you'd make," Conway later explained to NJ Advance Media. And Conway was nothing if not quick and hungry.

Like Dannenfelser, her career took off in the early 1990s, as the Year of the Woman took off in Washington, and any hope of overturning Roe seemed impossible. But Ruth Bader Ginsburg, Hillary Clinton, Senator Dianne Feinstein, and the other newly elected women in the Senate were not Dannenfelser's or Conway's kind of women. As action causes reaction, political change prompts political backlash. And 1992—the seminal year for Democratic women who supported abortion rights—sparked a band of conservative women devoted to the opposite.

Dannenfelser and Conway were at the forefront of this new, if much smaller, young sisterhood—fresh out of college, against abortion, and determined to make space for conservative women in politics. Young and idealistic, white and mostly Christian, these women saw themselves as the true champions of women and their babies. They hoped to expand the definition of being a woman in politics, to create a conservative womanhood where professional advancement and abortion rights were not synonymous. They had a lot of work to do. The political power against them—Planned Parenthood, EMILYs List, and other organizations that supported Democratic women who backed abortion rights—started years earlier, giving them a significant head start.

The question was how to push back. Dannenfelser, who had left her job as a House aide to take care of her young daughter, connected with Rachel MacNair, a vegan Quaker in Missouri who led a group called Feminists for Life. MacNair viewed being "pro-life" as also being against the death penalty and nuclear war, and had conceived her son through artificial insemination, something she said her Catholic friends just did not understand. MacNair, Dannenfelser, and others believed the antiabortion cause needed its own version of EMILYs List, so they started a new group to promote female candidates who opposed abortion rights. They named it for Susan B. Anthony, the suffragist, who they believed had once described abortion as "child murder" in an article from 1896. The article was signed only with a single "A.," and there was no contemporary evidence that Anthony opposed abortion. But she became a symbol to them of a powerful woman on their side.

In 1994, SBA's first, small class of candidates was lifted into office as part of the wave that swept the Republicans to unified control of Congress. For the first time since Roe, a party that opposed abortion controlled both chambers of Congress. That year became a beginning for antiabortion women, their own miniature 1992.

When MacNair left to pursue a PhD in psychology, Dannenfelser raised her hand to become SBA's executive director. Dannenfelser turned a closet in her home in Arlington, Virginia, into the group's office. One of her first actions was perhaps her most consequential: they would no longer support only female antiabortion candidates. SBA would back anyone who opposed abortion, male or female. The cause came first. If a woman who supported abortion rights was running, they would back an antiabortion man running against her.

Conway came on as an early pollster for the Susan B. Anthony List. She hosted one of Dannenfelser's earliest fundraising events, a tea for the spouses of members of Congress. With Republicans in power, brazen young conservative women were getting their moment. The media couldn't get enough of them. As Conway put it, they were "Young. Lively. Stylish. Opinionated. Thin." What they were certainly not was feminists, a phrase Conway and her crew dismissed as outdated, anti-male, and pro-abortion. "You can't appeal to us through our wombs," she told *The Atlantic* shortly after opening her polling firm. "We're pro-life. The fetus beat us. We grew up with sonograms. We know life when we see it."

Soon Conway had Washington currency, making regular appearances on cable news shows. Still, it wasn't always easy. The men at *The Weekly Standard* dubbed her part of "a new class of Washington-bred cigar-and-martini bimbos," along with Ann Coulter, Laura Ingraham, and other "policy babes," as another piece put it. And then there were the unwanted sexual advances from powerful men. Back then it was better to pretend they didn't happen or were your fault or wouldn't happen again, Conway later told *Cosmopolitan*, the women's magazine. Her political rise, after all, was sandwiched between two seminal episodes of male sexual misconduct in Washington: Clarence Thomas's alleged harassment of Anita Hill, and Bill Clinton's sexual relationship with White House intern Monica Lewinsky. Conway learned quickly that trying to make some "federal case out of somebody who was in a huge position of power" would only embarrass the woman making it. She wanted power to push her agenda in Washington, and she understood the rules conservative women had to follow to get it.

By the time she addressed the Republican retreat that chilly week in 2013, she had married George Conway, the prominent conservative lawyer and star of the Federalist Society, had four children, and enjoyed a successful career as a political strategist. As the Republican men jotted down her advice in their notebooks, she knew her party's problems ran deeper than just talking about rape. The Democratic strategy painting Republicans as waging "war on women" had worked. The gender gap in 2012 was substantial, with Obama winning female voters by twelve points—as the autopsy pointed out.

But it was wrong to think that Democrats had won on the abortion issue itself, argued Conway. Yes, Democrats jumped on Akin's "legitimate rape" comments to cast Republicans as disconnected and tone-deaf. But they used the misstep to bolster a broader, more effective political rallying cry—that they were the party of women's health care and empowerment. In surveys before the election, only a minority of Democratic and independent voters had said abortion would be very important to their vote. To them, abortion seemed secure. But health care was near the top of their list of concerns. "Part of the hijacking of the lexicon this year has been, instead of talking about abortion, then it was choice, now it's women's health," Conway had said a month before the election, when she sat on a stage with Richards for a panel on the women's vote in the coming election. What Conway saw was that Democrats had transformed attacks on abortion into an attack on women's health, a far more energizing issue.

In her own presentations, Conway often argued that women were the "chief health care officers" for their families—the ones who made the appointments and nagged everyone to go to the doctor. They were motivated by health care issues, even if they didn't think much about abortion. Tying those issues together made for a far more potent message than simply being "pro-choice." And for the Democrats in 2012, it had worked. Obama was again in the White House.

Unless Republicans reclaimed the issue of women's health with their own message, their own infrastructure, even their own set of facts, they would lose again, Conway believed. Women should take the lead in delivering the conservative case against abortion. And when their men talked about the issue, they needed to do so with empathy and care—and not be scared to defend their position. Democrats used words like *health*, *freedom*, and *choice*. Conway would work with Dannenfelser to do the same thing, and purge their movement of words like *rape*.

They took their advice on the road. At the party's quarterly meeting, Dannenfelser and Conway set up in a discreet conference room at the Peabody Memphis, away from the live ducks in the fountain and the reporters who roamed the ornate lobby. Their sessions were kept quiet, not listed on the event's public schedule—a secret abortion boot camp.

Candidates and congressmen rolled through, eager to win elections and female voters. The two women offered blunt advice: silence on abortion isn't an option. Unlike Democratic voters, Republicans were likelier to list abortion as important to their vote.

Republicans lost when Democrats attacked them for being too extreme and they did not fight back, they argued. Their party's silence on abortion allowed liberals to define what conservatives believed.

Dannenfelser and Conway pointed a video camera at each man and asked a simple question: "Why do you believe abortion is wrong?" Then they all reviewed the tape. It didn't always go well. The men rattled on for too long or struggled to find the right words. Or, worst of all to Conway, they used the "R-word." Simpler was better, they advised. "Two sentences is really the goal," said Dannenfelser. "Then stop talking."

Flip the script, said Conway. Challenge Democrats when they try to trot out their message about women's health. "Women's health issues are osteoporosis or breast cancer or seniors living alone who don't have enough money for health care," said Conway, not abortion. Polling showed that voters were more supportive of restrictions later in pregnancy, once women were in the second trimester. So ask your opponent, "Exactly when in a pregnancy do you think abortion should be banned?"

These "murder boards," as Dannenfelser called them, were a central part of a new mission: "Project Lifeline." The stakes were too high for their candidates to approach a podium or camera unprepared, so SBA offered them a "lifeline." Major statewide candidates got one-on-one, in-person training sessions. Others could do them online through a password-protected site. Any politician who wanted SBA's endorsement was required to participate, though the group made some exceptions.

The overall goal, of course, was much bigger than simply fixing how their politicians talked about abortion. It was part of a longer-term strategy to regain power and end abortion. Dannenfelser had transformed her anger in Norquist's conference room into something more effective: a plan. She envisioned fixing it all. She would reshape media coverage in their favor, with their own experts and testimony. She would push new restrictions as far as they could through the House, where Republicans were in control. And she would win enough seats in the Senate to put an antiabortion majority in control.

They needed data, their own science, to more credibly push back against the statistics coming from what they saw as "hostile sources," such as the Guttmacher Institute, the research and policy center that originally started as part of Planned Parenthood in 1968. SBA expanded its nascent Charlotte Lozier Institute to become a research arm that hired its own ob-gyns and scientists, people who identified as "pro-life." (The group was named for one of America's first female physicians, who died from a hemorrhage after the birth of her third child.) Mainstream doctors disagreed with their findings. But Dannenfelser and the movement now had their own scientific reports and their own experts who could testify before Congress for abortion restrictions and produce research that supported their goals.

They jumped on opportunities to press their case. When Kermit Gosnell, a doctor who ran a West Philadelphia abortion clinic, was found guilty in 2013 of murdering preterm babies after they were born, Dannenfelser used the very public examples of infanticide to push for a federal twenty-week abortion ban. Gosnell's horrific actions and the gruesome images that emerged in his trial led to broad condemnation, and abortion opponents equated the murdered infants who were born early with fetuses aborted at a similar gestational age. "This is a visual argument that no one would ever want to have," Dannenfelser told *The New York Times*. "But if we're going to have it, let's go ahead and have it. What are the limits? What are we as a society willing to forbear?"

Dannenfelser realized they could use the shifting media and technology environment to their favor. It was the new journalistic era of the "micro-scoop," the blog, the tweet. The internet was endless, and media outlets were desperate to fill it with their content. Suddenly, Dannenfelser seemed to be everywhere. Available for lunch or a coffee. Happy to dash off a quote to mainstream reporters, unlike so many others in her conservative circles. Her staff filed

Dannenfelser's quotes in binders by year and outlet: Christian and mainstream and women's magazines. They piled up in stacks and boxes against the wall of SBA's small office, a physical manifestation of their expanding influence to reshape the national conversation.

The number of her quotes—her flood of words—gave SBA an outsize voice and concealed the small stature of its actual operation. Even as a majority of Americans continued to support abortion rights, the saturation and digital spread created a sense that Dannenfelser's movement had more reach and public support than it actually did.

While SBA grew its reach and influence over how the party messaged its antiabortion positions, its allies in states like Texas pushed through the twenty-week abortion bans. When antiabortion lawmakers in the US House of Representatives passed their most far-reaching abortion bill in decades, a ban on most procedures after twenty weeks of pregnancy, they named it the Pain-Capable Unborn Child Protection Act. SBA and other antiabortion groups furnished the politicians with studies arguing that a fetus could feel pain at twenty weeks post-fertilization.

But the developing science of fetal pain was complex, and most scientists who had researched the issue said those claims were false. The American College of Obstetricians and Gynecologists, the main association for ob-gyns in the United States, pointed to research showing that a fetus could not perceive pain until perhaps the third trimester. But the antiabortion movement used the still-evolving and disputed science to point out doubt. "I am a bit concerned that if we just say we don't know, we may be causing quite a lot of suffering. I would rather err on the safe side and say, 'Well, the fetus may be suffering and so we ought to do something about it,'" said Vivette Glover, a perinatal psychobiologist, whom the Family Research Council, a social conservative group, cited in a pamphlet about fetal pain.

In reality, the bill had no chance of becoming law, given that Democrats controlled the Senate. Instead, it was constructed as a legal and political trap, designed to undercut the viability standard set in Roe and to force Democrats to defend the less popular position of permitting abortion later in pregnancy. The legislation was a continuation of the chipping-away strategy that had long been a template for their movement.

But they knew that seemingly futile bills could become law if they just persevered long enough. Back in 1995, the National Right to Life Committee began to refer to an abortion procedure called *intact dilation and evacuation* as "partial-birth abortion," using the language associated with birthing a viable baby to campaign against the procedure. Congressional Republicans took up the cause, crafting legislation that would ban it, and President Clinton vetoed those bills twice during his administration. But in 2003, after eight years, President Bush signed a ban into law. The Supreme Court affirmed the restriction four years later, and intact dilation and evacuation abortions became illegal. The ruling marked the first time since Roe that the court upheld an abortion restriction without an exception to protect women's health.

So when the twenty-week ban passed the House in June 2013 but failed to advance beyond that, antiabortion Republicans looked to the recent past for proof a win was possible if they just stayed in the fight long enough. In comments to reporters, Representative Trent Franks, who sponsored the twenty-week ban, cited the fight to ban partial-birth abortion as a model. "Everybody said, you know, it's not constitutional, it can't pass, it can't go anywhere," he told *Politico*. "It took time to do that and it even had to succeed a presidential veto. But it eventually did."

In story after story about the twenty-week legislation, SBA was presented as a powerful force, equivalent to its opponent, Planned Parenthood. But in reality, SBA was a minnow in a city of sharks. Its whole operating budget in 2013 was $7 million, according to internal documents. (Planned Parenthood that year would spend nearly $400 million on its programs and operations, excluding the medical services that made up the bulk of its more than $1 billion budget.) Project Lifeline had a budget of about $264,000, according to SBA's private business plan.

Still, for all the binders of her press coverage, Dannenfelser knew the best way—really, the only way—to claim power and push back on the dismissal of their movement in the autopsy would be by showing the antiabortion message could win elections. SBA needed proof of concept that went beyond its work in smaller House races.

SBA had never run a statewide campaign before. There was no way that the group, with its tiny staff and shoestring budget, could participate in every competitive Senate race. It would have to be selective and pick its best opportunities for success. For now, it would start small, with three statewide elections in 2014. SBA targeted three incumbent Democrats in states with strong antiabortion electorates—Arkansas, Louisiana, and North Carolina—and aimed to make those campaigns directly about abortion policy. Republicans needed to gain six seats to win control of the Senate; Dannenfelser's three could put them halfway there.

SBA designed a door-knocking campaign, with year-round field offices, to increase direct contact with voters it believed could be influenced to cast their ballots based on their opposition to abortion. It was a tactic learned by studying the Obama campaign's winning strategy in 2008: start early and use the new flood of data now available about voters online to target those most open to your message.

But to do all that, Dannenfelser needed money. More money than the sisterhood of women volunteering at pregnancy centers and running the local antiabortion benefits for their church could give. Dannenfelser tapped her network of believers in Washington, including the kind of influential conservatives who attended the Falls Church, an evangelical congregation in the Northern Virginia suburbs. Its congregants included Republican power brokers like Marc Short, a close ally of Pence's from Capitol Hill who was now the head of Freedom Partners, an umbrella organization for donors allied with the conservative billionaires Charles and David Koch.

The brothers were part of a new class of megadonors whose political operation rivaled the Republican Party itself.

The Kochs and many of their libertarian donors didn't particularly care about ending abortion. David Koch was open about his support for abortion rights, even boasting about his position in interviews. But Short positioned Dannenfelser and SBA as a force that could drive the party's conservative base to the polls, a useful tool for the Kochs' aims of winning a Republican majority that could lower taxes and cut regulation. Freedom Partners would eventually give SBA around a million dollars, a rare seven-figure donation for the small group, according to two people familiar with the donation.

The sum was small by Washington standards. But the symbolism was big. To Dannenfelser, it felt like validation, a sign that their plan to gain power just might work.

6

The Pendulum

The night the Texas twenty-week abortion ban passed, Cecile Richards couldn't sleep. She was confident that the law could be overturned at the Supreme Court, where Roe was the law of the land, but she kept thinking about the people she'd met, the effort they had mounted, the experience of it all. These people, all these women who showed up, who left work early and brought their daughters and told their stories and cried and screamed and shouted—those people were voters. And they were energized by abortion rights, Richards thought. They had lost this particular battle, but still Richards believed Wendy Davis had ignited something new.

The filibuster rocketed Davis to fame and helped create space for a more open national conversation about abortion. Davis devoted pages in her memoir to her experience with Tate, and Richards told her abortion story in *Elle*. The abortion "wasn't a difficult decision," Richards wrote. "When politicians argue and shout about abortion, they're talking about me—and millions of other women around the country."

Davis was a heroine for the abortion-rights movement, expanding the values of Obama's America. And in a heroine's story, the fact that she lost one battle wasn't the main point. It was the uprising she caused that mattered. Davis showed Democrats a new political opportunity, a chance to take Texas back or at least send a serious message that even in conservative ranchlands—the heart of Republican America—liberal views could gain momentum.

Vogue invited Davis to pose in its pages, and top party strategists in Washington urged her to run for governor. Democrats brought her to Congress for meetings and celebrations. Davis raised $1 million and launched a national tour, building her network of financial supporters. Her effort was a long shot: no Democrat had won statewide office in Texas since Ann Richards did in 1990. To win, she would have to run a near-perfect campaign.

Ann Richards's election in conservative Texas was, Richards admitted, close to a political "miracle." But she was hopeful it could happen again. Planned Parenthood promised to spend $3 million on the race as Richards anointed Davis with the image of her mother. "Mom was an authentic Texan, just as Wendy is," Richards told the magazine *Texas Monthly*. "And Wendy's story is the Texas story."

Yet there was another story happening in Texas too. Planned Parenthood sued to stop the new requirements on clinics and abortion doctors. But its litigation did not address the part of the law that prohibited abortion at twenty weeks. The case, the lawyers suspected, would eventually be taken by the Supreme Court, where Justice Anthony Kennedy would likely be the crucial swing vote. They worried he might uphold a twenty-week ban. In *Gonzales v. Carhart*, the case over banning partial birth abortion, Kennedy the court's swing vote on abortion rights, wrote critically about abortion later in pregnancy, describing graphic details and speculating that some women might regret their decision.

Contesting the twenty-week ban could lead Kennedy "to view the whole case in a negative light," said Stephanie Toti, the lawyer from the Center for Reproductive Rights, who was leading the case on behalf of Planned Parenthood, the American Civil Liberties Union, Whole Woman's Health, and the other organizations involved with the litigation. They decided to leave the twenty-week ban part of the law unchallenged to avoid turning Kennedy against them. "We would take an incremental approach," said Toti. "Then we could circle back using the precedent that we created to go after the twenty-week ban and other restrictions that had been in Texas law." Besides, the twenty-week ban was dated to a woman's last menstrual cycle, meaning that in practice it was actually closer to a twenty-two-week ban. A larger percentage of fetuses could possibly survive outside the womb at twenty-two weeks than could at twenty weeks, making the Texas law a less clear-cut violation of Roe's viability standard.

As the case proceeded, the law took effect and abortion providers were powerless to stop the real impact on women in Texas. Republicans held a trifecta of power in the state—control of the House, Senate, and governorship—meaning no legislation undoing the restrictions would be likely to become law. Their case against this law could take years, a long road of appeals and filings. The number of clinics began dwindling. Before the law went into effect, there were forty-one facilities providing abortions in the state. Four months later, the number had dropped to twenty-two.

The diverging narratives—one planning for legal victory at the high court and another facing losses in Texas—revealed the central paradox of this new decade on abortion. At the national level, abortion rights were strong, protected by the Supreme Court and backed by the Democratic Party. But in Republican states across the country, they were growing weaker by the year.

For national Democratic leaders, the political stakes felt, if not low, certainly not existential. Roe loomed so large in American life that it was almost impossible to imagine that it could disappear. Every election Democrats and their allies in the abortion rights movement warned voters about the potential consequences to abortion rights, should they vote Republican. But truthfully, almost no politician, strategist, or official on either side of the aisle really believed Roe would fall. It was an established legal precedent for forty years. Yes, the court had been chipping away at it since then, with cases like Webster and Casey. But aside from a persistent group of antiabortion believers, who were on a spiritual mission to undo the decision, Roe was simply part of American identity.

Even Nancy Northup, the former prosecutor who headed the Center for Reproductive Rights, which had joined Planned Parenthood in the case against the Texas law, didn't think Roe was directly at risk. Her group was filing brief after brief, challenging the new restrictions popping up across the country. It was impossible to keep up—as soon as one law was challenged, another appeared. And Northup, who rarely minced words, knew that they couldn't keep up. As far as she could tell, the antiabortion movement's strategy was to chip away at abortion rights until there was nothing left, rather than strike directly at Roe. She offered a solution to her Democratic allies in Congress. They could codify Roe into federal law, protecting women in conservative states from these kinds of restrictions. She wanted to call her new bill the Roe Restoration Act. But polling showed the case didn't resonate with voters, who didn't really see it at risk. Better to put the words *women* and *health* in the title, her political strategists said. The title became the Women's Health Protection Act.

It wasn't an easy case to make: Democrats didn't see the new state restrictions as a priority in a world with Roe. And anyhow, even though they controlled the Senate, there weren't enough Democrats who favored abortion rights to pass the bill. The proposal died in committee, never even making it to a vote. Democratic strategists largely saw Northup's legislative effort as a waste of time. They didn't see the value of pushing abortion rights as a message, if it wasn't the issue that motivated their voters in elections. Besides, at least five Democrats were shaky on abortion rights in the Senate, and making them take a vote on the issue could come back to hurt their chances in the coming midterm elections.

In the summer of 2014, with the midterms looming, Richards faced a setback. The Supreme Court ruled in *Burwell v. Hobby*

Lobby that the Christian-owned craft store and other for-profit companies were not, in fact, required to provide contraception coverage to their employees against their religious objections, despite what President Obama promised Richards in that phone call a year earlier. The ruling undercut the victory Richards described as her proudest professional moment. It was upsetting, she said, but even with this loss, more than thirty million women already had access to the free contraception benefit in Obama's health care law. The law, she wrote, remained "the biggest step forward for women in a generation."

Still, another moment that had seemed like a victory had become another defeat. Like the Texas law, the ruling was a hairline crack, one that seemed so small it could be hard to see clearly, given the left's sense of Roe's inviolability. And it wasn't the only one.

Where Richards saw the health care law as a big win, another smaller coalition of activists argued they had given up too much ground. The abortion-rights movement was dominated by four big organizations. Planned Parenthood was the health care arm. The Center for Reproductive Rights functioned as the law firm of the movement. NARAL was the political operation. And EMILYs List funded Democratic candidates who backed abortion rights. All were run by white women. Each had more money than SBA and the other antiabortion groups.

But there was also a constellation of far smaller, largely Black and Hispanic abortion-rights organizations, part of the reproductive justice movement that orbited Planned Parenthood. These activists believed existing rules restricting abortion access made Roe already an illusion to many low-income women. They saw the new health care law—which did not undo the most onerous of those restrictions—not as a generational win but a generational defeat. To get enough votes to pass the health care bill, top Democrats had made a deal with the antiabortion wing of their party. The new law would reaffirm the Hyde Amendment, a 1970s policy that banned federal funding for abortions to women insured by Medicaid and had been reaffirmed for decades as part of the federal budget. The Hyde Amendment had a big impact on low-income women, who were disproportionately likely to rely on Medicaid for their healthcare coverage. About 75 percent of abortions were among low-income women, and of those, just more than half of the patients were non-white women. For some of these women, the cost of an abortion was prohibitive. The median out-of-pocket cost was $575, one study found, more than a third of the monthly income of most women insured by Medicaid.

Richards knew that Democrats didn't have the votes to end Hyde. With the dozens of antiabortion Democrats in their ranks in 2009, they'd barely been able to keep their coalition together to pass the health care law. "You always wish you could have done more," Richards later acknowledged. But she insisted that their best opportunity during the Obama administration had been to get birth control covered and ensure that abortion coverage wasn't banned entirely under the new law. Still, the disagreement over what, exactly, constituted a victory for their movement weakened the coalition. To the Black and Hispanic reproductive justice activists, the new health care law, which left the Hyde Amendment intact, was a sign that the biggest organization in their world was willing to trade away their rights.

Three years later, more fissures surfaced when Planned Parenthood launched a new messaging campaign that dumped the decades-old terminology of *pro-choice* for a broader approach. "When it comes down to it, we just don't know a woman's specific situation. We're not in her shoes," read Planned Parenthood's new tagline, in a video released to mark the fortieth anniversary of the Roe decision. "So the next time you talk about abortion, don't let the labels box you in." The new messaging frustrated reproductive justice movement activists who had always believed that the fight for abortion rights couldn't be severed from the economic, justice, housing, and maternal health care struggles that disproportionately affected the reproductive lives of women of color. Now, it felt like

Planned Parenthood was stealing their approach and acting like it was its own.

"If we don't stop this now, our organizations are going to disappear. They're going to close," said Monica Raye Simpson, the executive director of SisterSong, a collective of abortion-rights organizations run by women of color. "They will be absorbed into this white feminist agenda."

Some establishment Democrats, too, rejected the new approach. "Pro-choice" might be a dated rallying cry, but it fit on a campaign sign. Planned Parenthood's new approach lacked the clarity of its opponents' tactics, which cast the issue in starkly black-and-white terms. Even Richards, at her press conference unveiling the new messaging, acknowledged that the group's new approach wasn't quite "bumper-sticker ready." The simmering frustrations—both from the reproductive justice movement and Democrats—revealed that Planned Parenthood, the largest organization standing between the antiabortion movement and the American people, had critics even within its own coalition.

At the time, these fractures seemed like small setbacks in a war that abortion-rights activists were winning. Even with the Hobby Lobby ruling, abortion rights still had their movement's champion on the court: Justice Ruth Bader Ginsburg, who had responded to that decision with one of her signature dissents. In a sign of the depth of her concern, the senior member of the court's liberal bloc read portions aloud from the bench. Approving only some religious claims for accommodation risked the court favoring one religion over another. "The court, I fear, has ventured into a minefield," she wrote.

At eighty-one, Ginsburg was a feminist icon who had reached the peak of her profession. Since her nomination to the bench in the wake of the "Year of the Woman," she had risen to become the "Notorious RBG," a nickname first coined by a blogging law student that exploded into the popular consciousness. Her face was emblazoned on pins and magnets, feminist greeting cards and coffee mugs. Mothers even dressed their daughters as "baby Ruthie" for Halloween.

Ginsburg herself was never all that fond of Roe. Fundamentally, she agreed that there should be a constitutional right to an abortion. But she disagreed with how it happened. "The political process was moving in the early 1970s, not swiftly enough for advocates of quick, complete change, but majoritarian institutions were listening and acting," she wrote in 1984. "Heavy-handed judicial intervention was difficult to justify and appears to have provoked, not resolved, conflict."

She also believed the court had made the right ruling based on the wrong argument in 1973. Abortion rights weren't about privacy, she argued, but rather should be rooted in gender equality. Ginsburg wished the court had established a right to equal protection for women. The justices could have done that, she thought, if they had taken up a different case also from the early 1970s. Back then, Ginsburg represented Captain Susan Struck, a nurse who was serving in Vietnam when she became pregnant. The US military at the time required women to leave the service if they became mothers. Struck, a Catholic, wanted to carry the pregnancy to term and keep her job. Ginsburg appealed to the Supreme Court on Struck's behalf, which eventually agreed to hear the case. Then, the Air Force relented, rendering the issue moot. The fact that the case did not reach the high court meant the justices did not examine how pregnancy affected women's equal protection under the Constitution.

A few months after Hobby Lobby, shortly before the midterm elections, Ginsburg explained how grounded Roe had become in American life. Between questions about her workout routine and what she watched on television in an interview with *Elle* magazine, Ginsburg opined on the permanence of the decision. In fifty years, she said, no one would be able to understand how the court could have ruled against contraception. The right to an abortion, she believed, would remain standing because America had come to see it as foundational.

"One of the reasons, to be frank, that there's not so much pro-choice activity, is that young women, including my daughter and my granddaughter, have grown up in a world where they know if they need an abortion, they can get it. Not that either one of them has had one," she said. The state restrictions, she noted, were mainly an issue for poor women. Eventually, those would also fall. "The country will wake up and see that it can never go back to [abortions just] for women who can afford to travel to a neighboring state."

Ginsburg didn't plan on going anywhere. Obama gingerly hinted at the possibility of retirement in a private lunch with her right after Davis's filibuster and raised the prospect that Democrats could lose control of the Senate in the midterms. The political map favored Republicans, with control of the body hinging on races in conservative states, and the party of incumbent presidents typically lost seats in midterms. If the Senate flipped, Obama would not be able to appoint a justice to the court who could continue the liberal legal project for decades.

Ginsburg responded with the court's version of a public reprimand. Even if she retired, she said in a rare interview, Obama was more likely to appoint a compromise candidate than a true liberal like she was. "There will be a president after this one, and I'm hopeful that that president will be a fine president," she told *The New York Times*.

Presidents would come and go, Ginsburg implied, but the Supreme Court was for life. While Washington descended into partisan warfare, the court remained set apart, a lone bastion where comity still reigned. Ginsburg was known for her friendship with Justice Antonin Scalia, her ideological opposite in most every way. Debate and disagreement would happen on the bench. But the acrimony could be left there. Their much-lauded friendship was a symbol of a political world where bipartisanship was possible and ideological differences were not moral failings.

That was certainly not the world of Texas or the other conservative states where the antiabortion movement was charging forward.

But Ginsburg did not believe the restrictions on abortion would continue. The pendulum, she said, had swung "about as conservative as it will get."

THE MIDTERMS WERE the Democratic bloodbath that Obama feared. Democrats lost control of the Senate, lost seats in the House, and lost closely contested races for governor. No president, in more than fifty years, suffered as big a defeat to his party's political standing in the Senate.

Davis, the woman perhaps more associated with the cause of abortion rights than any Democrat in the country, ended her campaign with the worst showing by a Democratic gubernatorial candidate in the state since 1998, when George W. Bush was on the ballot. It was clear that Davis hadn't been running in Ann Richards's Texas. Attorney General Greg Abbott, her opponent, didn't make Clayton Williams's mistakes; in fact, it was Davis who faced personal attacks over her past and was branded "Abortion Barbie" by conservatives. And none of her tough Texas gal attitude was enough to overcome the state's sharp shift to the right or Abbott's barrage of negative ads. Democrats explained away her loss as the result of a bad candidate with a muddled campaign strategy and disorganized operation. Davis started as Joan of Arc, charging into the Senate chamber in her salmon-pink sneakers. In a sense, she ended that way too. Joan of Arc was eventually burned at the stake in 1431, accused of heresy for flouting female decency and disseminating beliefs contrary to the Catholic Church.

Another Democratic candidate, Senator Mark Udall—or "Mark Uterus," as his opponents called him—focused so heavily on abortion that a local reporter joked that if the race were a movie, it would be set in a gynecologist's office. Like Davis, Udall was defeated that fall, making him the first incumbent from Colorado to lose a Senate race in thirty-six years. The depth of those losses reinforced a lesson for many Democratic officials: abortion could go viral, but it didn't win them elections.

The Democratic defeats provided some evidence that Marjorie Dannenfelser and Kellyanne Conway's training had worked. Their candidates avoided Todd Akin's high-profile missteps on abortion and when the issue did come up, they successfully moved the conversation onto politically safer ground. After the Hobby Lobby decision, Democrats attacked Republican candidates as against access to contraception. In response, Republicans rolled out plans to make birth control available over the counter. Of course, without the insurance coverage guaranteed in the health care law, which Republicans wanted to repeal, the pills would be prohibitively expensive for many women. Still, it was a strategy, Conway boasted in September, that would "neutralize and defang" the liberal attacks. Democrats, she said, "think that they've got a monopoly on talking to women from the waist down."

The Susan B. Anthony List won its three test case Senate races in Arkansas, Louisiana, and North Carolina, flipping all three seats from Democratic control. In total, SBA sent out 750 canvassers, knocked on 520,050 doors, and made 536,742 phone calls, according to an internal document. They spent nearly $3.5 million on campaigns, just about half of Planned Parenthood's $6 million that cycle.

Those Republicans could have certainly won without Dannenfelser's help. Many of the key races happened in conservative states, giving Republicans an advantage from the start. History, too, was on their side. The party in the White House had lost seats in nearly every midterm over the past eight decades. Republicans turned the race into a referendum on the economic stewardship of Obama, whose approval rating hit the lowest level of his presidency two weeks before Election Day. Exit polls showed voters far more worried about the economy and health care than abortion, which barely ranked as a concern.

But for Dannenfelser, the Senate victories were proof that her plan had worked. She had changed the tenor of the conversation around abortion for her party, laying a path that avoided the pitfalls of the 2012 race. The new strategy helped her cause fight its way back into the heart of the Republican Party. Its candidates would enter office as antiabortion champions. After twenty years, SBA could play in the big leagues.

And through it all, just below the radar, their allies in the states were taking a more aggressive approach toward Roe with a deluge of laws. Cases over admitting privileges continued in Alabama and Oklahoma. In North Dakota, the state's sole clinic stopped providing medication abortions to avoid further lawsuits. And in Texas, the lawsuit brought by Richards, Northup, and their allies was slowly winding its way to the Supreme Court.

Dannenfelser and the antiabortion movement had even grander ambitions for the next president. Now that they had proven they could win, they could aim even bigger, at a presidential election. The race to replace Obama was just getting started. But first, they needed to go after a different, but no less symbolic, target: Planned Parenthood.

7

The Radical Post-Roe Generation

Cecile Richards did not see the strike coming. The secret plan started two years earlier, in 2013, with a little-known twenty-four-year-old Catholic antiabortion activist, who was driving cross-country with his pet six-foot black-throated monitor lizard named Rocky, and couldn't stop thinking about Planned Parenthood and what he called "fetal trafficking." As he made his way to California, his trip became a pilgrimage of sorts, with stops to seek advice and mentorship from some of the antiabortion movement's more radical outside actors.

In Wichita, Kansas, David Daleiden briefed Troy Newman, president of Operation Rescue, on his ideas. He wanted to infiltrate Planned Parenthood and surreptitiously videotape what he believed to be crimes of selling fetal tissue after an abortion. Or, as he often put it, selling "baby body parts." And then he would expose the women's health organization to the world.

Newman's group was known for its aggressive protests of abortion clinics, actions that frequently resulted in arrests and jail time, but even he wasn't sure this plan would work. Daleiden would have to go deep, create an alternative identity, a fake company, employees, and a website. It would need to be flawless to survive Planned Parenthood's system of background checks.

In Denton, Texas, Daleiden brainstormed with Mark Crutcher, who had taped similar undercover videos inside Planned Parenthood years earlier. Crutcher became a full-time antiabortion activist the same year his daughter Jackie died hours after she was born. But his videos gained little long-term momentum. Even Republicans seemed not to care, he told Daleiden.

But Daleiden was undeterred. He drafted an eight-page proposal, marked "confidential," and circulated it to antiabortion donors. Under "GOALS," he wrote "catch fetal traffickers, especially Planned Parenthood clinics, violating laws, regulations, and common decency." The estimated cost of his operation: $120,000. He called it "The Human Capital Project."

Some donors doubted that any new national abortion restrictions could pass, with Obama in the White House and Democrats controlling Congress. "We simply do not believe that the environment is right for anything meaningful to come from this project or most other stings," Raymond Ruddy, a Catholic philanthropist, emailed Daleiden in 2013, in response to a fundraising request. Daleiden pushed them, fashioning himself as an investigative journalist conducting an undercover sting. He sent over a partial transcript of a secretly recorded conversation with a procurement manager of a fetal tissue company to illustrate the kind of footage his team was capturing.

Daleiden, who joined the antiabortion cause as a teenager after googling images of aborted fetuses, described himself as the child of an unplanned pregnancy. A devout Catholic, he had worked as a researcher for Lila Rose, a young antiabortion activist who pioneered her own undercover video operation that infiltrated Planned Parenthood in 2007. Rose created her videos with James O'Keefe, who went on to start Project Veritas, a conservative group that would spend the next decade using similar misleading tactics and falsified identities to "expose" people he saw as liberal enemies in media and politics. Abortion was O'Keefe's training ground, an early foreshadowing of how he would later attack Joe Biden,

The New York Times, and Pfizer, the manufacturer of one of the leading COVID vaccines.

O'Keefe, Rose, and Daleiden represented a new cadre of antiabortion activists, part of a generation that were children in 1992 when the movement lost Casey—a post-Roe generation. They grew up in the world the first generation of antiabortion activists had created—the children of the religious right—and had only known an America with Roe. They didn't plan on waiting another four decades for it to end. Raised and catechized almost entirely in the internet era, fluent in Facebook, Twitter, and YouTube, they weren't interested in the incremental approach of the generations of Christian activists that preceded them. Their goal was to set the system on fire. Burn it down and burn it down fast. The more established power brokers of the antiabortion movement needed the younger post-Roe generation to continue the mission they started in the 1970s and 1980s. And over time, Daleiden convinced them to support his project.

The attack landed on YouTube on a Tuesday morning in July 2015, in the form of a professionally dressed woman picking at her salad in an airy Southern California restaurant.

"A lot of people want intact hearts these days," Dr. Deborah Nucatola, the senior director of medical services for Planned Parenthood Federation of America, said in the video as she twirled her fork in her lettuce. "Some people want lower extremities, too, which, that's simple. That's easy. I don't know what they're doing with it, I guess if they want muscle?"

Nucatola chuckled lightly, noting that fetal livers seem to be particularly in demand. Between sips of wine, she described how a doctor could conduct an abortion to preserve the organs of the fetus. "We've been very good at getting heart, lung, liver, because we know that, so I'm not gonna crush that part, I'm gonna basically crush below, I'm gonna crush above, and I'm gonna see if I can get it all intact," she said.

It was a clip Daleiden had worked for years to get. The implication of the footage, however unfair, was unmistakable: Planned

Parenthood was a horrifying and criminal organization, whose employees were laughing as they harvested fetal organs for profit. "Hold Planned Parenthood accountable for their illegal sale of baby parts," flashed the glowing white text as the screen faded to black.

Within hours, the video headlined national news, playing on a loop across cable television. It was bad, Richards's communications director warned her that morning before she saw the footage. Really bad. To Richards, it felt like a terrorist attack. Reports flooded into Planned Parenthood's Manhattan headquarters that Daleiden and his team had infiltrated the group's clinics, laboratories, and conferences. He had even secretly taped a brief conversation with Richards herself. Despite all their power and money, Planned Parenthood had been played.

More videos with even more explosive footage were coming, Daleiden promised. One new video, every week, for months. Richards didn't know exactly what they had, just that they had hours of it. Her staff lived in a state of fear for months, not knowing whether the next morning would bring another video that would unleash another wave of harassment on their doctors and staff. Her kids worried about her. Friends recommended she start meditating. If the attack was intended to intimidate, it accomplished its mission.

The reality was much more complicated than Daleiden's video portrayed. Research using tissue from aborted fetuses had been commonplace since the 1960s, funded by the National Institutes of Health for decades and supported by both parties. The tissue offered a uniquely fertile source of the stem cells that generate tissues and organs, providing particularly useful scientific material for advancements in the treatment of eye diseases, diabetes, and muscular dystrophies. Typically, the tissue was collected, with full consent from the women carrying the fetuses, by biological research companies who processed it before selling it to researchers. The practice was legal, as long as no one profited from the tissue itself. And it was rare in the Planned Parenthood network, with only one clinic each in Washington state and California providing tissue from aborted fetuses to researchers.

In the full, nearly three-hour tape Daleiden recorded at their lunch, Nucatola repeatedly tried to explain that Planned Parenthood does not profit when it provides fetal tissue to medical centers, researchers, or the companies that act as middlemen for those institutions. It charged thirty to one hundred dollars, she said, to cover expenses like preservation, transport, or shipping—legally permissible fees for costs. The full explanation of her statements was not included in the nearly nine-minute video that Daleiden released, an editing decision that transformed tonal missteps into the appearance of federal crimes.

Those facts were no match for powerful political backlash that followed almost immediately. Conservative media and Republican lawmakers pounced on the explosive footage, touting the videos as proof of Planned Parenthood's alleged crimes. "I could talk about the video but I think I'd vomit," said House Speaker John Boehner. "It's disgusting." A House bill that would have raised money for Komen's breast cancer research—a measure that was expected to easily pass—was pulled from the floor after abortion opponents linked the charity to Planned Parenthood. Four congressional committees soon announced separate investigations into Planned Parenthood, demanding thousands of pages of confidential documents. And Republican governors launched their own investigations against Planned Parenthood's state affiliates in Texas, Louisiana, Georgia, and Indiana.

Democrats, including allies Richards spent years and tens of millions of dollars cultivating, were largely silent. Even Hillary Clinton, already on the campaign trail for the coming 2016 presidential election and long one of Planned Parenthood's most stalwart supporters, said nothing about the videos for days.

Yet even as antiabortion movement leaders publicly celebrated, relishing the news that Richards could soon be forced to testify before Congress, it was not widely known just how radical the video sting operation truly was. It was an all-out assault, reliant on a deeply intertwined network of allies, from fringe activists to the highest ranks of the federal government, that few in the mainstream fully understood.

The day after the video landed, a private email chain circulated among top leaders across all sectors of their movement, from Marjorie Dannenfelser to Leonard Leo, one of their movement's most powerful lawyers, who was connected to seemingly every conservative lawyer, politician, and judge. Some on the chain had only learned of the project just before it went live, and were eager to capitalize on the fresh publicity for their cause. Others had worked for weeks, months, or years to maximize Daleiden's potential for success.

Autumn Christensen, the staff director of the Pro-Life Caucus in Congress, congratulated Daleiden for "doing a great job of working with folks on the Hill to grease the skids so we could respond appropriately quickly." Dannenfelser commended the fast political impact. "Just expressing gratitude again. God is good and you guys planned this masterfully," she said.

"But let's remember the talking points," Newman from Operation Rescue reminded the group. "This is about Planned Parenthood. Putting them in jail. Defunding them. Taking down their empire. Blessings and thanks to all."

FOR THE ANTIABORTION movement, taking down Planned Parenthood was about more than just ending abortion. It was about striking at the biggest symbol of the sexual revolution in America over the past one hundred years, and it required doing things differently to leverage the technological tools of this century. The footage was as evocative as those old photographs of mangled fetuses that activists once carried at their rallies and that John C. Willke put in his early books. But it was supercharged for an online era, able to travel far wider and faster than their posters and pamphlets.

The video was unlike attacks of the 1980s and 1990s, when antiabortion activists posed as patients to get into clinics and chain themselves to operating tables, or firebombed and vandalized clinics, or murdered doctors and clinic staff. This was an online firebombing, a nonviolent action that could be mainstreamed into national politics. And unlike the violence of their past, this action was one that could win support from the most powerful players in the highest ranks of the Republican Party.

It was a new strategy for a new generation of antiabortion activists, digital natives able to harness the power of the internet for maximal impact. The post-Roe generation was pushing their movement into a new era of American politics, adopting more aggressive techniques that were rewarded on social media platforms powered by political polarization. They used the tenets of American democracy to their advantage. Daleiden claimed his operation was undercover journalism, protected by the First Amendment.

But Daleiden built his project on falsehoods. After his road trip with Rocky the lizard, he filed with the IRS to gain tax-exempt status for a nonprofit named the Center for Medical Progress to collect donations. The group qualified under a category for "Diseases, Disorders, Medical Disciplines: Biomedicine, Bioengineering"—not the grouping that applied to antiabortion organizations. Then he made a fake persona, Robert Daoud Sarkis, complete with a falsified driver's license. After that, a front company, BioMax Procurement Services, described in paperwork filed with the state of California as a corporation that "provides tissue and specimen procurement for academic and private bioscience researchers." CMP staffers pretended to be officers and employees of BioMax, complete with pseudonyms and credit cards that they used to attend closed conferences held by Planned Parenthood and the National Abortion Federation. They leveraged contacts they made at those events into private meetings at Planned Parenthood affiliates across the country. They filmed for thirty months, wearing police-grade hidden cameras, and taped thousands of hours of footage of doctors, medical assistants, and top staffers.

Daleiden's project became something much more formidable after his efforts caught the attention of the Alliance Defending Freedom, the hard-charging and well-connected Christian law firm that had supported Lila Rose during her video sting. ADF, which has been called a "religious ministry" by its leadership, was started by a group of men on the religious right in Arizona after Bill Clinton's 1992 election. Their original mission was to push back against liberal efforts to expand sexual freedoms and "radically reshape America." Both a law firm and a Christian ministry, ADF aspired to "keep the doors open for the Gospel," and it often did so by leveraging the First Amendment to roll back laws that expanded rights for abortion and same-sex marriage.

Dannenfelser was on ADF's board, invited to join for her work against abortion. Unlike Dannenfelser and much of the antiabortion movement, ADF was rooted less in Catholicism and more in conservative evangelical Christianity. Lawyers for the group signed a statement of belief that included principles found on many evangelical church websites, like the primacy of the Bible and Jesus Christ, and agreed to pray and participate in Christian worship services in and outside of work.

ADF had built a practice defending Christians, with a track record of victory at the Supreme Court. The group successfully represented clients fighting against the contraceptive coverage mandated by Obama's health care law. It got involved in lower-court cases over laws banning what it called "partial birth" abortion and protecting the rights of antiabortion protesters at clinics. The ADF team also won major Supreme Court cases on things that seemed small, like overturning laws to limit the size of church signs, but in doing so established significant constitutional precedent.

The Alliance Defending Freedom specialized in tightly packaged projects. It was not only the legal strategy that mattered but an entire marketing component too. In 2013, the group offered its expertise to Daleiden. A series of documents later revealed in court proceedings gave insight into Daleiden's plan and the help he received from ADF and the wider universe of antiabortion organizations. Casey Mattox, a lawyer at ADF, flew to California to meet Daleiden "to talk about maximizing the legal impact of the project," according to an email Daleiden sent to Ruddy, the Catholic donor. Over the next two years, a small fleet of ADF lawyers joined the effort, giving legal advice on recording laws and other matters. Daleiden's campaign was part of their much larger effort to end abortion and change American culture. And for Daleiden, ADF's support helped him connect with the broader constellation of antiabortion power.

Americans United for Life, one of the oldest antiabortion policy organizations, became involved in his operation in 2015, according to email logs. Daleiden contacted Kellyanne Conway, too, in May to collect data about how the videos were received, according to court testimony. Both were Catholic, and Daleiden later extolled Conway to the National Catholic Register as an example of what Pope John Paul II called the "feminine genius," describing her as "indispensable" to his movement. "It's to their own detriment and, ultimately, defeat, that people underestimate her," he said.

Daleiden also contacted an even more powerful player: Leonard Leo, the head of the Federalist Society, the conservative legal network, and a passionate opponent of abortion. According to court documents, Leo advised on how to successfully prosecute "the criminal actors" that Daleiden's video exposed. He connected Daleiden with state and local law enforcement officials in Arizona, Louisiana, Texas, and Michigan, Daleiden said, so that he would not have to "cold call" to share his findings before they were publicly released. Leo said later he never watched the videos, and that he spoke to Daleiden once after they were released to recommend a pro bono lawyer. A close associate of Leo, Greg Mueller, whom Daleiden described as a mentor, helped coordinate media around the release of the videos.

Students for Life, a post-Roe generation group on whose board Leo served, paid Mueller's bills for Daleiden's messaging work. The group's leader, Kristan Hawkins, had trained Rose and other young activists through internships, boot camps, and other programs run by their group on college campuses, where they recruited the new foot soldiers of their movement. Hawkins, who was just four years older than Daleiden, saw abortion as the human rights atrocity of this moment in history and their fight as akin to the civil rights movement. Hawkins opened the Students for Life handbook, a guide for her activists featuring testimonials of "serious abortion abolitionists," with a quote from Martin Luther King Jr.'s *Letter from Birmingham Jail*. The book—a mission statement of sorts—cast Christians who opposed abortion as heroes in epics of human injustice, comparing the issue to slavery and the Holocaust. "Ask God how he can use you, and I'm sorry if the results are a little radical for you," she urged young antiabortion activists at a gala in Indiana alongside Governor Mike Pence.

Like Daleiden, Hawkins had been focused on Planned Parenthood. Three years earlier, she hired Conway to learn her supporters' attitudes toward Planned Parenthood, to better attack the organization on college campuses.

Perhaps most important, Daleiden's operation built advance support in congressional offices. Before the videos were released, Daleiden and his allies contacted a series of allied elected officials to brief them on their findings. In Oklahoma, Daleiden's legal advisers corresponded with top lawyers in the attorney general's offices months before they released anything publicly. In Congress, Daleiden worked directly with Christensen at the Pro-Life Caucus to line up political support. At least two Republican congressmen saw the videos several weeks before they were released, including Representative Trent Franks, who had sponsored the bill for a national twenty-week abortion ban, and Representative Tim Murphy, another outspoken abortion opponent and the chairman of an Energy and Commerce subcommittee that quickly announced an investigation into Planned Parenthood. When Murphy was asked by reporters why he didn't take action immediately after privately viewing the footage, he stumbled for an answer. "Um, I don't know why. All I know is I saw it and he said he was going to post it eventually, so that's all I know," he said, abruptly ending the conversation. (Murphy resigned from Congress two years later after allegations that he encouraged a woman, with whom he was having an affair, to have an abortion.)

By the project's launch day, nearly all the most powerful forces in the antiabortion movement were involved somehow with Daleiden's operation. The upstart plan that seemed crazy just two years earlier was poised to make major gains for their cause.

There was only one thing left to do. Daleiden requested that a priest say a Mass in the old Latin for Nucatola, the Planned Parenthood doctor he secretly recorded, to intercede for her soul to God.

8

The Symbol of Sanger

Republicans did not always revile Planned Parenthood as a criminal enterprise. Nor did they always see its mission as a partisan one. For the early decades, in fact, they were some of the organization's strongest champions.

The early seeds of Planned Parenthood were planted in 1898, when Margaret Sanger, a nineteen-year-old first-grade teacher, returned home to Corning, New York, to care for her ill mother, who was wasting away from tuberculosis. The sixth child born to Irish Catholic immigrants, Sanger saw her mother's ability to fight the disease weakened by her eighteen pregnancies—eleven childbirths and seven miscarriages. When her mother died, Sanger lashed out at her father, who would live until age eighty.

"You caused this," she said, standing over her mother's coffin. "Mother is dead from having too many children."

Sanger was determined not to die the same way. She dreamed of a magical pill that would prevent pregnancy. After nursing school, she worked as a visiting nurse on the Lower East Side, one of the poorest parts of New York City, where women begged her for contraception. She watched others die from abortions induced by drinking turpentine or infections after visits to illegal abortionists. Sanger came to believe that the only way to liberate women from poverty was to give them control over their reproduction.

"Enforced motherhood," she wrote in 1914, "is the most complete denial of a woman's right to life and liberty."

She opened her first clinic in Brooklyn three years before the passage of the Nineteenth Amendment, the constitutional amendment granting women the right to vote. Her clinic, where she provided women with items like diaphragms and information about what she started calling *birth control*, was the first of its kind in the country. A flyer, printed in English, Yiddish, and Italian, advertised her services. "MOTHERS! Can you afford to have a large family?" it read. "Do you want any more children? If not, why do you have them? DO NOT KILL. DO NOT TAKE LIFE, BUT PREVENT."

Women pushing strollers and clasping the hands of their children lined the block on the day Sanger's clinic opened. The first day, she saw one hundred women. The first week, four hundred women. And after nine days, authorities arrested her and shut down the clinic. Sanger had violated the Comstock Act, a law that criminalized the mailing of things deemed "obscene, lewd, or lascivious," including information about contraception, as well as devices and medications. But her arrest turned her effort into national news. Sanger was convicted after the judge concluded that women did not have "the right to copulate with a feeling of security that there will be no resulting conception"—tantamount to arguing that women shouldn't have sex unless they were willing to face all the possible consequences of childbirth, including death. Sanger was sentenced to thirty days in jail.

After two years of litigation, a judge ruled that doctors could prescribe contraception to married people for the prevention of disease. Sanger opened more clinics, and in 1921, she founded the American Birth Control League. The group's mission focused on one cause: contraception. Abortion was illegal throughout Sanger's lifetime. She didn't condone the widespread use of the procedure. "It is an alternative that I cannot too strongly condemn," she wrote in 1932. "Although abortion may be resorted to in order to save the life of the mother, the practice of it merely for limitation of offspring is dangerous and vicious." Sanger believed that if contraception were widely available, abortion would become obsolete.

At the time, widely available birth control was a radical idea. Sanger courted anyone who would help make her vision a reality, including eugenicists. Sanger calculated she could give her cause greater legitimacy by allying with that movement. The theory of selective breeding—weeding out the "mentally and physically defective," as Sanger put it—was a mainstream idea in the 1920s and 1930s, though it was later condemned as racist, classist, and ableist.

Yet Sanger's strategy to expand political support for her cause may have worked too well. A year later, she was pushed out of her position as president by members who found her brand of socialist feminism too radical. And in 1942, over her objections, the American Birth Control League, which had become the Birth Control Federation of America, adopted a totally new name as part of an effort to move away from the more controversial phrase of "birth control": Planned Parenthood Federation of America.

Prominent Republicans embraced the cause of birth control. These men were interested in contraception not to liberate women, as Sanger once dreamed, but because they worried about overpopulation. At the time, prominent political figures worried about how a higher birth rate could stress the world's resources. Birth control like condoms or diaphragms, "family planning" as they called it, offered a solution. Prescott Bush, the father and grandfather of two future Republican presidents, was the treasurer for the group's first major fundraising campaign, his name next to Sanger's atop the organization's letterhead in 1947. His son, George H. W. Bush, later took up the mantle of federal family planning, earning him the nickname "Rubbers." Barry Goldwater backed the group, and President Eisenhower and President Truman served as cochairmen of a Planned Parenthood committee after their presidencies.

Sanger was frustrated by the conservative shift of her organization. "If I told or wrote you that the name Planned Parenthood would be the end of the movement, it was," she wrote to a former national director, after she was no longer president. "The movement was then a fighting, forward, no fooling movement, battling for the freedom of the poorest parents and for women's biological freedom and development. The P.P.F. has left all this behind."

Still, Sanger kept pushing. In 1953, she convinced a little-known scientist, Gregory Pincus, to develop a new form of contraception—a birth control pill. In the years that followed, the final hurdles to Sanger's vision were overcome. The U.S. Food and Drug Administration approved the pill in 1960. Five years later, the Supreme Court ruled that married couples had a right to contraception in *Griswold v. Connecticut*. The case grew out of the arrest of Estelle Griswold, the executive director of Planned Parenthood League of Connecticut, who was violating state law by distributing contraception to married women. And in 1970, legislation creating Title X, the program that contributed millions of federal dollars to Planned Parenthood to help fund contraception, cancer screenings, and other types of women's health services, passed with bipartisan support. It was championed by then representative George H. W. Bush and signed into law by President Nixon. In 1972, the decision in *Eisenstadt v. Baird* created a right for single people to access contraception.

And in 1973, Roe made abortion legal. At first, only a handful of Planned Parenthood's affiliated health centers, like its clinic in New York, offered abortion services. But slowly, those who were uncomfortable with the procedure left the organization and Planned Parenthood embraced abortion care as central to its mission.

By the time Faye Wattleton, the organization's first Black president, took over in 1978, the political environment had grown more hostile to abortion rights. Wattleton, a nurse and the only child of a Pentecostal female preacher, came from a local Planned Parenthood in Dayton that didn't provide abortions; it faced attacks from the Catholic Church nonetheless. She believed Planned Parenthood would have to adopt a more aggressive defense of abortion rights. "It was prophetic that I felt this was the direction we would have to go, without knowing we were nearing the Reagan years," she later said. "But I saw the growing political opposition on the local level."

At her first press conference as president, Wattleton announced that she was "putting the world on notice" that Planned Parenthood would fight for abortion rights. Its legal victories in the 1960s and 1970s had made many in the movement "complacent," Wattleton said. But efforts like those of Henry Hyde to severely limit access to abortions for women on Medicaid showed that the battle was far from won. "What has happened is that we've allowed them to have center stage," she said of the new "right to life" movement. "I'd like to say those days are over."

Like Cecile Richards, Wattleton expanded Planned Parenthood's political profile, setting up a Washington office to lobby Congress and launching a political action committee to endorse candidates. She hired pollsters and media experts and created a team to streamline national policymaking. Under her leadership, Planned Parenthood grew fast, adding clinics and expanding services. Income and operating budgets skyrocketed. The organization grew from serving 1.1 million patients in 1978, when she became president, to about 5 million by the time she left in 1992 to become the host of a daytime television show.

As Planned Parenthood grew, the conservative attacks on the organization escalated. The Reagan administration targeted Planned Parenthood for funding cuts. The antiabortion movement dubbed Planned Parenthood public enemy number one. It was "the single largest child killer in the United States," said Randall Terry, the head of Operation Rescue, the group Troy Newman would eventually lead.

As antiabortion activists pushed Republicans to make opposition to abortion a central plank of their party, a right-wing fringe grew more powerful within their movement. Operation Rescue became known for blockading clinics and screaming at patients through bullhorns, organizing thousands of antiabortion activists in chaotic protests that sometimes resulted in criminal charges.

"Rescue as often as you can," Terry instructed his supporters from a jail cell in 1989. "Go to jail as often as you can." Violent actions spread throughout the 1990s, as antiabortion extremists firebombed clinics and gunned down doctors.

By the time Richards took over Planned Parenthood in 2006, almost all Republican support for the group had vanished. A year later, a staunchly antiabortion little-known Republican congressman debuted a new way to undercut its operations. Representative Mike Pence sponsored the first bill in Congress to strip Planned Parenthood of its federal funding. "If Planned Parenthood wants to be involved in providing counseling services and HIV testing, they ought not be in the business of providing abortions," he said. "As long as they aspire to do that, I'll be after them."

His effort marked a new strategy for antiabortion lawmakers. Previous fights over abortion focused on procedures—like so-called partial-birth abortion—or direct federal funding of abortion as with Hyde. They didn't attack Planned Parenthood, which provided health services to millions of American women annually. "There was some unwritten agreement that we had arrived at, an unstated truce between pro-abortion and pro-life legislators that the debate would happen within certain parameters," Pence later told *Politico*. "When we introduced this, it was a completely different element in the equation."

Pence reintroduced his legislation three times before the new Republican majority, fueled by Tea Party conservatives, passed the bill in 2011. The defund rallying cry was embraced across the party, championed from the presidential primary debate stage to the halls of Congress. The new attack amounted to a striking twist of history: Republicans were now actively working to dismantle the same family-planning programs their party founded three decades earlier.

From the invention of Sanger's pill to its support for abortion rights, Planned Parenthood led and championed the changes that reshaped women's reproductive and sexual lives. Yet, where abortion-rights advocates saw themselves as driving the country toward greater equality and freedom, conservatives like Pence saw national decline, a chipping away of what they believed were the core values of American life: traditional marriage, religious faith, and family.

The story of Planned Parenthood was intertwined with the broader cultural transformation of women's rights and sexual freedom. When Planned Parenthood was founded in 1921, as the American Birth Control League, birth control was criminalized, abortion was banned, and gay sex was illegal. By 2015, when Daleiden unveiled the results of his sting, contraception was not only no longer controversial but covered by insurance. Abortion had been a federal right for more than four decades. And two weeks before the videos exploded into public view, the Supreme Court legalized same-sex marriage.

To social conservatives, Planned Parenthood had come to represent the diminished power of traditional religion, gender roles, and families in American life. The fight was about abortion, of course, but also taking down an entire liberal social agenda and the threat of Hillary Clinton as president. In more than two decades in Washington, Clinton had proven to be not only a champion of women's reproductive rights, but also liberal feminist ideals. "I think Cecile Richards has now become the puppetmaster for Democrats in Congress," said Carol Tobias, president of the National Right to Life Committee. "There is no doubt that Cecile Richards wants to influence a President Clinton and control the Supreme Court."

Over time, the symbolism of Planned Parenthood had far outpaced the reality of its services. Planned Parenthood was the country's largest abortion provider. But the vast majority of its work involved far less controversial health care like testing for sexually transmitted disease, screening for cancer, and providing contraception. Only about 12 percent of patients came to its clinics for abortions in 2013, according to PolitiFact. In 2015, when the videos were released, Planned Parenthood operated 661 health care centers across the country and saw 2.5 million patients. Its clinics performed 324,000 abortions—nearly half of the total recorded by the federal Centers for Disease Control and Prevention—but those were a fraction of the nearly 9.5 million services it provided that year.

Despite Republican claims, taxpayers funded a very small number of those procedures. Hyde blocked most federal money from being spent on abortions. In total, the federal government contributed funds to pay for just 160 abortions in 2015, spending a total of $490,000 out of a more than $1 trillion federal budget.

Still, Republican efforts to defund Planned Parenthood posed an existential threat to the organization. About 43 percent of its total annual revenue—approximately $550 million—came from federal funding. Losing that money would make it difficult, if not impossible, for many clinics already operating with tight margins to remain open.

An irony of the Republican defunding efforts was that they could end up costing taxpayers more. An analysis by the Congressional Budget Office in 2015 found that defunding Planned Parenthood would increase federal spending by $130 million over a decade. Nearly 2.5 million low-income women got their contraceptives at Planned Parenthood centers. If those centers closed, some of those women would go to other providers. But others—the Congressional Budget Office estimated several thousand annually—would have children. Those pregnancies would cost the federal government more than contraception, given that the prenatal care, labor, and delivery would likely be paid for by Medicaid. And then, potentially, those children could qualify for Medicaid and other federal programs—costing even more taxpayer dollars.

That cost was well worth it to abortion opponents, who saw an opportunity to shut down the biggest abortion provider across America and strike a blow at the liberal worldview the group represented. Targeting Planned Parenthood had become a proxy for conservative America to project its anxieties about gender dynamics and families in a changing and increasingly secular country.

And Richards, preparing to testify to Congress, was about to experience the full force of their fears.

9

The Hearing

All summer, David Daleiden's videos kept coming. In late July, footage showed Dr. Savita Ginde, vice president and medical director of Planned Parenthood of the Rocky Mountains, poking at bloody bits in what looked like a Pyrex dish. She narrated what she saw: "Here's some stomach, a heart, kidney, and adrenal. I don't know what else is in there. Arms?"

"Another boy!" exclaimed her medical assistant as the ominous music rose and the video cut to black.

Planned Parenthood struggled to convince even some of its own donors that it had, as Cecile Richards saw it, been scammed. Its "fight back" effort, as the group called it, was extensive. It bolstered security to protect the staff and doctors in the videos and protect against increasing threats of cyberattacks. It hired Anita Dunn, a former adviser to Obama and Biden, to help with crisis communications, targeted key senators with an ad campaign, and brought on white-shoe lawyers to defend them in the state and congressional investigations. None of that came cheap; the lawyers alone cost nearly $3 million. The campaign quickly blew through the group's lobbying budget, prompting an emergency appeal for another $1.5 million from the Soros Foundation, a civic society organization founded by one of the country's biggest Democratic donors.

Eventually, Planned Parenthood brought on its own investigator—Fusion GPS—to examine the veracity of the videos. The forensic analysis concluded that the videos had been edited in ways it deemed misleading, but it found no evidence that the antiabortion group made up dialogue. David Daleiden attributed the gaps to "bathroom breaks" and "waiting periods between meetings."

But there were other manipulations too. A shot of a fetus included in one of the videos with the implication that it was aborted was later found to be an image of a child born at nineteen weeks, whose mother took the photo two years earlier to memorialize her son. The cuts and edits, investigators concluded, meant the videos had "no evidentiary value in a legal context and cannot be relied upon for any official inquiries." The footage was real but the packaging of the videos didn't tell an accurate story. The framing created by Daleiden and his allies across the antiabortion movement gave the false impression that Planned Parenthood was breaking the law.

As the congressional investigations proceeded, Richards spent weeks preparing to testify, poring over thousands of pages of documents with her lawyers. When the big day arrived, she wrapped herself in her mother's legacy. She put on her dark blue suit and stuck on her lapel the gold pin of Ann's that always reminded her of a sheriff's badge—the one she wore when doing hard things. Taped inside the cover of the thick binder of research assembled by her team was another talisman of support, a photo of her three kids when they were toddlers. As she walked into the room, Richards checked her phone one last time. There was a final blessing from a friend: "May the rage of women through the centuries center you as you go into this," texted Terry McGovern, an expert in women's health at Columbia University.

The support of antiabortion leaders had given Daleiden's guerrilla tactics greater impact. But in Congress, they had to cede control to their Republican allies. And despite all of Marjorie

Dannenfelser's trainings, the party squandered the opportunity that the antiabortion movement had worked so hard to create. In the early moments of the hearing, Representative Jason Chaffetz, the chairman of the committee, made clear that he planned to focus on Planned Parenthood's finances, rather than the morality of the procedure itself. His first line of attack was over Richards's salary, and he fumbled, overstating it by $70,000. She corrected him: "I think we've been extremely forthcoming with all of our documents."

When Chaffetz flashed a chart that he claimed was based on Planned Parenthood data, Richards called him on the mistake, pointing out that the information was pulled from Americans United for Life, the antiabortion group. "I would check your source," she said. Chaffetz appeared deflated: "Then we will get to the bottom of the truth of that," he said.

When other Republicans attempted to compare Richards to a criminal, she "respectfully" disagreed. And when they interrupted her responses, again and again, she calmly asked for a chance to answer the question, leaving the complaints of misogyny to her Democratic allies on the committee. "I'm not clear on this: Do you defend the sale of baby body parts?" asked John Duncan of Tennessee, after suggesting Planned Parenthood was taking federal funds that could have gone to Boys and Girls Clubs. "No, and I think that is really a total mischaracterization," Richards replied in a tone that reflected the fatigue of hours of polite endurance.

It was a performance so skillful that even some conservatives couldn't help but offer damning praise of Richards's handling of the more than four and a half hours of questioning. "Masterful evasiveness," Kristan Hawkins, of Students for Life, told reporters. As for the Republicans, "there's always room for improvement," Daleiden said.

Hillary Clinton called that evening to congratulate Richards. Once Clinton spoke out, about two weeks after the first video, she never wavered in her support for Planned Parenthood. She called the tapes "disturbing," but she also added a new line to her campaign stump speech. "I will defend Planned Parenthood," she told voters in Iowa and New Hampshire.

Clinton watched Richards's testimony as she herself prepared to testify before a House committee a few weeks later about the 2012 attack on a US diplomatic outpost and CIA annex in Benghazi, Libya. "You were wonderful," she told Richards. "I'm going to be up there myself soon. Good for you for standing up to them."

Clinton knew who they were fighting. She remembered being personally attacked by the local conservative Christian groups in Arkansas in the 1980s, and fighting the religious right in Washington in the 1990s. "I don't know how best to convey the really extraordinary hostility that I personally experienced being pro-choice in certain political settings," she reflected later. "And I just saw how determined they were."

The weeks of controversy over the videos appeared to have little impact on public opinion. Planned Parenthood was still viewed more favorably than not by most Americans. A *Wall Street Journal* / NBC poll released the day before Richards's testimony found that the organization was viewed positively by 47 percent of people, a percentage largely unchanged from the 45 percent who said the same in July.

After years of litigation and millions of dollars in legal fees, Planned Parenthood was cleared of the cloud of wrongdoing. Two weeks after Mike Pence launched an investigation in Indiana, his state department of health cleared its state Planned Parenthood affiliates. The investigations in nineteen other states and in Congress failed to find significant evidence that Planned Parenthood profited off fetal tissue. The efforts of House Republicans to defund the organization stalled in the Senate, making it no further to becoming law. In 2016, agents dispatched by Kamala Harris, then the California attorney general, searched Daleiden's apartment, confiscating his computers and hard drives. Years later, the courts would find that Daleiden had broken the law, holding him and the Center for Medical Progress liable for more than $2 million in damages.

In the end, Planned Parenthood was vindicated. The assaults did not come from true concerns over the work of her organization, Richards concluded. They came from people "who resent that women actually have the legal right to make their own decisions about their pregnancies," she told the magazine *American Prospect* a few months after she testified. "That's what they're mad about, and they're really mad."

Once again, the country faced a crossroads over abortion rights, and Richards believed that the future would favor her side, the side of Roe. "I believe this country is not going to go backwards," she said.

Yet the videos also made clear that Planned Parenthood's opposition had entered a new, more aggressive phase. A fringe of the antiabortion movement was interwoven with the mainstream. Though the sting was nonviolent, the unfounded accusations of criminal activity were repeated by more radicalized opponents. In November, a mass shooting occurred at a Planned Parenthood clinic in Colorado Springs. Three people were killed, and nine others were wounded. In a rambling interview after his arrest, the shooter said the phrase "no more baby parts."

The video campaign proved effective where it needed to be. The antiabortion movement was now powerful enough to convince conservative Tea Party lawmakers in the House to threaten to force a government shutdown unless Congress defunded Planned Parenthood, effectively holding the government hostage over abortion—one unpopular position building to another even more unpopular stance. That effort even led to the ousting of House Speaker John Boehner, the devout Catholic congressman from southern Ohio. For years, he was seen as the strongest antiabortion lawmaker ever to hold the speaker's gavel. But now, even he couldn't compete with this new class of more radical social conservatives who would accept no compromise on the issue. It was a sign of how the antiabortion movement had regained its national political grip. Its agenda could force the resignation of the second in line to the presidency.

Daleiden also saw another win. His videos focused on abortions in the second trimester. Up to that point, much of the public focus had been on abortion later in pregnancy. With the controversy started by his footage, antiabortion activists were shifting the country's attention to fetuses prior to viability. "It was progress," he said.

The antiabortion movement had come so far from just three years earlier, when the autopsy called for their expulsion from the Republican Party. When Republicans passed yet another bill to repeal Obama's health care law, they added a measure to defund Planned Parenthood. It never became law, of course: Obama vetoed the legislation and Republicans lacked the votes to override the president. But the fact that the bill passed Congress was a sign that the antiabortion movement had gained traction, and just in time for a coming critical juncture. Only the president now stood between them and their goal. And the Republican field looked more promising to them than it had in years.

Weeks after the videos dropped, Dannenfelser sat in the audience of the very first prime-time Republican primary debate and watched as the candidates practically tripped over one another to be the strongest ally of her movement. Mike Huckabee, the former governor of Arkansas, argued for giving a zygote, from conception, rights as a full person under the Fourteenth Amendment. Wisconsin governor Scott Walker said he wanted a complete ban on abortion even in cases of rape, incest, or to save the woman's life, a position he said was "in line with everyday America," even as the Fox News debate hosts pushed back that the majority of Americans did not agree. And minutes after Jeb Bush, the former Florida governor, touted his "completely pro-life" record, his home state senator Marco Rubio outdid him, saying that "future generations will look back at this history of our country and call us barbarians for murdering millions of babies who we never gave them a chance to live." Only one man on stage, a political novice named Donald Trump, was an outlier, offering what Dannenfelser and her allies saw as an inadequate answer, particularly when compared to his rivals.

The antiabortion movement may have lost the fight to defund Planned Parenthood, but it had powerfully advanced its cause. "We may be at a political crossroads where the right has a resurgence," warned Ellen Chesler, a former Planned Parenthood board member and Sanger biographer, in an interview with *The New York Times*. "The politics is so totally unpredictable and unknowable."

PART II

THE POLITICAL WAR

JUNE 2022

Cincinnati, Ohio

Jocelyn opened her sonogram for a moment and then folded it back up. She knew that if she stopped taking birth control, she could get pregnant, but she didn't really think it could happen so fast. She took a pregnancy test. And then a second one. Both were positive. Still she wasn't sure she was really pregnant. The weeks passed. She started to call around to doctors' offices, but had trouble getting an appointment, she said. One doctor had availability, but not for weeks.

So she went to Pregnancy Center East and discovered that she was sixteen weeks along. Jocelyn was not considering an abortion. At this point, she just wanted any information about her pregnancy and any material assistance. She had not paid much attention to the Supreme Court case, and did not know that Roe had fallen during her appointment.

"My sister actually told me about this place," Jocelyn, twenty-nine, said as she sat down in a consultation room after her ultrasound. Her older sister, also pregnant, sat down next to her and smiled. "She's like my firstborn," she said of Jocelyn.

Jocelyn couldn't get medical care at PCE, but she watched videos about topics like parenting and breastfeeding and got free diapers. "They took their time with me trying to understand my situation and if I wanted to continue with this pregnancy," she said.

When they asked if she wanted an ultrasound, Jocelyn hesitated. But that was free too.

Like most antiabortion pregnancy centers, PCE's goal was to stop women like Jocelyn from having abortions and then support them throughout their pregnancies. PCE provided a range of free services, including pregnancy testing, limited ultrasounds, and supplies like clothes or formula for infants. It led chastity classes in local schools, teaching students not to have sex outside of marriage, and parenting programs and mentorships for men. It promoted what many in the antiabortion movement called an "abortion pill reversal," a procedure that purports to stop a medication abortion or Plan B, but is considered "unproven and unethical" by mainstream medical associations. PCE did not offer contraception or prenatal testing for birth defects or genetic conditions. If clinicians noticed an ectopic pregnancy, they directed the woman to the emergency room.

The clinic's offerings were not unusual: in 2019, only 5 percent of centers offered prenatal care, and just 2 percent offered well-women exams, according to the Susan B. Anthony List's own research arm. But in recent years, Laura Curran, the clinic director, had started a partnership with a midwifery program at TriHealth, one of the largest health care systems in the Cincinnati region, to help its patients get into the medical system.

Jocelyn was already in the queue at TriHealth, so the center's new partnership didn't move things faster for her, she said. Still, everything about the experience felt so welcoming, Jocelyn said. Here she did not need to worry about insurance or credit cards, or paying at all. Appointments at PCE could be as long as a client needs, fifteen minutes or three hours. The clinic had more than one hundred volunteers who answered a hotline, greeted walk-in clients, and sorted donations. After her first appointment, Jocelyn kept coming back.

"When you go into the doctor's office, you are tense about the situation, because you know there is something as far as payment," she said. When you are a new mother, you have to focus on new things, she said. "I have to manage my money way better now."

About half of PCE's clients were on Medicaid, Curran estimated. In 2021, about 25 percent of its clients came because they needed proof of pregnancy to apply for Medicaid or wanted to sign up for parenting classes where they could earn a free crib or car seat, she said.

The other 75 percent were what they called "abortion-vulnerable"—women they saw as likely to get an abortion. "We want the woman who feels like [abortion] is her only choice. We don't shy away from that," she explained.

They looked at factors that might make a woman choose abortion and then advertised to reach those women, on radio, on billboards, and online. Curran said that about three-quarters of those women, or about half of their total clients, decided to give birth.

The clients had so many needs. On this day, one woman said she got no maternity leave, just one week of paid vacation. Curran could not give them maternity leave, but she wanted to be there for those women.

As news spread that Roe had been overturned, it wasn't just new clients making their way to the pregnancy center. Former clients arrived. One woman brought a bouquet of yellow roses.

As she walked out of her office into the hall, Curran bumped into Barbara Momper, one of the founders of Pregnancy Center East forty years ago. "I've just been crying all morning," Momper said.

She had rushed over to the center after going to the 11:45 a.m. Mass at her Catholic parish. As news of the court's decision trickled out, people had spontaneously come to the church to celebrate—including Katherine, she said, nodding to the woman walking toward them.

"She was one of my clients," Momper said. "I got to cut the cord."

Curran grabbed Momper's arm. "You're her Katherine?" she gasped, greeting the woman. "I remember you now."

Katherine's voice was low and strong as she told her story.

It was ten years ago, and she was a young woman from Pennsylvania who had come to Cincinnati at age eighteen to attend art school. "I was very terrified," she said. "Because I was all by myself."

Momper had brought Katherine into a room, and they talked by the light of a small lamp. The father didn't want the child, Katherine said. When she finally found him to tell him she was pregnant, he was in jail, and when he got out of jail, he lost his job. He told her to just have an abortion, she said. Momper had listened and asked her what she wanted to do.

Katherine put her hands over her heart and pressed in. "I knew that I couldn't kill my child. I just couldn't," she remembered. "I have to carry that burden, that sin, of, I killed my baby."

Her own mother's situation had been similar, she said. Katherine had found out who her father was only two years earlier. Her mother and grandmother raised her, but they were gone. No one in her mother's family believed in abortion, she said.

"I don't have an option but to have the child," she said. "I had the fear of the Lord. And I had the fear of my grandmother." She gave her new baby girl a name that reminded her of divine mercy. "I look back over my life, and I say, look at where I came from. I was just a little old eighteen-year-old," she said. "Came down here with like three or four trash bags of clothes."

Momper became her mentor, invited her to Thanksgiving dinner, took her to the grocery store, and made sure her daughter had clothes that fit, she said. But still, it was not easy. To get through college, she relied on government programs and day care services. She applied for WIC, the government's supplemental nutrition program for women, infants, and children. Now, she had built a career in digital marketing and was pursuing a master's degree. Over time, she moved from a studio to a one-bedroom apartment to a three-bedroom town house.

She pulled out a photograph of her daughter. "Nine years old, and she is thriving," she said. "Straight-A student."

She pointed to the lapel pin Momper was wearing on her jungle-green jacket—it was an image of the tiny soles of a fetus's feet, a symbol for the antiabortion movement. "She wears it every day," Katherine said.

It was already well past 1:00 p.m. when Curran closed up for the day. She had heard that an abortion-rights group called Jane's Revenge had declared a coming "night of rage" in response to the Supreme Court decision.

"I have to call the police in a minute," Curran said, "see if I've got security tonight."

In the months ahead, Curran would get estimates for panic buttons and add more security cameras. The FBI would investigate arson and vandalism crimes against pregnancy centers in Colorado, Tennessee, Oregon, and elsewhere. She would also change the center's name for the new era: Pregnancy Center Plus.

Curran believed that no woman really wanted to have an abortion. "It's not because she has the choice," she said. "It's because she feels like she doesn't have a choice that leads her to abortion."

Curran saw this in many other clients over the years, women like Jocelyn and Katherine. But outside her walls, there was a rising backlash. Women were angry. Many seemed to hate centers like hers, and Curran couldn't understand why.

Her center would stay safe. But that first night, two men Curran knew volunteered to keep watch. They set out lawn chairs in front. As the hours passed, one prayed the rosary, rolling the beads between his fingers.

Hail, Holy Queen, Mother of Mercy,
our life, our sweetness, and our hope.
To you do we cry,
poor banished children of Eve.
To you do we send up our sighs,
mourning and weeping in this valley of tears
Turn then, most gracious advocate,
your eyes of mercy toward us,
and after this exile
show unto us the blessed fruit of thy womb,
Jesus.

2016–2017

10

Titans and Saints

Leonard Leo bowed at the altar and ascended the marble pulpit of the Basilica of the National Shrine of the Immaculate Conception in Washington. The casket below was draped in a white pall, lying beneath the blue and gold neo-Romanesque-Byzantine dome.

It still felt surreal, even seven days later. Justice Antonin Scalia was dead, found in his bed in the El Presidente suite of a luxury ranch in West Texas. He had been quail hunting with elite members of an exclusive fraternity for hunters, the International Order of St. Hubertus, and did not show up for breakfast. Leo was so close to Nino, as his friends called him, that he heard the news before it became public.

Leo's voice echoed over the packed pews. "The souls of the just are in the hand of God, and no torment shall touch them," he said, reading from the Catholic scripture. "Chastised a little, they shall be greatly blessed, because God tried them and found them worthy of himself."

Through his horn-rimmed glasses, Leo could see all eight remaining justices of the Supreme Court, seated before him in the front. Normally, the basilica was filled with pilgrims. A million people came each year to pray at the site, the largest Roman Catholic church in North America, dedicated to the Virgin Mary. Now he saw hundreds from the conservative legal world who had revered

Scalia as their unofficial leader. There were a host of high-level dignitaries—Vice President Joe Biden, former vice president Dick Cheney, the Vatican's ambassador to the United States, and dozens of Catholic priests.

Scalia was a titan of conservative law. But few Americans had ever heard of this short, round man in a finely tailored three-piece suit with a pocket square, who led the Federalist Society. Leo preferred it that way, out of the public eye and the press, easier to maneuver behind the scenes. He was building power with the small group of people who mattered for his mission, and many of them were here, too: law clerks and attorneys and federal court judges who shared a vision to shift American law and culture along with it.

Leo wasn't a litigator. He wasn't a registered lobbyist. He had never worked for a major law firm. Leo was a power broker, a networker, the kind of pivotal Washington player who could navigate his way through the morass of politics to advance a mission. His connections at the court were deep: he met Samuel Alito in 1989, Clarence Thomas in 1990, and Antonin Scalia in 1991. He could get billionaires to donate enormous checks to further his causes, in service of the network of conservative Catholic and judicial organizations he was building, and presidents to rely on him. It made him one of the best-connected Catholics and conservatives in America, or, as Thomas once joked, "the third-most powerful person in the world." And even on this day, there were hints that Leo's legacy might prove, in the end, even larger than Scalia's.

Leo's rise to power began after law school when he took a job with the Federalist Society, which was established in 1982 with a goal to train, credential, and grow a generation of elite conservative lawyers who could ascend to the highest levels of American government. Its vision was long-term: to build a strong network that over decades would create a pipeline for conservative lawyers and law students to government, academia, and the judiciary, even the Supreme Court. It was a secular group, not connected to any broader Christian vision, and some of its members supported abortion rights.

The Federalist Society helped steer promising conservative law students into clerkships, jobs, and eventually judgeships, making sure they got jobs in places of influence across the entire legal landscape. And it helped expand the intellectual class of government officials, academics, and advocates who could create the scholarship and legal theories that would provide a foundation for upending decades-old decisions—like Roe.

Scalia had been one of the group's early advisers, and he infused the Federalist Society with his method of legal interpretation called *originalism*. Originalists argue that judges should hew as closely as possible to the original intent of America's founders in the Constitution and interpret laws based on the meaning they had for the people who wrote them. In practice, it meant that if America's founders did not believe they were establishing a right to abortion or gay marriage or limiting assault weapons, then modern judges should not either when interpreting the Constitution. Legislatures should be in charge of writing laws, and justices should simply interpret them.

Roe symbolized the kind of legal thinking the originalists wanted to change, a decision they believed veered from how the Constitution was understood when the founders wrote it. Another related school of legal theory called *textualism* also raised objections to the decision, arguing that there was no clear text in the Constitution providing a right to privacy, which the judges used to ground abortion rights.

Leo and other conservative lawyers saw those problems of legal interpretation as far more sweeping than just Roe. The left had a choke hold on American legal culture, Leo believed. The result was so-called rights that were not really rooted in the Constitution and cases that were wrongly decided, he once explained to students at Hillsdale, an evangelical college in Michigan. The Griswold decision, which legalized contraception for married women, had wrongly instituted a right to privacy "so general and vague that its application is purely subjective," he said. That led to Roe "and a long line of cases affirming a right to abortion with ever narrowing exceptions," and then came Obergefell, which "announced a right to same-sex marriage." The problem extended to cases that limited a state's authority to restrict material it found obscene, as was allowed under the Comstock Act, or that protected against religion in the public square, or that permitted affirmative action, he explained. "Such an exercise of power by nine mortals, given lifetime tenure is, in my view, unjust and deeply, dangerously undemocratic," Leo told the students.

If Leo and the Federalist Society could get originalist judges on the bench, the decisions themselves would be different. While Leo cast his goals in legal terms, arguing that he wanted to restore the original intentions of the Constitution, the impact of his strategy was to push back against the cultural change that had swept the country since the 1960s and 1970s. "Law is something that obviously signals to people what is acceptable or unacceptable in a society," he said. "The perspective that the right has about Roe is, 'Well, there isn't anything in the Constitution on this issue, the Supreme Court made it up.' And by making it up, the court is trying to put its thumb on the scales of social and cultural decision making."

Over time, Leo built a large network to advance his conservative mission, an intertwined web of legal activism, Republican politicians, rich donors, and Catholicism that reached from parish churches to the Supreme Court. Groups like the Susan B. Anthony List and Students for Life, where Leo offered advice or served on the board, represented the outer tentacles of his reach.

Leo worked to galvanize Catholic voters for George W. Bush's 2004 reelection campaign against John Kerry, and to turn ethnic Catholic voters, who often voted as Democrats, into ideological Christian voters who would support Republicans by appealing to their socially conservative views on issues like abortion. Once Bush won, close allies of Leo—Ann and Neil Corkery, along with

Republican donor Robin Arkley II—helped found a new nonprofit called the Judicial Confirmation Network (later renamed the Judicial Crisis Network), or JCN, to influence public opinion on Supreme Court hearings and other judicial elections. The group was tax-exempt and could spend unlimited funds without disclosing its donors, and it set up its offices on the same hallway in a downtown Washington building as the Federalist Society.

Leo was soon leading the campaigns to support Bush's Supreme Court nominees and raising the money from conservative donors to fund them. In 2005, he helped usher Chief Justice John Roberts onto the bench. Less than a month later, Federalist Society members helped sink Bush's nomination of White House counsel Harriet Miers and persuade the administration to replace her with Samuel Alito, who had ties to the organization.

Leo and his justices remained close. After Alito was confirmed to the court, Leo connected him with ideologically aligned businessmen, some of whom had cases before the court, strengthening the pipeline between conservative money and legal ideology. In 2008, Leo organized a fishing trip to Alaska for Alito, where they stayed at Arkley's luxury lodge. He spent time with Thomas at Camp Topridge, a private lakeside resort owned by a major Republican donor, Harlan Crow. Their visits were memorialized in a painting hanging inside the lodge, depicting Crow, Thomas, Leo, and two other conservative lawyers deep in conversation and smoking cigars.

LEO'S FATHER HAD died when he was young, so he was raised by his mother and looked up to his grandfather, an Italian immigrant who had worked his way up from a tailor at Brooks Brothers to a vice president of the company. His grandfather and parents, he said, were "faithful Catholics." Leo served as an altar boy and had close relationships with his local priests and parish. From his early days in elementary school, Leo believed abortion was "an abomination," he said, due to his devout Catholicism.

As Reagan nominated Scalia to the Supreme Court in June 1986—the same summer Marjorie Dannenfelser first came to Washington—Leo was a rising senior at Cornell University and one of thirty-seven students nationwide to get a special government grant to study the Constitution. He chose to focus on religion and what the founding document intended for prayer in public schools and taxation of religious entities.

Leo met Thomas during a clerkship on the DC circuit, where Thomas had recently joined the bench.

They discussed a book by Paul Johnson, a British historian admired by conservatives, about the role of Christianity in Western civilization, Leo recounted. At the time, Thomas was a lapsed Catholic, who had moved away from the faith of his childhood.

Later, Leo noticed a small statue on the justice's desk: Saint Jude, the patron saint of seemingly hopeless causes. His great-grandmother had a similar one, and she would tell Leo to look to Saint Jude as a reminder of how the human spirit can triumph over the struggles in life. "Perhaps it should not have been a surprise then that Justice Thomas would play some of the same inspirational role that my great-grandmother did," Leo would say, at a talk with Thomas hosted by the Federalist Society. "Justice Thomas demonstrates a tremendous abiding faith in the capacity of the human spirit to rise above adversity."

When his clerkship ended, Leo accepted a job with the nascent Federalist Society, pushing off his official start date to help Thomas with his confirmation hearings for the Supreme Court, as Thomas navigated the accusations of sexual harassment by Anita Hill.

Around that time, Leo's wife, Sally, was pregnant with their first of seven children. The joy turned to anxiety when testing revealed the developing baby's spine was splaying and the head was taking the shape of a lemon. The diagnosis was myelomeningocele spina bifida, a severe form of the neurological disorder. The doctor encouraged her to undergo further testing. "My next question was, 'What do I do about it anyway?'" Sally said. "His answer was that many people decide to abort. That was out of the question." It was a view shared by Leo's mentor. Scalia, a father of nine, once told his biographer, "Being a devout Catholic means you have children when God gives them to you, and you raise them." The Leos arranged for a neurosurgeon to be ready to do surgery once their daughter was born—and a priest to baptize her in case she died.

They named her for Margaret Mary Alacoque, a French saint born in 1647, who as a child was paralyzed and grew to have visions of Jesus revealing his Sacred Heart to her. The Sacred Heart was a mystical sign, Catholics came to believe, of the long-suffering and divine love Jesus has for humanity, and was often symbolized with an image of a human heart wrapped in a crown of thorns like the one Jesus wore as he was crucified. Her visions inspired devotion in Europe and eventually an official Catholic holy day, the Feast of the Sacred Heart.

The Leos adored their Margaret and recounted her story once to a Catholic writer in a small book about spiritually strong children, called *Littlest Suffering Souls*. Her physical life was difficult. She was paralyzed from her midsection down, and had cognitive challenges and shunts to drain spinal fluid from her skull. When doctors put titanium rods in her back to try to keep it straight, her body bent them.

Yet she was a happy child, with a quick smile and an ability to charm everyone around her. Her parents marveled at her ability to love. She shared a room with her younger brother, whom she adored, and she loved stickers and chocolate ice cream. Sally took her to daily Mass, and Margaret delighted in seeing the priests, participating in the Eucharist, and for over a year counted down the days until she would be confirmed. Leo remembered bringing her several times to the March for Life in Washington, the antiabortion movement's annual protest of the Roe decision. Her parents believed she had a "sensitivity to evil," they later recounted, and pure and simple love for anyone around her. It was Margaret who urged her father to go to daily Mass, after a brief period when he had stopped. The morning she died, he was on his way there. She was fourteen.

They buried her in a garden cemetery near the cathedral in Arlington, her headstone a simple pink granite. "Always rejoice. Pray without ceasing. In all things give thanks," the stone read, quoting Saint Paul. Justice Thomas was one of her pallbearers, and Chief Justice Roberts came to the funeral, where Father Paul Scalia, the justice's son, helped to celebrate the Mass. Thomas kept Margaret's drawings under the glass on his desk, and, on top, a picture of her in a frame she had made with Popsicle sticks. Leo saved her titanium rods and kept them in his office at the Federalist Society.

After her death, the Leos, and some of their friends, came to see Margaret as a divine intercessor, with an ability to alleviate the suffering of others. They spoke of miracles, small and large, that they saw when they asked Margaret, in prayer, to intercede for them to God.

It started after Margaret's death, when Sally asked her to ask God to silence some noisy birds while she was trying to pray and, she said, they immediately went quiet. Weeks later, Sally became pregnant with their son, Francis, who was diagnosed with the same myelomeningocele as Margaret. When doctors said he would need an operation, she took the baby to Margaret's grave and asked for her late daughter's help, the Leos said; and the need for that procedure disappeared. The Leos also believed Margaret intervened to protect another one of her brothers, Anthony, during a health crisis. Ed Whelan, one of Leo's lawyer friends and then-president of the Ethics and Public Policy Center, a group that aims to apply Judeo-Christian values to public policy, asked Margaret to intercede for his father, who he thought was dying. His father suddenly recovered.

Then there were the Sacred Heart medals—the medallions they would find in unexpected places, like the house on a California ranch where they were staying shortly after Margaret's death that belonged to Robin Arkley, the megadonor who would fund the

Judicial Crisis Network. No one knew how they appeared. For Leo, the hearts were a sign of God's "playfulness," and a "reminder to have hope that all of that human suffering is permitted because there's good that comes of it." Watching his daughter struggle strengthened Leo's faith, pushing him to embrace a view of suffering as a sacred part of the human experience. Catholics like Leo seek to embrace suffering like Jesus embraced his crucifixion, as a means to achieve salvation. Catholicism teaches that life on Earth and the pain it brings is a small part of an eternal journey that continues after death with Jesus in heaven. That attitude infused Leo's beliefs about abortion, guiding his view that women should not end pregnancies as a way to avoid what he saw as temporal suffering.

"I saw firsthand the dignity and worth of a human person, even in a broken state, and I understand better than I ever otherwise could have the way in which human suffering can provide redemption not only for the individual who's suffering it but for mankind, humanity at large," he said. "That has enormous impact on my view of why our society, our culture, and our political and legislative arenas ought to embrace human life and reject abortion."

Leo's beliefs on the value of suffering were also reflected in the ideas of a Catholic community he was close to called Opus Dei, Latin for "work of God," a small international network of believers whose mission was to use their daily lives—the work of their days—to sanctify the world for Christ. Leo said he had no formal role in the group but was an admirer of "the work." He had served on the board of the Opus Dei–run Catholic Information Center, a spiritual and professional networking group near the White House, along with other prominent conservative lawyers like William Barr and Pat Cipollone. The official rolls of Opus Dei were a closely guarded secret, and the network, a relatively new devotional practice in Catholicism, had only about three thousand members in the United States and ninety thousand globally.

Years after Margaret's death, a famous oil-on-canvas artist, who had painted portraits of popes, presidents, and Justice Samuel

Alito, painted Margaret, smiling with a broad grin as Jesus blessed her from above. The portrait of *Margaret Leo of McLean*—a nomenclature used for saints—hangs in a gold frame in the Catholic Information Center. She was, in a way, Leo's own saint. She was a baby they did not abort, who, they believed, interceded with God to bring miracles on Earth, leaving Sacred Hearts behind as a divine sign. She led her father down a professional path with a spiritual goal.

IT WASN'T DISCUSSED at Scalia's funeral Mass, of course, but Scalia did not like the idea that his legal opposition to abortion might somehow be connected to his Catholicism. As a judge, he opposed Roe on legal grounds, not moral ones. After the Supreme Court upheld the Partial-Birth Abortion Act in 2007, a University of Chicago professor pointed out that every justice in the majority was Catholic. Scalia was furious and refused to speak at the school until the professor was gone.

Catholics in the United States were divided on abortion, with polling showing them nearly evenly split between supporting and opposing abortion rights. But the views of the Catholic Church were clear: abortion was a grave sin, punishable by excommunication. That theology was not always static—for centuries, the church taught that the soul entered the fetus only later in pregnancy, but in 1869, as the scientific revolution took hold, the church decreed that a human life begins at conception and expressly forbade abortion at any stage of pregnancy.

Leo stood firmly with Catholic orthodoxy. "I believe that abortion is an affront to the dignity and worth of a human person, and I think we have a moral and ethical obligation to preserve and defend human life from conception to natural death," he said.

He also looked to the church as a model for his conservative legal goals. Leo pointed approvingly to Thomas and compared his actions on the court to the Catholic Church during the Middle

Ages, building a philosophy slowly and over time. The church then was "laying the foundations for future Catholic thinking and Catholic thought to sort of grow the church and preserve its traditions," Leo told *The New York Times*. The idea was "tilling the ground," Leo said, something he saw Thomas do by staking out strong if lone positions on issues like abortion restrictions and gun rights, to prepare the field to one day be ready for "things to blossom or flourish."

At Scalia's funeral, Leo listened as Father Paul Scalia preached the homily in remembrance of his father. The priest had helped return Clarence Thomas to the Catholicism of his childhood in 1997. Leo was used to seeing him at his home parish, St. John the Beloved in McLean, Virginia, where he was a priest and where the Leos sat two rows in front of Eugene Scalia, the second-oldest of Scalia's children, and his family.

This day, they were all gathered to honor one man, Father Scalia told those in the pews, and it was not his father. It was Jesus of Nazareth. His father "knew well what a close-run thing the founding of our nation was," he said. "And he saw in that founding, as did the founders themselves, a blessing, a blessing quickly lost when faith is banned from the public square, or when we refuse to bring it there. So he understood that there is no conflict between loving God and loving one's country, between one's faith and one's public service."

Also in the basilica was the man who threatened to tip the court away from Leo's grasp—Merrick Garland, the man Obama would nominate as Scalia's successor.

11

The List

The moment of mourning in Washington was as fraught as it was sad. The 2016 election to replace Obama was well underway, and the future of the Supreme Court suddenly became a live issue. Just hours after the funeral, Donald Trump clinched the South Carolina primary, cementing his place as the Republican front-runner for president. If he won the nomination, he would almost certainly face off against Hillary Clinton, the longtime enemy of the anti-abortion movement. In an extraordinary break of congressional norms, Mitch McConnell, the Republican Senate leader, had already decided to take no action on the open seat, refusing to hold hearings and effectively blocking Obama from filling the spot with one of his nominees. The next Supreme Court justice, vowed McConnell, would be chosen by whichever candidate—likely Clinton or Trump—won the election.

Before Scalia died, the court was tilted toward justices who generally leaned toward a constitutional right to abortion by a 5–4 split. To Leonard Leo, the outcome of the election could herald the continuation of America's decay, or it could be the seed of the court's rebirth. If Clinton won, her Supreme Court nominee would presumably secure an abortion-rights majority—a wall of support for Roe that would be difficult to overcome for at least a generation. If America picked a Republican president, conservatives could maintain the current divide and maybe, over the course of his term, get another seat or two that could flip the court more starkly in their favor.

As Marjorie Dannenfelser watched Trump's poll numbers rise, she began to worry. Somehow this reality television star had transformed from a laughingstock to a candidate who dominated polls, cable news coverage, and the debate stage, dwarfing all her preferred options. She and other antiabortion leaders did not know Trump well. But what they did know, they did not like.

His position on abortion had shifted repeatedly over the years. In 1989, long before he seriously entered politics, he hosted a dinner at his Plaza Hotel honoring a former president of NARAL. He ultimately didn't attend, saying his family received death threats. Four years later, his then girlfriend, Marla Maples, had an unplanned pregnancy that resulted in his youngest daughter, Tiffany. "I'm not the kind of guy who has babies out of wedlock and doesn't get married and give the baby a name," he told *Vanity Fair* the night before his second wedding, to Marla, and two months after Tiffany was born. "And for me, I'm not a believer in abortion."

In 1999, as he flirted with a presidential run, Trump declared himself "very pro-choice," adding that he would not support a ban on the procedure in the later weeks of pregnancy. In 2011, Trump publicly reversed his position. "Just very briefly, I'm pro-life," he told attendees at the Conservative Political Action Conference, the annual gathering for the conservative movement.

At the time, Trump framed his change of heart in language familiar to religious Christian voters: a conversion story, marketed to the evangelical masses. When the topic of abortion came up, he often told a story of unnamed friends who planned to end a pregnancy. "He ends up having the baby and the baby is the apple of his eye. It's the greatest thing that's ever happened to him," Trump said in an interview with the Christian Broadcasting Network, two months after his CPAC speech. "And you know, here's a baby that wasn't going to be let into life. And I heard this, and some other stories, and I am pro-life."

But by the time he ran in 2015, Trump rarely talked about abortion. Instead, his campaign was dominated by one shocking moment after the next. He told voters he intended to bar Muslims from the country and deport undocumented immigrants, and he boasted that he could shoot someone on Fifth Avenue in New York City without losing voters' support. When he did mention abortion, Trump often contradicted Dannenfelser's desired talking points, like when he praised Planned Parenthood after David Daleiden's videos were made public, telling CNN that "they do some things properly and good, good for women." Trump, a twice-divorced casino owner, who framed his *Playboy* cover and boasted about a threesome, did not share their Christian values, the antiabortion leaders believed. Nor did he seem interested in publicly adopting their socially conservative mores or promoting their antiabortion cause. He was operating from his own playbook, one shaped not by their movement or even the Republican Party but by the rough-and-tumble politics that shaped his rise in liberal New York City.

With his every stumble, every inflammatory statement, Dannenfelser, leaders of the antiabortion movement, and establishment Republicans hoped Trump's candidacy might be finished. Their skepticism only deepened after Trump floated his sister Maryanne Trump Barry, a federal judge in New Jersey, as a "phenomenal" Supreme Court nominee. Trump said he was joking, but for conservatives who remembered her decision in 2000 that called banning late-term abortions "unconstitutionally and incurably vague," the remark was enough to confirm what they already believed: Trump wasn't an ally. He didn't seem interested in improving, either. When Penny Nance, president of Concerned Women for America, tried to organize an abortion briefing for Trump, his campaign was uninterested.

As the nominating contests approached, things were starting to feel desperate. Their only real shot at halting his rise was in Iowa, the first stop in the primary calendar. So in January, just days before Iowans would caucus to decide their preferred candidate, the super

PAC for Senator Ted Cruz, which Kellyanne Conway was running, released an attack ad focused on Trump's 1999 statement declaring himself "pro-choice." Dannenfelser organized ten antiabortion leaders to sign an open letter urging Iowa caucus-goers to pick "anyone but" Trump. The next president would be responsible for potentially four Supreme Court justices, the women argued, and Trump's vision so far "does not bode well" for overturning Roe.

"America will only be a great nation when we have leaders of strong character who will defend both unborn children and the dignity of women," they wrote. "We cannot trust Donald Trump to do either."

A moment of hope came when Cruz won Iowa by six thousand votes, powered by support from evangelical Christians, who were a significant portion of the state's primary electorate. But Trump surged back in New Hampshire, bolstered by voters who felt anxious about the changing country and betrayed by the Republican establishment on issues like immigration. Then he won South Carolina, where more than seven out of ten Republican primary voters were evangelical. Turnout for Republican primaries was higher than at any time since Reagan's run in 1980, an increase that could be attributed largely to evangelical voters. The leaders of the antiabortion movement had made clear that Trump was not the best champion of their cause. A large portion of their voters supported him anyway.

Trump understood something about these voters that Dannenfelser and her allies had missed. Like Dannenfelser, Trump believed the Republican autopsy of their losses in 2012 underestimated the power of an energized conservative base. "Does the GOP have a death wish?" he had said when the report was released, railing against the call for immigration reform included in the document. Unlike Dannenfelser, Trump believed the best way to channel the anger of the party's base was through a new kind of culture war. His vision was not based in traditional opposition to abortion rights and gay marriage but in a broader, angrier populism that was superheated by anti-immigrant rhetoric, a hatred of elite urban liberals, and a racial backlash to Obama.

Trump channeled broader evangelical anxieties about conservative white Christianity's declining numbers in a changing nation. Christians, these conservative white evangelicals believed, could soon become a persecuted minority, drowned out by what they saw as the forces of secularism, a diversifying nation, and an elite class—Hollywood, media, academics, and even Wall Street—that had turned against them. In just a matter of years, support for same-sex marriage had gone from a fringe position to one widely supported across the country. They watched several high-profile examples of people who shared their views—Christian wedding cake bakers, Hobby Lobby, Catholic nuns, county clerks—being required by the government to follow nondiscrimination laws, or to certify same-sex marriages or provide contraception coverage under the new health care law, things they said violated their beliefs.

But just as these conservative Christians believed they had been, Trump was rejected and dismissed by the Republican Party establishment. In an irreligious Manhattan businessman, many of them somehow saw themselves. And he promised them a restoration.

Trump made these voters a pledge bigger than conservative vows to ban abortion, stop same-sex marriage, or end racial preferences like affirmative action. "Christianity will have power," he declared before the caucuses to evangelicals gathered at a Christian college in the conservative northwest corner of Iowa. "If I'm there, you're going to have plenty of power. You don't need anybody else."

For much of his primary campaign, Trump had largely circumvented the traditional social conservative leaders of the movement—people like Leo and Dannenfelser. Instead, he relied on the more populist elements of evangelical Christianity. The televangelists and Pentecostal preachers with large followings online or on television, who did not have the strong political apparatus that the social conservatives did, made his case directly to primary voters. But now he appeared headed to the nomination and a difficult general election contest. To unify the party after a divisive primary, Trump would need the support of those conservative power brokers. And behind the scenes, some of his top aides had already been working out a deal to bind Trump to the conservative legal establishment, and with it, the antiabortion cause.

The day Scalia died, Don McGahn, a longtime Federalist Society member who was representing Trump's campaign, called Leo. The ninth Republican debate was in just a few hours, and Trump would certainly be asked about the sudden Supreme Court vacancy. Were there any judges, people who were "downright edgy," that he should be sure to mention as possible replacements, McGahn asked. Standing on the stage that night, Trump gave the public its first glimpse of his type of Supreme Court. He named two judges whom Leo had suggested—Diane Sykes and Bill Pryor, a favorite of conservatives for his views on Roe, or as he once put it, "the day seven members of our highest court ripped the Constitution and ripped out the life of millions of unborn children."

Shortly after the funeral, McGahn called Leo again, with an audacious proposal. Trump would release a public list of potential Supreme Court nominees and commit to appointing one of them should he win. The idea marked a startling break with political and legal norms. Previous presidential candidates had been purposely vague about their favorites—fearing the names could be leveraged against them in the campaign or, if they won, by interest groups during their administration. Even President George W. Bush, a champion of the antiabortion cause, spoke about a judicial litmus test for judges on Roe only in the most coded terms. When asked about judicial selection at the second presidential debate in 2004, he cited Dred Scott, the 1857 decision that ruled slaves remained the property of their owners, as an example of a bad ruling. The mention of such an old case baffled many viewers. But the antiabortion movement heard his meaning: Bush would never appoint a Supreme Court justice who supported Roe—a decision they often compared to the Dred Scott case.

Trump would adopt a far more transparent approach. In March, a month after Scalia's funeral, Trump attended a lunch at the Washington office of McGahn's corporate law firm, Jones Day, with two dozen prominent conservative lawmakers and lobbyists, people like Senators Tom Cotton and Jeff Sessions. McGahn told Leo to come to the meeting, and arrive prepared. In a private moment with Trump and McGahn after the larger discussion, Leo pulled out a list of names. It would take a few months to iron out the details, as various factions of the party fought over who would make it onto Trump's list of potential nominees. In May, his campaign released the first version of his list: eleven judges, including Pryor and others hostile to abortion rights. A second list would follow four months later that included Neil Gorsuch. They omitted another favorite, Brett Kavanaugh, a former lawyer in the Bush White House and circuit court judge in Washington, DC, who was suggested by allies at the Heritage Foundation and had long coveted a Supreme Court seat. He was too much of a Washington insider, and Trump was running on a "drain the swamp" message. If Trump won, Leo figured they could always supplement the list later.

Trump would later describe his picks as "pro-life judges," a term Leo repeatedly argued against in private conversations. "You're not nominating pro-life judges, you're nominating pro-constitutional judges," he said. The issues were broader than just abortion rights, Leo explained, and besides, judges were supposed to impartially rule on legal principle—not their preconceived political or religious beliefs. Trump didn't listen.

Regardless of how the judges were described, the roster of names signaled to conservatives that Trump would make promises no one else would. He was willing to go further than any other Republican candidate in modern history. Many conservative rank-and-file voters were already with Trump. But *the list*, as it would soon come to be known, would work as intended, providing the ultimate guarantee to conservative politicians and other elites—many of whom were Federalist Society members themselves. It "reassured a whole lot of Republicans," Mitch McConnell would explain years later at a Federalist Society event in Kentucky with McGahn, "that, okay, maybe he was doing fundraisers for [Democratic Senator Chuck] Schumer four years ago, but looks like he may be okay on something that's really important to us."

But the list wasn't enough to reassure Dannenfelser. While the male leaders in their movement flocked behind Trump, many of the women were horrified that Trump made headlines on abortion for all the wrong reasons. Just days after his meeting at Jones Day, Trump said women who have abortions should face "some form of punishment." It was Todd Akin all over again, gutting the credibility of female activists like Dannenfelser who had spent years trying to frame their movement and party as pro-woman. Conway, in an interview with *The New Yorker*, called it "a great example of him just undoing decades of work." Dannenfelser took a more tactical approach, and publicly excused Trump's comment—just as she once stood by Akin. "As a convert to the pro-life movement, Mr. Trump sees the reality of the horror of abortion—the destruction of an innocent human life—which is legal in our country up until the moment of birth," she said. "But let us be clear: Punishment is solely for the abortionist who profits off of the destruction of one life and the grave wounding of another."

Democrats, too, noticed the list. Already, they were enraged by the fact that McConnell and Senate Republicans refused to move forward with Garland. Now, the list marked another democratic norm being shattered by a man whose candidacy seemed to break every unwritten rule of politics and Washington.

But on some level, abortion-rights advocates did not believe the list of names really mattered. They felt confident that their own presidential candidate could not lose.

12

Hillary

Cecile Richards couldn't believe the moment had finally arrived. When Planned Parenthood was founded, almost a century ago, women didn't have the right to vote. Now, the group was about to make its first presidential primary endorsement. For a woman.

And not any woman. A feminist icon, a history-maker. First female partner at the oldest law firm in Arkansas. First wife of a major presidential candidate to have her own career, not to just "stay home and bake cookies." First Lady with an office in the West Wing. First female senator from New York. First major female candidate for president. And Obama's secretary of state.

In the early months of her campaign, Hillary Clinton wondered whether her life story was compelling enough to power a presidential candidacy. The forty-three men who held the job had fashioned their personal histories into narratives that reflected heroic national myths. Her husband's journey from the small town of Hope, Arkansas, to the White House was a triumph of the American meritocratic dream. Obama's multicultural journey, placed squarely in the civil rights tradition, spoke to progress toward a post-racial America.

The daughter of a middle-class couple from suburban Chicago, Hillary Rodham was the first in her family to attend college. A lifelong Methodist, she met Bill Clinton in law school, and her future became intertwined in his. Little seemed remarkable about that story, a common one for women of her generation, she believed. What grand narrative did her personal history tell about America, she wondered, as she prepared to launch her campaign.

But over time, Clinton came to realize that her life was a revolutionary story. One that started at home, exploded into the workplace, and then, finally, entered the halls of American power. Her mother was born on the day Congress took final action to give women the right to vote. Now Clinton, part of the very next generation, would vie to lead the nation. But that narrative—one of women's advancement in American life—lacked a political tradition with the same public resonance as Obama's civil rights struggle or her husband's meritocratic climb. Even in 2016, a female presidential nominee remained a novelty, an idea with a long history but little real-life precedent.

In the years that followed, analysts would describe the historic campaign between Clinton and Donald Trump as a referendum on immigration, racial fears, income inequality, distrust in government, and countless other issues. They would blame Clinton's lackluster political skills, muddled message, or the failures of her campaign operation for her eventual defeat. But what was also inescapable was the intertwining of this particular electoral matchup—a contest between an experienced female politician and a male celebrity—with the country's complicated feelings about women and their place in a changing nation.

Clinton, with her unique position on the front lines of American gender politics for decades, became an avatar for the past fifty years of gender progress. Unlike during her first run for president in 2008, when she largely ceded the mantle of making history to Barack Obama, Clinton now leaned into her gender. Her crowds were mostly female, as were most of her donors. Out of the eighty-four slogans considered by her team, "I'm with her" became the one chanted at her rallies. Trump's "Make America Great Again," meanwhile, carried an implicit promise to undo the sexual revolution and return the country to an idealized version of 1950s America. A time before sexual mores shifted, before second-wave feminism, before women flooded into professional life. A time before Roe.

Clinton was old enough to remember that earlier America. She was twenty-five years old when the Roe decision was issued, finishing Yale Law and working to defend the legal rights of children. From the time she arrived in Washington as First Lady, on the heels of the 1992 Year of the Woman, she fought openly for abortion rights. She used her platform to declare "human rights are women's rights, and women's rights are human rights." Later, when she became a senator, she voted against the partial-birth abortion ban, unlike more than a dozen of her Democratic peers. Then, as Obama's secretary of state, she made a mission of expanding reproductive health across the globe.

Early in her tenure, she offered a defense of abortion that became legendary.

"Does the United States' definition of the term reproductive health or reproductive services or reproductive rights include abortion?" Representative Chris Smith, the chair of the Pro-Life Caucus in Congress, asked her during a 2009 House hearing, clearly thinking he'd found the question to make her squirm.

"You are entitled to advocate, and everyone who agrees with you should be free to do so everywhere in the world. And so are we," said Clinton, sitting still in a white suit jacket and pearl necklace, before launching into a three-minute defense of abortion rights.

"So we disagree," she finally concluded, "and we are now an administration that will protect the rights of women, including their rights to reproductive health care." Then, as Smith glared, she lowered her eyes, ever so slightly pursed her lips, and leaned back against her chair, in effect dropping the mic. Abortion-rights advocates circulated the clip for years.

Now, Planned Parenthood hoped that Clinton would bring that revolution to transform abortion rights all the way into the

White House. But first, there was one small issue her campaign had to handle.

For years, when it came to abortion, Hillary Clinton championed her belief in the words of her time: "Safe, legal, and rare." It was a phrase popularized by her husband during his 1992 presidential campaign as a way to position himself as a moderate and win support from Reagan Democrats—particularly working-class Catholic voters—who opposed the procedure. But nearly a quarter century later, younger abortion-rights advocates saw those kinds of words, and others used by supportive Democrats in the 1980s and 1990s, like *choice* and *women's health*, as euphemisms that stigmatized the procedure and made it more difficult to defend politically. Not saying the word *abortion* reinforced the view that it was different from any other kind of medical procedure—more shameful or wrong—and implicitly fed into their "opponents'" arguments that it should be banned, these activists argued.

Clinton realized the dynamics had shifted even since her previous run for the White House in 2008. She saw the restrictive laws passing in the states, and she had monitored the escalating attacks against Planned Parenthood. But while no one doubted her support, some on her staff worried that her words hadn't quite caught up to the moment. Before she formally accepted Planned Parenthood's endorsement in early 2016, campaign aides scheduled an internal call to brief Clinton on the new rules when talking about abortion.

The call was limited to a small set of aides, but the message was crucially important. When you mean abortion, say abortion, her staff urged. Not "women's health." And most of all, don't say "safe, legal, and rare" anymore, they argued. "Safe and legal" was still okay. But not "rare."

"What?" Clinton replied. She demanded the rationale for the change.

Aides explained that many activists thought calling for abortion to be "rare" would offer a political concession to their opponents.

Plus, with so many new restrictions in the states, abortion was increasingly difficult to obtain, particularly for poorer women, making "rare" the wrong focus for their message. Abortion should be "safe, legal, accessible, and affordable," they told her.

"Well, that doesn't make any sense," Clinton huffed. "That's stupid."

It was a small but meaningful conversation that illustrated a notable generational shift on the issue. Clinton's befuddlement reflected how her generation, the one that fought for Roe, understood abortion politics. But now women were beginning to speak about their miscarriages and abortions with more candor. This new generation of activists wanted to pull abortion out of the shadows. They could start by changing the language of their allies. Clinton erased the phrase from her vocabulary. And she never looked back.

What she and other Democrats had tried to do in 1992 with "safe, legal and rare" was "send a signal that we understand *Roe v. Wade* has a certain theory of the case about trimesters," she explained. But by 2016, the world had changed. "Young women did not understand the effort that went into creating the underlying theory of *Roe v. Wade*. And the young women on my campaign made a very compelling argument that making it safe and legal was really the goal," she said. "I kind of just pocketed the framework of Roe. Roe is there."

Led by one of their most stalwart champions, the abortion rights movement entered a new era. When Clinton took the stage in Hooksett, New Hampshire, in January 2016 to publicly accept the Planned Parenthood endorsement, her navy pantsuit drawing a sharp contrast against the hot-pink backdrop, she cut straight to the point. "I have stood with you throughout my life and certainly throughout my career, and I promise you this: as your president, I will always have your back," she said. "We will work and fight together."

She also issued a warning: "I shudder to think about what the Republicans would do if given the chance," she said, raising the possibility that the next president could make multiple appointments to the Supreme Court. "They are telling you exactly what they will do if they get elected. And you know what, we should believe them."

Still, the future seemed brighter than ever for supporters of abortion rights. Richards hadn't been this excited about a candidate since her mother announced she was running for governor more than a quarter century earlier. In her New York City apartment, she kept a go bag packed with a hand steamer and sensible shoes—so she could quickly travel the country building support for Clinton.

For her part, Clinton made good on her promise. She didn't just oppose the Hyde Amendment, advocating for the repeal of the decades-old policy to be included in the party platform for the first time in history; she actively campaigned on the issue. A right is "no right at all," she said, if you have to take "extraordinary measures to access it." She promised to appoint judges who would preserve Roe. A lawyer herself, her judicial thinking took into account societal changes, the opposite philosophy of the originalism of Leo. She dismissed any idea that fetuses had constitutional rights. And she opposed efforts in Congress to pass a twenty-week abortion ban.

The sense of possibility grew in late June, when the Supreme Court finally ruled on the abortion restrictions Davis had filibustered in Texas. Sitting in her office in Manhattan, Richards got a single-word text message from her daughter: "Yay!" On the steps of the Supreme Court, abortion-rights activists hollered, hugged, and cried joyful tears. It was the court's biggest defense of abortion rights since Casey in 1992.

Their confidence that the Supreme Court would eventually save them was, in this instance, proven correct. The vote in the case, *Whole Woman's Health v. Hellerstedt*, vindicated their belief that the Texas law was illegitimate. The majority ruled that the restrictions on doctors and clinics violated the prohibition set in Casey of placing an "undue burden" on the ability to obtain an abortion.

The vote was 5–3, the justices short one of their nine due to Antonin Scalia's death.

To Richards, the ruling showed the power of their protest in Texas. To her, it was a lesson in the role that organizing—not just litigation—could play in the abortion rights fight. They had failed, but not really, she thought, because they won at the Supreme Court. Justice Ruth Bader Ginsburg cited the very stories and research Davis had read aloud during her filibuster. "Organizing matters," Richards said. "You just never know and you just never can give up. And things happen that people say are impossible." But the reality was that their trust in the court carried a cost. The case took years and cost millions, and twenty-two abortion clinics in Texas had closed.

There was another cost, too, one that was harder to see at the time. A section of the law still stood. It was the very portion that most directly undercut Roe, the part that prohibited abortion after twenty weeks, several weeks earlier than Roe's viability standard. Abortion groups had not asked the Supreme Court to review that provision in the law. It had been a strategic choice: Why risk alienating Justice Anthony Kennedy and causing the court to uphold a twenty-week standard, they reasoned, if there was the possibility of an even stronger 6–3 majority after Clinton won and got to fill Scalia's old seat? After all this litigation, they could end up with a future Supreme Court that was even more favorable to abortion rights.

Within days, Planned Parenthood announced legal campaigns to repeal similar laws mandating restrictions on doctors and clinics in eight states. It was a first salvo in a longer plan to challenge the 286 other abortion restrictions passed by conservative state legislatures across the country since 2010.

Stephanie Toti, the Center for Reproductive Rights' lawyer who argued the case, made plans to form a new organization that would leverage the new precedent created by the case. Her new group planned to challenge abortion restrictions across the country, taking advantage of the "golden age of reproductive rights" that would begin once Clinton reached the White House. It was, she thought at the time, "a moment of great potential and great promise."

No one doubted that Trump was a threat. Days after the ruling, Justice Ginsburg took the extraordinary step of speaking out against the Republican candidate. She called him "a faker" to CNN, and wondered about the need to move to New Zealand if he won. "I can't imagine what the country would be with Donald Trump as our president," she told *The New York Times*. "For the country, it could be four years. For the court, it could be—I don't even want to contemplate that."

As she campaigned across battleground states, Clinton continued to offer warnings about the court, pointing to the originalist jurisprudence a Trump-appointed justice would likely embrace. "In a single term, the Supreme Court could demolish pillars of the progressive movement," she said in a speech at the University of Wisconsin in Madison. "What kind of justice will a President Trump appoint?"

But few of her supporters believed he could actually win. To many on the left, Trump, a neophyte who stayed busy breaking every rule of politics, seemed practically unelectable. A more feminist future seemed ascendant. In Los Angeles, a feminist graphic design studio began printing THE FUTURE IS FEMALE on shirts, reclaiming a 1972 radical lesbian slogan and donating 25 percent of the proceeds to Planned Parenthood. The shirt started appearing on women and their daughters in liberal enclaves from Silver Lake to Hyde Park, Park Slope to Burlington.

For the first time in history, the Democratic National Committee platform included a call to repeal the Hyde Amendment and the Helms Amendment, which prohibited foreign aid from being spent on abortion. When Richards took the stage at the Democratic convention that year, once again in a navy suit and her mother's gold sheriff-badge pin, she couldn't help but remember her mother addressing the 1988 convention. Standing under the bright lights, in a prime-time speech broadcast across the country, Richards said *abortion*, the word once considered politically unsayable, three times in five minutes. As the red warning light telling her she was over her time blinked, Richards said with a smile: "Tonight, we are closer than ever to putting a woman in the White House, and I can almost hear Mom saying, 'Well, it sure took y'all long enough!'"

When Clinton finally accepted the nomination on that final evening, in her white suffragist pantsuit, even some of the strongest Trump supporters couldn't deny the power of the moment. "I won't be voting for her, but there's no doubt that today is a historic day as one of America's major parties nominates a woman for president," said Lynn Fitch, the Mississippi state treasurer, who stood behind Trump, in a gleaming white blazer, clapping and cheering at his rally in Jackson that evening. But, she added, "having the same sex doesn't mean her policies are best for women."

The cultural moment, the political winds, and the electoral momentum all seemed to be propelling abortion rights forward. Polls predicted a historically large gender gap, even bigger than in Obama's race against Mitt Romney four years earlier.

Liberal women everywhere thought they glimpsed the future. A President Clinton would prioritize women in their policies across the globe. Supreme Court Justices Stephen Breyer and Ruth Bader Ginsburg would retire, and Clinton would get to appoint at least three liberal replacements, stacking the court in their favor for a generation. Champions of their movement—women like Richards—would be placed in influential posts across her administration. They would expand the availability of contraception and repeal Hyde. Planned Parenthood would be protected. And the promise of Roe would become a reality.

After she won the election, Clinton would expand Obama's liberal vision into a new era, one where abortion rights were not just protected but expanded. The arc of history that Obama was so fond of mentioning would bend even further toward equality and diversity, her supporters expected, with at least a dozen straight years of Democratic governance. America would be remade by the first woman president. It was only a matter of waiting until Inauguration Day.

13

The Oddest Couple

The night that Indiana governor Mike Pence introduced himself to the world as Trump's running mate, onstage at the Republican National Convention in Cleveland, he attacked Clinton thirteen times by name. But he made just one passing reference to the issue that had been the heart of his career: the "sanctity of life." The politics were obvious. Hatred of Clinton energized Republican voters like perhaps no other Democratic politician could. Still, it was a notable omission from a politician so zealously opposed to abortion that he had been making the case with the exact same phrases for some three decades. Again and again, in campaign speeches and official events as governor, Pence expressed his desire to send Roe "to the ash heap of history, where it belongs." Yet on this night, Pence spoke with far less passion about his core cause. Instead, he described himself with another saying he was fond of using: "I'm a Christian, a conservative, and a Republican, in that order."

Most Americans had no idea just how much opposition to abortion underlined Pence's political work. The myriad controversies around Trump meant there was little public scrutiny of Pence's record or how he carried the antiabortion mantle like few other politicians since Reagan. As a congressman, he was an antiabortion and anti–gay marriage firebrand, and his broader policy agenda represented such a minority view that none of his bills ever made it to a full floor vote. He served on the House Judiciary Committee, and shared an originalist philosophy with his longtime friend Leonard Leo, whom Pence first met when he was invited to speak at a Federalist Society event while serving in Congress. As governor, Pence signed a law prohibiting abortion based on the gender, race, or disability of the fetus—a measure activists hoped would wind its way to the Supreme Court and, eventually, end Roe. Days before Trump asked him to join the ticket, an Indiana court put the law on hold while challenges were considered.

Pence's allies in the antiabortion movement could read between the lines of his convention speech and catch his more coded references to their mission. "Every American should know that while we are filling the presidency for the next four years, this election will define the Supreme Court for the next forty," Pence said. "Elect Hillary Clinton, and you better get used to being subject to unelected judges using unaccountable power to take unconstitutional actions." But for the general public, those mentions were easy to dismiss as standard political lines.

From the start, Trump and Pence were an odd couple. The crass, thrice-married tabloid playboy who rarely attended church, and the doctrinaire archconservative Christian who would not eat alone with a woman who was not his wife. Even some social conservatives weren't totally convinced that the ticket would hold or that Trump would win.

Pence was born Catholic, the third of six children, who all had names of saints. His mother was a Democrat who supported John F. Kennedy. He and his siblings attended the parish's parochial school, where a young Pence was a favorite of the nuns for his public-speaking skills. The four brothers were all altar boys. And when tornadoes touched down in their neighborhood of Columbus, Indiana, his mother would sprinkle them all with holy water from the local parish for divine protection, as they did not have a basement. The Pences felt the small Catholic community there faced prejudice, a vestige of the Ku Klux Klan's anti-Catholic ambitions.

The family called little Mike "Bubbles," because he was "chubby and funny," one of his brothers told *The New Yorker*. He was also ambitious. In high school during the years immediately after Roe, he lost fifty pounds and was elected senior class president. But he told friends the election he really wanted to win was the presidency of the United States.

The country's growing evangelical fervor drew him when he started as a freshman at Hanover College, a small liberal arts school on the banks of the Ohio River. In April 1978, he drove with friends two hours south to the Ichthus Music Festival in Wilmore, Kentucky, home to Asbury University and its spiritual revivals. Ichthus, named after an early Christian symbol for Jesus, was started as an alternative to Woodstock—its focus on spiritual ecstasy, not the joys of rock and roll and sex. Saturday night in light rain, his story goes, Pence came forward in the crowd and made a personal decision to trust Jesus. From then on, he would be born again. It was a classic conversion story reflecting the populist Christianity of his time.

But Pence did not immediately leave the Catholic Church or the Democratic Party. He voted for Jimmy Carter in 1980, when the white evangelicals of the new religious right threw their support behind Reagan and helped boost him into the White House. After college, Pence briefly pursued becoming a Catholic priest. Instead, he went to law school, and attended Mass at St. Thomas Aquinas. The church was one of the most progressive parishes in the entire archdiocese of Indianapolis, known for its acceptance of gay people at the height of the HIV crisis and permission to let women serve as lay eucharistic ministers. There, he saw a woman playing guitar during worship, a second-grade teacher named Karen Whitaker, who had also gone to Catholic high school. She was slightly older, and divorced from her high school sweetheart, who was not Catholic and who said they simply "grew apart" after several years of marriage. Pence was smitten. They married at St. Christopher's Roman Catholic Church, and the priest who officiated was Father James W. Lasher—a gay man who came out and left the priesthood soon after marrying them, and went on to lead Indy Pride. It was an irony of history: a gay man made possible the marriage for one of America's fiercest opponents of same-sex marriage.

All Karen ever wanted was to be a mom but for more than five years, pregnancy test after pregnancy test came back negative. In vitro fertilization was just starting to become mainstream during the 1980s, changing the way couples imagined they could have children. But the Catholic Church strictly opposed IVF and most fertility treatments. The problem, the church taught, was that fertility treatments substituted for sexual intercourse, which it believed to be the expression of the sacrament of marriage. Cardinal Joseph Ratzinger, who went on to become Pope Benedict XVI, linked the IVF procedure to abortion: "The abortion-mentality which has made this procedure possible thus leads, whether one wants it or not, to man's domination over the life and death of his fellow human beings and can lead to a system of radical eugenics," he wrote in *Donum Vitae*, his "Instruction on Respect for Human Life."

For years, the Pences did not publicly discuss their fertility challenges. But Karen later spoke about their decision to try fertility procedures. The Pences used a less common procedure called Gamete Intrafallopian Transfer, or GIFT, according to *Slate*. The Catholic Church remained undecided about GIFT, because the procedure could still include intercourse, so some devout Catholic couples turned to it when they wanted to pursue medical treatment while technically staying within the teaching. In GIFT, sperm is collected and put in a test tube with an egg, separated by an air bubble, all of which is then injected into the woman's fallopian tube in the hope that fertilization will happen there.

The Pences grappled with a different vision for their lives, one where perhaps they would not have children, and began to pursue adoption. Then, Karen's pregnancy test came back positive. In what felt like a miracle, they soon had three children under age three.

Like Marjorie Dannenfelser and Leonard Leo, the Pences experienced a kind of pregnancy-related loss and suffering that set a backdrop to their views about issues like abortion and adoption. Dannenfelser had a daughter with cognitive challenges, Leo's Margaret had spina bifida; and the Pences struggled with infertility. Kristan Hawkins, the Students for Life leader, had two children with cystic fibrosis. Fighting abortion—protecting what they viewed as complete, full babies—was one way to give meaning to their suffering and could provide solace and purpose amid pain.

It was during these periods of infertility that Pence first ran for Congress, as a graying twenty-nine-year-old in 1988. Abortion was a central political mission from the start. He supported a constitutional amendment that would ban abortion, with exceptions for rape and incest and to protect the life of the mother. Pence lost, twice, and became a conservative talk radio host.

Pence's departure from Catholic practice was slow, and also overlapped with his and Karen's infertility challenges—it was 1995, after the birth of his three children, before Pence publicly said he was attending an evangelical church. He was eventually elected to Congress five years later, where he argued that protecting human life at conception was the foundation of America's moral integrity. Roe was "legally poorly conceived and morally wrong and should be overturned," his campaign website said. He supported legislation to make clear that the protections of the Fourteenth Amendment applied to a fertilized egg. Karen Pence attended one of Kellyanne Conway's earliest fundraising tea parties to support the Susan B. Anthony List.

Pence led the charge for the Partial-Birth Abortion Ban Act, introducing the bill by quoting the Bible, "Whatsoever you do for the least of these, you do to me," and used graphic language to describe the procedure: "forcibly turning the child to a breech position, pulling the living child out of the mother by the leg, stabbing the child in the base of the skull, removing its brains with a vacuum, and pulling the dead child out of the mother."

His ethic was uncompromising and at times contrary to scientific fact. "Condoms are a very, very poor protection against sexually transmitted diseases," he argued to Wolf Blitzer on CNN in 2002. "The only truly safe sex, Wolf, as the president believes, is no sex."

Onstage at the 2003 March for Life, where the Pences often came as a family, Pence squinted in the bright sun and declared it was time for President Bush to put "principled pro-life judges" onto the court and "end *Roe v. Wade* forever." He smiled as he paraphrased Billy Joel:

"'You may be right, I may be crazy,'" he said to a cheering crowd. "But it just may be a lunatic America is looking for."

Pence went to Trump Tower for the first time in 2011, to ask Trump to financially support his 2012 run for governor. They'd met just once before, briefly at a fundraiser at Mar-a-Lago a year earlier. The dynamic was transactional from the start, and it centered on women. Trump was fixated on gossip about Indiana governor Mitch Daniels's marriage, divorce, and remarriage to the same woman. He told Pence he would never take back a wife who had been unfaithful. Pence bristled at the awkwardness of the conversation. But he accepted the $2,500 check.

Dannenfelser had asked Pence to run for president that year, but he told her he would only ever do it if he felt called by God. Tom McClusky of the March for Life even bought a website for him in hopes that call would come against Obama. But Pence ran for governor of Indiana instead.

In the summer of 2016, Trump was pondering whom to pick as his running mate, and Pence was running a tough reelection campaign in Indiana. His net approval rating was lower than thirty-three other governors'. His signature 2015 law on religious freedom unleashed a deluge of nationwide criticism for the leeway it gave businesses to not serve LGBTQ customers. He supported a constitutional amendment to ban gay marriage before the Supreme Court ruled to legalize it. But Conway, who had just joined the Trump campaign and who had done polling for Pence in 2009, believed that he could be a political asset. She had made the case for Pence without using his name, arguing that Trump needed to shore up Middle America. Pence could speak to the Rust Belt states they needed to win. He had strong relationships with Republican governors in places like Kentucky and Michigan.

Trump's polarizing style and divisive statements turned off moderate swing voters. To win the general election, Trump would need to compensate for those losses with historically high turnout from the party's white conservative Christian grassroots. Pence could boost their numbers with that key demographic. And critically for the campaign, he was a key point of contact for conservative billionaire donors like Charles and David Koch.

Trump liked the idea that Pence, unlike some of the other vice presidential hopefuls, such as Chris Christie or Newt Gingrich, could never upstage him. His supporters liked that too: "I'd say he is like the very supportive, submissive wife to Trump. He does the hard work, and the husband gets the glory," was how an evangelical female Trump supporter in northwest Iowa later put it.

Days before the Republican National Convention in Cleveland while Trump was visiting Indiana, his plane got a flat tire. He was stuck there overnight and met Pence for dinner at the Capital Grille in Indianapolis. Trump was still toying with the idea of the other possible picks. But he asked if Pence would say yes.

Pence had three words: "In a heartbeat."

THE TICKET THAT came out of Cleveland wasn't perfect for the antiabortion movement. Trump still rarely mentioned abortion on the campaign trail, focusing far more on promises to "drain the swamp" of Washington corruption and build a wall along the southern border to keep undocumented migrants out. But short of the presidency, Pence was as close a guarantee as the movement could get. He was a known quantity, on the straight and narrow. And realistically, social conservatives no longer had the power to win the White House. Since George W. Bush, none of their preferred candidates had broad enough appeal in the Republican Party to win the presidential nomination. Their movement had been losing power, within their party and the nation, as the Republican autopsy had pointed out. But now, they had found another way. They fused themselves to a candidate who needed them and whom they could use. If they could get in the door, they could figure out how to leverage power. Pence could be their man on the inside—the man with the conviction that Trump lacked to push their cause.

The newly approved GOP platform included a twenty-week abortion ban, defunding Planned Parenthood—explicitly citing the 2015 congressional investigation that grew out of David Daleiden's video sting—and appointing Supreme Court justices who would overturn Roe. Then, soon after the convention, Trump named Conway his campaign manager. It all represented an incredible feat for Dannenfelser and her cohort of antiabortion women, another indication that their movement was no longer cast out of the party but at its very center.

In September, Dannenfelser secured a letter from Trump that she could use to grow the campaign's Pro-Life Coalition, which she led. Like the list, she saw the letter as a public promise, a way not only to drum up support for Trump now but also to hold him accountable later, if he won the White House. Trump signed the letter on his way to the funeral of the anti-feminist activist Phyllis Schlafly, on his campaign plane, with Conway by his side. He made four promises: to nominate only "pro-life justices" to the Supreme Court, to sign into law a bill that would make abortion illegal after twenty weeks, to defund Planned Parenthood if it continued to provide abortions, and to make the Hyde Amendment permanent.

While they worked to harden Trump's views, advisers worked to publicly soften Pence's to avoid alienating female voters and more secular white working-class supporters. As Pence prepared to debate Clinton's running mate, Tim Kaine, Pence's daughter Charlotte reviewed his answers about women and abortion with him at the kitchen table. Her father could not talk about the issue without talking about his faith—the driving force of his views. They worked to frame his answer to sound more inclusive, not exclusionary, as if it were only motivated by his Christianity. The strategy was new, but old, grounded in John C. Willke's instruction to make abortion more than just a "religious question."

In the debate, Pence sold his opposition to abortion as love, urging Americans to "welcome the children into our world." The country, he said, "can be judged by how it deals with its most vulnerable, the aged, the infirm, the disabled, and the unborn. I believe it with all my heart. And I couldn't be more proud to be standing with a pro-life candidate in Donald Trump."

The Trump-Pence marriage was a pairing of opposites. One man was not supportive enough of the antiabortion cause for social conservatives. And the other was too pious for secular working-class white voters, another necessary faction of the coalition. But with their forces combined, they hoped to have the makings of a winning political campaign.

14

"Grab 'Em by the Pussy"

When the *Access Hollywood* tape tore across the internet orders of magnitude faster than David Daleiden's Planned Parenthood videos, Mike Pence went home to Indianapolis to talk with Karen and pray. Campaign aides wanted him to defend Donald Trump before Trump even said a word. Other Republicans were pressuring him to get off the ticket and disavow Trump, as they were doing. But this mess was not his to clean up, he thought. Trump was the one who said it:

"Grab 'em by the pussy."

Trump bragged about assaulting women on an *Access Hollywood* video from 2005 that was suddenly playing on every channel. And at first, he refused to address the issue on video, releasing only a statement dismissing his words as "locker-room banter" and apologizing "if anyone was offended."

If Pence could publicly grant Trump grace, he could show the way for their conservative Christian base to do so too. But Pence would not speak publicly until Trump did. And even then, Pence refused to defend or condone the remarks. His followers in the antiabortion movement were left to make their own peace with the deal they had struck.

For more than a year, the antiabortion movement had tried to skirt the moral choice on Trump. They found ways to justify his coarse behavior, his curses, botched Bible references, and insulting words. They were electing a president, not a preacher, and policy mattered most, went their argument. But the reckoning had come. It was not just the video. Multiple women had come forward accusing Trump of unsettling sexual advances, groping, and even sexual assault, charges Trump denied.

Marjorie Dannenfelser saw herself as a defender of women. In her mind, and in those of women like her, opposing abortion was a way to save women from what she saw as a choice that destroyed their lives and left them crippled with regret. She had made a calculation that Trump, with all his faults, would be better for their cause than Hillary Clinton. Even as she and others in her movement believed Trump would lose, they had planned for the courts and captured the vice presidential spot on the ticket, in hopes that somehow, if he did win, they would be in place to act. That was what it meant for them to act in faith. But now, all of that was at risk. The choice was suddenly so stark.

Some donors pressured her to back out. Trump was going to lose, they argued, and supporting him would ruin the future of the antiabortion movement as Todd Akin had threatened to do. But the Susan B. Anthony List had a single mission, and only Trump gave her a chance of achieving it. "Which of the two paths would result in overturning *Roe v. Wade*?" she asked herself. It would be at least a generation before they had another chance to turn the Supreme Court in their favor, she thought. One candidate would lock Roe in forever, and the other could overturn it.

The hardest cost was the most personal: her daughters. Dannenfelser's oldest told her she could not support her if she continued to help Donald Trump. "My daughters saw a snapshot in time and were right to be appalled," Dannenfelser later wrote. "But I saw the evil that had been wrought in the decades since Roe v. Wade, which had ended the lives of more than 50 million pre-born babies." By the time she called into NPR's *Morning Edition*, a few days after Trump's apology, her answer was clear.

"It is not to be set aside, the assault and offense of women," she said when the interview started. And then, "I am still with Trump."

Top Republicans like Senator John McCain, the party's 2008 nominee, withdrew their support. Some even called on Trump to leave the race. Dannenfelser stood by her man once again, committed to her strategy now as she had been with Akin, even if all signs pointed to Trump's defeat.

The controversy over the tape focused on his history of assaulting women—not abortion rights. But in another sense, Trump's words revealed exactly how far he would be willing to go.

THE FULL ABSOLUTION finally came under the bright lights of a debate stage twelve days later. When asked about the Supreme Court, Clinton said the country must not reverse marriage equality or Roe. Trump gave a very different response. Under his presidency, Roe would fall because he would appoint "pro-life" judges from the list. "If we put another two or perhaps three justices on, that is really what will happen. That will happen automatically in my opinion," he said. Then he fired off a quote Dannenfelser could have only dreamed of when she was training the scores of Republican men. "If you go with what Hillary is saying, in the ninth month, you can take the baby and rip the baby out of the womb of the mother just prior to the birth of the baby."

In a viewing room backstage, Kellyanne Conway jumped out of her chair and squealed with delight. It was a "decades-in-the-making zinger," she crowed. Trump's "ripping" description didn't account for the medically complicated and emotionally painful reality of late-term abortion procedures. But that didn't matter. No one had ever heard a presidential nominee talk so graphically about abortion from the debate stage. They had always been too worried about alienating mainstream America, losing the moderate voters they needed to win a national election. Trump had turned the tables, and Clinton was now cast as the "extremist" in America's culture wars, at least in Conway's eyes.

In some ways, Trump's comment about abortion was an outward sign of an inward, more invisible gift. His words were a message to white conservative Christian America, much bigger than Bush's remark about Dred Scott. Trump's opposition to abortion rights mattered to them, of course. But what mattered more was that Trump would be their weapon against an America fighting against them on a host of issues, from transgender rights to the place of religion in public life. It was another version of the message he delivered those months ago in Iowa, "Christianity will have power." Trump would take up their language, their anger, and wield his power in their broader war.

In their own backstage room, Clinton's campaign aides jotted down Trump's prediction that he would overturn Roe on a large whiteboard, where they were tracking the key moments of the debate. They knew that the idea was out of step with the majority of Americans and offered an opportunity for a political attack.

But quickly, a different Trump line gained notoriety, overpowering the first. Asked whether he would accept the results of the election if he lost to Clinton, Trump refused to commit. "I will tell you at the time," he said. "I'll keep you in suspense."

The Clinton aides had a frenzied discussion: What message should they elevate in the spin room to define the narrative of that final debate? The voters they most needed to pull from Trump—suburban women and moderate Republicans—weren't worried about Roe, a legal ruling that seemed cemented in American life, they decided. There was little evidence the issue resonated beyond Clinton's most ardent supporters. They chose his comments about the election results.

Yet as Stephanie Schriock, the president of EMILYs List, walked out of the debate, she couldn't shake a sinking suspicion that they had witnessed a pivotal moment. The line about the babies "ripped from the womb" felt rehearsed to her. Clearly, it was a political tactic to boost his numbers with evangelical and conservative Catholic voters. But the donors around her buzzed with excitement over what they saw as Clinton's killer performance. They were all but celebrating victory.

Schriock was right, even if no one understood precisely why yet. Democrats lasered in on Trump's words about the election itself. But conservative Christians heard something else that night—the unchecked power Trump promised them.

A FEW WEEKS after the votes were counted, a missed call and voicemail popped up on Dannenfelser's phone. She didn't recognize the number. But the voice was unmistakable.

Hearing from Trump was an unfathomable turn from where she was just four years earlier, relegated to the sidelines of the party. It was a sign that her movement was now entrenched in the seat of political power. With the groundwork they had laid, antiabortion activists could go straight to the top. Against all odds, Trump had won with Pence as his vice president. Republicans had not just captured the White House but kept control of the Senate and the House. Trump would be the one to fill Antonin Scalia's old seat.

The victories were an extraordinary stroke of luck. The antiabortion movement leaders had plotted and positioned where they could at every turn along the way, gotten their lists, pledges, and vice presidential pick from Trump. But even as they executed their plans, many of them didn't think they would actually win the White House. Trump's victory shocked not just them but the nation. He won by fewer than eighty thousand votes, combined from just three states. As liberal America reeled, the antiabortion activists celebrated. Now, they could hold the formerly pro-choice, soon-to-be president to a new set of promises.

In his first prime-time interview after the election, Trump reiterated the pledge he made from the debate stage. "I'm pro-life, the judges will be pro-life," he told *60 Minutes*. If Roe were ever overturned, he added, "it would go back to the states." Women would "have to go to another state," he said. "We'll see what happens. It's got a long way to go, just so you understand."

Dannenfelser's movement hadn't changed Americans' hearts and minds, which had long been what she said was the ultimate goal. Just as they had for decades, a majority of Americans still supported Roe, saying they did not want to see the court overturn the decision. White conservative Christians were becoming more of a minority in America with every passing year. But they had shown that it was not size that mattered—it was power. And now, with Trump about to move into the White House, political momentum was on their side. If they played it right, this was their opportunity to change generations of American life.

Dannenfelser listened to the familiar voice coming through her phone, the voice of the candidate she had stuck with for a larger prize. She could draw a line from her choices with Akin to Trump. Once again, many in the Republican establishment fled from a man her cause needed because of his controversial comments about sexual assault. But this time, the conservative grassroots boosted him to victory. It was a sign that Republican politics had changed. Dannenfelser believed back then that an energized conservative base could overpower the demographic trends working against them. And four years after the autopsy argued otherwise, she was proven right. Despite the early skepticism of elite Christian leaders, including Dannenfelser, when November came, her people had stood by Trump en masse. Eighty-one percent of white evangelical Christians voted for Trump in 2016, their highest support for a presidential candidate in at least a dozen years, if not longer. But Dannenfelser wasn't correct about everything. She didn't need the power of the party establishment. She just needed to find someone who could overtake it.

Dannenfelser and the antiabortion movement may have set out to reclaim power in the Republican Party, and they succeeded. Without their support, Trump wouldn't have won. But their efforts did more than just elect a new president. They were at the forefront of reshaping the Republican Party into a new coalition, one that mirrored the more populist and radical priorities of the new president. And that shift would become a turning point for American Christianity itself, as the new conservative politics roiled and remade churches across the nation.

"I want to just thank you and thank all of the people that were with you, and we will never forget. You are incredible. Everybody's talking about you," the president-elect said in his voicemail. "You keep in touch."

Of course, many of those in the conservative grassroots wanted to overturn Roe. It had been a goal of the religious right for decades. But in this race, abortion was revealed to be more than moral outrage over a medical procedure that they believed murdered babies. Abortion was a symbol of their place in America. To them, Trump and his slogan of "Make America Great Again" represented a promise to restore the country to a time before Roe, when the values of conservative Christians on the relationship between women and men were prevalent and powerful.

Most voters did not realize those potential consequences when they cast their ballots in 2016. When voters were asked to rank their top concerns, abortion rights were low on the list, below even the Supreme Court. Other topics—Trump's fitness to serve, the economy, immigration—dominated the thinking of voters, strategists, and media observers. Young voters, who didn't know a time before Roe and never imagined it was at risk, turned out in lower numbers for Clinton than just four years earlier, unmotivated to vote for either candidate. To some more moderate white women, Clinton was too divisive, even if they agreed with her that abortion rights should be protected. And to many Republicans who backed Trump, the contest was largely about immigration, economic concerns, and a desire to put their party back in the White House.

Clinton saw her defeat as inextricable from her gender. She blamed former FBI director James Comey's last-minute reopening of the investigation of her private email server—after clearing her of wrongdoing—for her immediate defeat. "But once he did that to me, the people, the voters who left me were women," she said. "They left me because they just couldn't take a risk on me, because as a woman, I'm supposed to be perfect. They were willing to take a risk on Trump, who had a long list of, let's call them flaws, to illustrate his imperfection, because he was a man, and they could envision a man as president and commander in chief."

But it was more than just the old double standard. Clinton was shocked by how little impact the reports of Trump's sexual misconduct and assault seemed to have on the race. They didn't disqualify him from the presidency, at least not among most Republicans and conservative Christians. "I also saw the way women were devalued and ignored as the revelations about Trump came out," she said "The belittling, the demeaning."

That moment in the third debate, she realized, had been a "set-up," a way to claim that she was "not just pro-choice but pro-abortion" in more conservative parts of key swing states. And it had succeeded. "Politically, he threw his lot in with the right on abortion and was richly rewarded," she said.

Looking back, the story of the 2016 election was not just about a man who won an unexpected victory. It was a referendum about women and the debate over their place in a changing nation. The election had been a battle between liberal feminism and conservative Christianity—and the Christians won.

Republicans hadn't just secured the White House. During Obama's tenure, Democrats had failed to cement their power beyond Washington. They neglected state races, losing more than 1,030 seats in state legislatures, governors' mansions, and Congress. Democrats were left holding total control in only five liberal states: Oregon, California, Connecticut, Rhode Island, and Delaware. But Republicans had twenty-five, giving them power over much of the country. Their increasing state power allowed antiabortion legislators to continue passing a deluge of abortion restrictions as they gained full control of the federal government in Washington.

"This is the strongest the pro-life movement has been since 1973," Dannenfelser said in the weeks after Trump won. "We are dealing now with a president who has not been playing the game in the way that other presidents, including Republicans, have."

With Trump, their movement jumped on a bullet train. It didn't travel on a predictable schedule. And it wasn't the most reliable service. But it was powerful enough to defeat one of the most iconic figures in the history of American feminism. And now it was headed directly toward the White House.

15

The New Giants

It started almost by accident, over cocktails. Exactly the kind of accident that Leonard Leo intended to happen at the Federalist Society's annual conference.

Just nine days after Donald Trump won the 2016 election, the event was part victory party and part job fair for the incoming administration. Leo arrived after spending the day at Trump Tower in New York, talking about turning the list into legal reality with the president-elect and some of his top aides. Trump was very clear that he had not changed his mind—if someone was not on the list, they were not being considered. Inside the Mayflower Hotel, the list came to life. At least nine judges of Trump's twenty-one possible Supreme Court nominees were slated to speak, and most of the other hopefuls attended at various points.

The halls were abuzz with all the possibilities in a future that had changed overnight. So, the young solicitor general of Wisconsin, Misha Tseytlin, was surprised when he overheard someone say that Roe would never be overturned. Tseytlin had clerked for Justice Anthony Kennedy and had long opposed abortion for moral reasons, though he was not particularly religious. His family had come to the United States when he was a child as Jewish refugees from the former Soviet Union, where communism had long suppressed religious practice.

To Tseytlin, the sentiment that Roe was infallible was frustrating and defeatist. But what neither he nor Americans on either side of the abortion debate could have imagined was the role that thought would have in pushing the court in a new direction.

There was no reason to think overturning Roe was impossible, especially not now, Tseytlin believed. Republicans had the White House, an open Supreme Court seat, and legislatures passing innovative laws in states across the country. If there really was no right to abortion in the Constitution, this was the time to prove it.

It wasn't lost on Tseytlin that Planned Parenthood and its allies had challenged the Texas law, but not the twenty-week limit included in the law. By 2016, nearly a third of states had twenty-week bans. Most had not been challenged by abortion clinics, leaving them in effect in places like South Carolina, West Virginia, and his own state of Wisconsin. Across the country, a twenty-week ban was now normalized, even though it was roughly three weeks shy of the viability standard set in Roe, which with advancements in prenatal care had shifted earlier than the original twenty-eight weeks.

Some states, led by activists who had grown tired of the national groups' incremental strategy, had tried to shrink the time frame of when abortion was allowed, moving to twelve weeks in Arkansas or six weeks in North Dakota. But the court struck those down. So if twenty weeks stood, but twelve and six weeks did not, Tseytlin wondered, was there a magic cutoff in those middle weeks?

What would happen if a state tried to pass a limit at, say, fifteen weeks? An ever-so-slightly earlier restriction could force the court to examine the viability rule and shake the very foundations of Roe. Could they push the number of weeks back just to the point where their opponents would challenge it?

Kennedy, his old boss, had ruled in favor of abortion rights in the landmark cases of Casey and Whole Woman's Health. But he had also criticized abortion later in pregnancy in *Gonzales v. Carhart*, where he wrote the majority opinion upholding a ban on so-called partial birth abortion. Tseytlin had a hard time believing that Kennedy, or

John Roberts, would strike down a ban that was just a few weeks earlier than twenty. Many restrictions in Europe were around twelve or fifteen weeks. It wasn't a totally equivalent comparison, given that national health insurance programs and more robust social safety nets made it easier for European women to detect their pregnancies faster and access an abortion more quickly if they wanted one. But those countries did present an earlier standard in developed nations. It was a piece of data they could use.

He had other ideas, too, including passing more laws that would prohibit abortion based on things like selection for race, sex, or disability. But no matter what, the priority needed to be on undoing the viability rule, he believed. Striking down that part of Roe would functionally undo the decision, even if the justices never wrote the words outright.

Tseytlin mused about all of this to a new acquaintance connected with the Alliance Defending Freedom, the Christian law firm that worked with David Daleiden during his video sting. Even during the political exile of the Obama administration, ADF had racked up some big victories, winning six cases at the Supreme Court since 2011. Leo, a man who spent his life cultivating legal power for the right, would call the firm "formidable," describing it as "a real major force in the conservative legal world."

And now ADF was looking to do something even bigger. The group saw a new opportunity to advance a body of law to attack abortion rights. It was an opening that its lawyers believed might not be available for more than a few years, and they were determined to take advantage of it.

Already, ADF had been developing a wide-scale approach to change laws around sexuality—first, writing model legislation to push back on expanding gay rights, then getting states to pass the bills, and then providing those states with legal defense in court when they were sued. It was a one-two-three punch that took full advantage of the Democrats' political weakness in the states, with those more than 1,030 seats lost during the Obama administration.

Since late 2014, ADF had been using that strategy to advance so-called bathroom bills, laws that required people to use the public restrooms of the sex they were assigned at birth. There was a state where those efforts had been especially effective: Mississippi. With its strong opposition to abortion, Mississippi could be fertile ground for ADF to run a similar play on Roe.

THE LEGAL IDEA was in motion. And the symbolic effect was too.

Penny Nance, the president of Concerned Women for America, looked out from backstage at the crowd gathered in the cold on the National Mall, as it had every year for the March for Life. For forty-four years, her movement had gathered on or around January 22 to protest the Supreme Court's ruling in Roe on that date.

Behind her was the Capitol. Ahead, the Washington Monument. And beside her, Marjorie Dannenfelser and other women of the small antiabortion sisterhood that got started that pivotal year of 1992, nearly a quarter century earlier.

Participants from Catholic churches and schools and antiabortion groups across the country broke into chants as they prepared to march toward the Capitol and the Supreme Court: "Hey, hey, ho, ho, *Roe v. Wade* has got to go!" They waved signs, flags, and banners that proclaimed the reasons they had come: "I am the pro-life generation." "We don't need Planned Parenthood!" "Babies can feel joy in the womb."

A week earlier, a far larger crowd descended on this same stretch—the Women's March, they called themselves—to protest Trump's election. Four million women had poured into the streets of Washington and around the country, a second suffrage protesting the new administration. They wore hot-pink "pussy" hats and waved signs with opposite messages from the ones that arrived on this day: MY BODY MY RIGHTS! THE FUTURE IS FEMALE! Some carried posters with quotes from Clinton's famous speeches. WOMEN'S RIGHTS ARE HUMAN RIGHTS, read one.

"We will not go back!" Cecile Richards shouted to the crowd, taking the stage in Washington in her hot-pink blazer. "My pledge today is, our doors stay open."

At a private party that night, Richards rocked out with the National, the band that had provided the unofficial soundtrack of Obama's campaigns, at a celebrity-studded celebration organized by Planned Parenthood long before Election Night curdled into a crushing defeat. "It ain't me, it ain't me, I ain't no fortunate son!" Richards sang from the stage, belting the Vietnam War protest anthem along with Planned Parenthood activists, donors, and supporters.

But the March for Life was not about celebrity or size. It did not matter if the Women's March had cooler music or got more attention. What mattered was that the antiabortion movement now had power. Not the power of broad public support. Nor the power of cultural cachet. But pure political power. They rose as a tightly connected group of unelected political actors, driven by undying belief, determination, and cunning. They were a minority that turned weakness into strength at the right places at the right time. What mattered was their network, the strong and weak ties and strategic positioning that could create the conditions for radical change.

It was difficult for many in the mainstream to see their force in the moment. Their view could be a minority view and still conquer the majority, through a combination of strategy, persistence, and pure luck. Or, what many of the people there would call Providence—the belief that God was acting in their favor and for their protection. They knew how to maneuver in Washington when Trump did not, giving them a strategic advantage even over him.

Standing in the cold, Nance watched as several black SUVs pulled up backstage. Mike Pence, now vice president, stepped out of the motorcade with Karen and their daughter Charlotte. For years, such a moment had been unimaginable. Never before had a president or vice president come to address the march in person.

When Pence told the story of his invitation to the march, and he retold it often, he recounted standing next to Trump in the Oval

Office. The new president said he had been invited but could not attend, so Pence volunteered to go in his place. What Pence did not say was that he had been invited first, months earlier.

Tom McClusky, the president of March for Life Action, had called Pence as soon as he heard that the Indiana governor was Trump's pick. No other elected official had likely ever spoken as often as Pence from the stage at the march, he thought. McClusky asked Pence to make a promise: Would he speak to the March for Life in January, win or lose? And when Pence won the vice presidency on Election Night, McClusky called his team to remind them. Trump was simply their Trojan horse, a vehicle to gain access to the White House.

One by one, officials of the newly minted Trump administration emerged from the black cars, each a longtime player in the antiabortion movement. Most people in America did not know them, but they had all known each other for years. There was Kellyanne Conway, now a White House adviser after becoming the first woman to run and win a presidential campaign, and plenty of staff from Pence's new office. They greeted the activists backstage as old friends, because they were. Pence locked eyes with person after person, close to tears.

Karen introduced her husband. Amid the excitement and blustering wind, Nance could not quite hear what he said. As soon as she got home, she put in earbuds.

More than four decades earlier, on another January morning in 1973, the Supreme Court had turned away from the unalienable right of life, Pence told the crowd. But three generations later, all that was over. "Life is winning again in America," he said. "We will not grow weary. We will not rest until we restore a culture of life in America for ourselves and our posterity." The crowd exploded in cheers.

Standing in her kitchen, Nance started to sob. She turned to her husband. "We won," she said. "We are going to change history."

Four days later, Nance and Dannenfelser headed to the White House, down the hall to the East Room, to witness Trump nominate

Neil Gorsuch to be the newest member of the US Supreme Court. It felt to Dannenfelser like the entire antiabortion movement had walked in after eight years of being shut out. Pence and Karen sat in the front row, in front of Mitch McConnell. Leo was also there in the East Room, sitting in an uncomfortable chair, and he marveled. The newest member of the Supreme Court would be a judge who ruled in favor of the *Burwell v. Hobby Lobby* decision while on the Tenth Circuit. He had now shepherded three nominations to the Supreme Court: John Roberts, Samuel Alito, and Neil Gorsuch, a third of the bench.

"Many are still trying to sort out all the lessons of 2016," Leo said a few months later. "But maybe one lesson is this: sometimes, in a good cause, your breaks take you by surprise as much as your setbacks."

No one knew how the next four years, or more, would go. For more than forty years, the antiabortion movement was David, fighting Goliath. But the country had shifted, and they were giants.

16

Stacking the Administration

The March for Life was but a flash in the lightning storm of the new administration. Within hours, it was practically forgotten by the wider public, when Trump announced that he was banning immigration into the United States from several majority-Muslim countries. Lawyers rushed to airports to defend incoming travelers, trailed by media covering the extraordinary scene.

America was unprepared for the intensity of Trump's early days. The president picked fights over the size of his inauguration crowd, railed against the "fake news media," and criticized his predecessor, Obama. He watched a steady stream of cable news, offering a bitter play-by-play of the coverage. He hired senior staff and ousted them. Protests erupted with rapid speed as liberals demonstrated weekly against everything from Trump's plans for a wall at the southern border to his denial of climate change. "Protesting is the new brunch" became a liberal mantra, invoked on podcasts and printed on T-shirts.

Yet just as in Texas, when protesters descended to support Wendy Davis, the most effective actions were happening not outside the halls of power but within them. Amid the chaos of Trump's Washington, one strategy was systematic and behind-the-scenes: the effort to make his administration the most airtight against abortion since Reagan.

Most of the effort had very little to do with the president. Instead, it had everything to do with Pence, the most powerful antiabortion advocate in the White House, who had a singular advantage—he was the only official whom Trump could not fire. What mattered, as Pence's team quickly realized, was not organizing mass protests but having the right people in the right slots on the organizational chart.

It was an extraordinary opportunity, a president who came into power with no political orbit of his own. Trump had few requirements for his staff beyond loyalty to Trump. There was a power vacuum, and abortion opponents filled it. Three days after the election, Trump fired the head of his transition team, Chris Christie, and asked Pence to run it instead. As the US attorney for New Jersey, Christie had successfully prosecuted the father of Trump's son-in-law, Jared Kushner, more than a dozen years earlier, sending him to jail for fourteen months. Now, as Christie saw it, Kushner got his revenge. And the antiabortion movement got one of its most stalwart champions as the new man in charge.

Pence saw his role as to surround the president with staff who opposed abortion. His team staffed the new administration in its image, reaching into the antiabortion ranks to fill roles deep in federal agencies with movement loyalists. Groups like the Susan B. Anthony List and the Heritage Foundation sent lists of staff recommendations for all sorts of positions, as is common for interest groups to offer incoming administrations, but in many cases, they didn't need to. The decision-makers had been in the movement for years. Everybody already knew everybody. And abortion opponents were among the earliest to take the professional risk of joining Trump's team.

In an administration that would be known for larger-than-life characters—people like incoming White House chief strategist Stephen Bannon, former New York City mayor Rudy Giuliani, Jared Kushner, and Ivanka Trump—the antiabortion cause would be moved forward largely by bureaucrats most Americans had never heard of who were ready for the moment. For these new staffers, it felt like everywhere they turned were former colleagues, friends, and mentors from the movement. They spread across nearly every part of the new administration from the White House to the Department of Justice to the State Department. They were delegates to the United Nations Commission on the Status of Women and populated the "spiritual advisory board" to the president.

It was not just staffing. In a campaign notably short on policy, allies of the antiabortion movement pushed forward plans before Trump even won his surprise victory. Aides like Andrew Bremberg, a Catholic lawyer who was policy director for the 2016 Republican Party platform before he joined the Trump team, sketched out language for executive orders against abortion before Trump won, giving them a significant head start compared to other interest groups. No one seemed to pay much attention—until the morning Trump won the White House, when they finally got their calls returned. To quote the old Latin proverb, they realized, fortune favors the bold.

Trump's abortion restrictions immediately went further than his Republican predecessors. Bremberg was hired to lead the Domestic Policy Council, making him responsible for coordinating and implementing all domestic policy inside the White House and across the administration. The Mexico City policy, which banned foreign aid to nonprofits that mentioned abortion as an option to pregnant women, was rescinded and reinstated by administrations for decades as control of the White House flipped. But Trump's version expanded the list of groups that would be ineligible—affecting fifteen times more funding than George W. Bush's policy did. The new administration repealed Obama-era protections for Planned Parenthood and began plans to defund the organization by changing Title X, the federal program that funds health care for poorer women. They readied "conscience protections" to make it easier for doctors and nurses to refuse to perform health services, like abortion, that conflicted with their beliefs. They canceled the grants to the Teen Pregnancy Prevention Program that the Obama administration had issued, forcing some school districts with high teen pregnancy rates to shutter their sex education programs.

To ensure those policies survived the inevitable legal challenges, the courts were another target. Under the leadership of Don McGahn and with help from Leonard Leo's Federalist Society network, allies would methodically stack the 120 openings on the federal bench, sending waves of conservative scholars and judges to the Republican-controlled Senate for confirmation. They were cranking out a wholesale reform of the federal judiciary to instill conservative ideology.

Few voters knew how to follow the complicated language of abortion policy—phrases such as "Mexico City policy," "Title X," and "conscience protections." Those policy terms had long served as a code that obscured the reality of abortion restrictions for non-experts. Few voters were paying attention to those details in this new administration anyway, because there was just so much else to focus on amid the chaos of those earliest days. And antiabortion leaders had long benefited from that kind of widespread confusion and an overwhelming crush of action through the hundreds of abortion restrictions enacted in state legislatures. The deluge, whether intentional or not, amounted to a strategy of distraction that worked to their advantage.

The drama Trump created became a sort of cover, allowing them to remake the government into an antiabortion machine, embedding their people at all levels of power and influence. Later in his term, Trump would frequently deride the "deep state," a moniker for the forces in government and law enforcement arrayed against him. But it was Pence, and the movement that had championed his political rise, that created their own deep state, a government apparatus with a shared goal: ending abortion in America.

At the highest levels, the cabinet was stacked with people—mostly men—who had made opposition to abortion central to their political careers. Conway became a senior White House aide. Marc Short, the former Pence aide who helped Marjorie Dannenfelser procure that crucial donation from the Koch brothers, became the director of legislative affairs. McGahn was picked as White House counsel.

Certain departments became power centers, like the Department of Health and Human Services, the nation's health department. It soon resembled a mini-Indiana, with leaders arriving from Pence's former orbit. Trump's first health secretary was Tom Price, a Republican congressman from Georgia who cosponsored bills in Congress that would have granted rights to zygotes and banned abortion at twenty weeks, and pushed to defund Planned Parenthood. A former lobbyist for National Right to Life, who criticized contraception methods and opposed mifepristone and the morning-after pill, came in to lead family-planning programs and oversee Title X. Matthew Bowman, a lawyer for the Alliance Defending Freedom who had a history of arrests at abortion protests, joined Health and Human Services as deputy general counsel. The department became like a "pro-life family," Dannenfelser told EWTN, a Catholic news network.

Roger Severino, a former lawyer with the Becket Fund for Religious Liberty, was named director of the department's Office for Civil Rights. His wife, Carrie, was a former Clarence Thomas clerk and the long-serving head of the Judicial Crisis Network, which was the front line of Leo's network to push conservative judicial nominees. The man who led the Republican congressional investigation into Planned Parenthood became Severino's chief of staff. They created a new entity—the new Conscience and Religious Freedom Division in 2018—that could protect doctors who refused to perform abortions or provide gender-affirming care on religious grounds. Severino saw their work as "institutionalizing" a change in government culture, where religious belief received equal protection along with race, age, sex, and national origin. "I knew how important civil rights were, and I noticed that the most important one, recognizing the right of unborn human beings to have protection, was not recognized," he said.

Their antiabortion options for cabinet posts were sometimes stacked three deep. Trump's first nominee for secretary of labor, Andy Puzder, whose company ran Hardee's and Carl's Jr., had helped write the Missouri law that the Supreme Court upheld in its 1989 Webster decision, which allowed states to impose abortion restrictions after Roe. When Puzder's nomination collapsed after old domestic abuse allegations resurfaced, Alex Acosta, a former Samuel Alito clerk on the Third Circuit, was confirmed. And when Acosta later stepped down following questions of how he had previously handled a sex crimes case involving Jeffrey Epstein, Eugene Scalia—the late justice's son—took the job.

The cohort's opposition to abortion was often part of a broader package of beliefs about marriage and sexuality. A primary goal was to eventually end abortion. But their larger mission was to shape the unit that governs most people's day-to-day lives: the family. For many, it was a way of carrying out Trump's promise to "make America great again."

They were evangelical and Catholic, a merging of two conservative religious movements that were growing stronger. There were so many observant Catholics in the new White House that Father Charles Trullols, an Opus Dei priest who led the Catholic Information Center two blocks away, quickly became an administration insider who regularly hosted a private Mass in the Eisenhower Executive Office Building. Other powerful Catholic legal players who once served on the Catholic Information Center board alongside Leonard Leo took top roles in the administration—William Barr eventually became attorney general, and Pat Cipollone would replace McGahn as White House counsel in December 2018.

For those on the inside of the antiabortion movement, everything felt different from the Obama years—and even the George W. Bush years—as their cohort reached new political maturity. Days after the inauguration, Pence invited their movement leaders into his ceremonial office for cheese and crackers. To Dannenfelser, it felt like a homecoming and a beginning: she was in the

White House seven times in Trump's first three months. At a dinner in the Blue Room with Trump and conservative leaders largely discussing tax reform, Dannenfelser sat between Leo and Short, one of three women in the room, the other two being Conway and Penny Nance. Evangelical pastors like Robert Jeffress of First Baptist Church in Dallas and Jentezen Franklin of Free Chapel outside Atlanta frequented the White House for photo ops and prayer meetings.

Younger staff of antiabortion organizations, who had never worked in Washington with a Republican in the White House, had their first taste of real influence. David Daleiden had meetings with Bremberg's team about policies to end "fetal experimentation" as a follow-up from his videos, he said. Emily Buchanan, SBA's vice president, could not get over what it felt like to walk into the White House for a meeting, amazed that the place had a bowling alley, that they would get White House candies and tickets to garden tours.

There were more significant—and more unusual—perks too. SBA held a briefing for donors in the Indian Treaty Room, the ornate hall in the East Wing of the Eisenhower Executive Office Building, in which Pence touted all the administration was doing for their cause. Donors remembered being especially moved in one such meeting when Sarah Huckabee Sanders, the first mother ever to be White House press secretary, grew emotional talking about her personal opposition to abortion.

They did not always get the allies they wanted in key spots in agencies like the National Institutes of Health or the Food and Drug Administration, which oversaw things like abortion medication. Trump, with the support of Ivanka, asked Francis Collins, Obama's director at the NIH who supported fetal stem cell research, to stay on, frustrating Dannenfelser and others. But out in the states, conservative lawmakers saw that this new regime meant Roe could go. Weeks after Trump's inauguration, a Texas state senator introduced a "trigger ban," a law that would automatically institute a state abortion ban if Roe were overturned.

Onstage at the SBA banquet nearly four months into the administration, where Leo was the honoree, Pence ran through the list of high-level officials who shared their ambitions. "Folks, this is the A-Team," he told the ballroom. "For the first time in a long time, America has an administration that's filled top to bottom with people who stand without apology for life."

Many of those at the bottom were part of the movement's newer flank, the rising, more radical post-Roe generation of activists. With Trump's victory, they were empowered like never before, placed in positions of great authority and control. True believers in the administration could implement the antiabortion mission, with enormous reach and effect.

One striking example was Scott Lloyd, a Catholic lawyer tapped early to lead an obscure office buried within the Administration for Children and Families at HHS. The Office of Refugee Resettlement appeared to have little influence over abortion policy. Its most high-profile purpose was to resettle child refugees seeking safe haven in the United States. Even Lloyd was surprised when he got the call tapping him for the position. He had worked his contacts, including Bremberg, for a job in the administration—but not this one. "It sounded very unexpected, but in the way that God does unexpected things," he said. He started the position within days.

Lloyd had no experience managing tens of thousands of migrant children being held in government custody. His most relevant work was as a lawyer for the Knights of Columbus, an antiabortion Catholic fraternal organization, where he focused on protecting Christians and Yazidis in the Middle East. What Lloyd knew better was abortion, and he brought that vision with intensity. Lloyd described his upbringing as that of a cultural Catholic and a political liberal. At nineteen, he impregnated his college girlfriend and she got an abortion. Even all these years later, he found the experience almost impossible to talk about. He found absolution in the forgiveness of the Catholic Church, he said. He later married, had eight children, and came to share orthodox Catholic views on abortion and birth control. He argued against contraception, writing that the pills and devices were "causing early abortions."

He crusaded against abortion, which he, like many other abortion opponents, described as a tragedy equivalent to the Holocaust—a fraught analogy that equated aborted fetuses with, or even elevated them above, adults and children who were murdered by the Nazi state. "The Jews who died in the Holocaust had a chance to laugh, play, sing, dance, learn, and love each other," he wrote in a paper for a course on Catholic social teaching during law school at Catholic University. "The victims of abortion do not, simply because people have decided this is the way it should be, not through any proper discernment of their humanity. Neither type of murder is more or less tragic, but don't fool yourself into thinking that they are not both tragedies, and they are not both murder."

During the Bush administration, Lloyd helped craft the "conscience protection" regulations that allowed medical personnel to refuse to provide abortions and contraception if it violated their beliefs. After Obama took office, Lloyd opened a "legal apostolate," a law firm and ministry in Front Royal, Virginia. He opened the firm officially on March 25, coinciding with the Feast of the Annunciation, a Catholic holy day sometimes called the Day of the Unborn Child. Exactly nine months before Christmas, it remembers the day that the angel Gabriel informed the Virgin Mary that she would become pregnant—reminding Christians that even Jesus was once an unborn child.

His views also represented the radical edge of the antiabortion movement that Trump had elevated to power. Lloyd saw his legal work as part of a much bigger religious project to enact God's kingdom on earth, a way to use the law to reshape the country around the tenets of Christianity. "Let's be blunt. The law is pagan territory. It is, in fact, one of the least Christian elements of our society," Scott said in a speech celebrating his apostolate's one-year anniversary. "Christ has already won for us victory over the culture we find in the law, the Culture of Death. It is ours to claim, but it will be a question not of our talents, our resources, our diligence, or our knowledge of the law, but of our faith."

Soon after starting the job, Lloyd reviewed what he saw as a critical piece of information: the number of pregnant migrant girls currently being held by the government. "The unborn child," he emailed his staff, "is a child [in] our care."

His office would keep spreadsheets tracking how far along the girls were in their pregnancies. A new policy was put in place: all requests for abortions would go directly to his desk—and he would work to block them. "It was a pro-life administration," Lloyd said, explaining his actions. "As a political appointee you feel an obligation to achieve what you think people are expecting out of an administration when they voted the way they did."

THAT PASSION FOR the antiabortion cause was not matched by the man at the top. Trump remained a lukewarm ally, with "pro-life" positions that seemed incidental at best. He mentioned abortion just once in speeches during his first year in office, a passing reference at a Republican retreat in Philadelphia.

In a meeting during those hectic first few months with Conway and Pence, Trump questioned whether to defund Planned Parenthood. His skepticism undercut a yearslong campaign waged by Pence, House Republicans, and the antiabortion movement—and echoed his comments that upset Dannenfelser during the Daleiden video sting in the earliest days of Trump's campaign. "I recognized immediately where that was coming from," Conway later wrote about the incident. "He had to be hearing from some of the registered Democrats on the senior White House staff. My guess was that some of them who had voted for Hillary over him months before doubted the sincerity of his pro-life conversion."

Pence and Conway closed ranks and made the case they knew could convince Trump: it would help him politically. They showed him state-by-state charts of Planned Parenthood centers, noting that most were in urban areas—where Mr. Trump's supporters were not. He pivoted back. "If anything, I think it could be a positive," he said, according to Conway's account.

That was how they worked in the new administration. The antiabortion faction would push its agenda and praise the president, appealing to his ego while also reminding him that this is what he owed his most loyal supporters. When they planned to make changes to Title X, a policy that would strip $60 million from Planned Parenthood annually, advisers reminded him that the policy of his administration was to defund Planned Parenthood and other abortion providers, and that his voters would love him for it.

They planned for Trump to announce the regulations himself at the upcoming SBA List Campaign for Life Gala. He was the first president to speak at the event and could push his upcoming agenda for the midterm election.

Backstage at the National Building Museum the day of the gala, Trump posed for a photo with one of SBA's special guests—Kathy Ireland, a *Sports Illustrated* swimsuit supermodel from the 1980s and 1990s, when Trump was at the height of his celebrity in New York City. She had converted to the antiabortion cause and was the night's emcee. Onstage, Pope Francis's ambassador to the United States, Archbishop Christophe Pierre, gave the invocation. The host committee of donors included the Leos, Eugene Scalia's wife, Trish, and more.

Trump paced back and forth backstage, watching on the monitor as Dannenfelser introduced him. A White House official later offered an explanation for why he seemed nervous: it was the first time Trump had ever spoken to such a high-profile, exclusively antiabortion gathering. It was a far cry from the dinner he cosponsored at the Plaza Hotel in 1989 to honor former NARAL president Robin Chandler Duke, the event he ended up not attending after antiabortion activists threatened his family—the year Ireland was first on the cover of *Sports Illustrated*'s swimsuit edition.

The reality was that what Trump truly believed about abortion didn't matter. Abortion opponents were integral to the entire ecosystem of his administration, their priorities woven into its very fabric, whether or not their cause was a priority for Trump. The machine was in motion.

Dannenfelser played a video before inviting Trump to the stage, functionally an ad for SBA's voter outreach project, with senators like Thom Tillis of North Carolina praising the group's turnout operation for helping boost him to victory in the 2014 midterms. They were on the verge of an even bigger revolution, the Dannenfelser voice-over said: "The most important thing that can happen in this election is that voters elect senators who will confirm a Supreme Court justice who will be the final vote to overturn *Roe v. Wade*."

Trump took the stage to cheers and put his arm around her. "All my friends are out here," he said.

When Conway rose to accept an award that night, she gave Trump all the credit for their accomplishments. And then she made clear that the ultimate work was not to simply win elections but to remake the country. "This is not a political calculus," she said. "This is a change in the culture. This is not about institutions. This is about the Constitution."

It was a remarkable flip from when Obama came to Planned Parenthood's national conference after his 2012 win, signaling to feminist progressives that their movement had national clout despite the rise of antiabortion state laws. "Cecile Richards was in the White House all the time during the Obama administration," Dannenfelser had said shortly after Trump took office. "It's our turn."

17

The Left's Denial

Cecile Richards certainly wasn't in the White House anymore. Instead, she was pulling into Bedminster, Donald Trump's club in New Jersey, on a cold Sunday morning, trying to find a way in to stem the damage.

The country had become almost unrecognizable to her in the days and weeks since Trump's victory. The feminist-led future that Richards and so many of her allies had thought was coming had vanished with the election results. No one had planned for this. There was no political response plan. No psychological preparation for Clinton's supporters. They were all plunged into a new reality. Now, Richards's top priority was to protect Planned Parenthood in this new world. Defunding Planned Parenthood, she believed, would be the "number one goal" of the new administration.

She knew her organization had support: donations and volunteers flooded their offices as women poured into the streets to protest Trump. Another hope, a friend in the fashion world had suggested, might be the rare people the president seemed to listen to—his daughter and son-in-law. The idea that the president's daughter and her husband would be negotiating over matters of national policy felt ridiculous to Richards, another politician's daughter. But, Richards realized, the threat to reproductive health care was enormous with the new administration. "I never want to turn down any opportunity to make our case," she said. She begged her husband, Kirk Adams, to join her as a witness to whatever might follow.

At the clubhouse, Ivanka Trump and Jared Kushner ordered breakfast. Richards couldn't stomach a meal; she could barely handle the meeting. Ivanka, a self-proclaimed feminist running a clothing brand built on hashtags like #womenwhowork, started by wanting to talk about her feelings. Her father, she said, was the only Republican during the campaign to say anything nice about Planned Parenthood, a message she personally pushed him to deliver from a primary debate stage. Why had Richards not complimented him in return?

Nursing a coffee on that bleak winter day, Richards couldn't believe she had to explain why Planned Parenthood wasn't excited to support a new president who had pledged to overturn Roe and wanted to defund her organization out of existence. "I did acknowledge those statements," Richards replied. "But he also said he was going to defund Planned Parenthood, so that's not going to be much help."

"Well, you have to understand, my father is pro-life," Ivanka responded.

Leaning across the table, Kushner explained to Richards what he saw as her big mistake—becoming "political." He proposed a simple solution: split Planned Parenthood in two, with a smaller arm for abortions and a larger one for women's health services. The ideal outcome would be a headline that read PLANNED PARENTHOOD DISCONTINUES ABORTION SERVICES. If that could happen, Kushner promised more federal funding for its health services.

Done, Kushner and Ivanka seemed to believe, Richards later recounted. Decades of abortion drama solved. The couple apparently thought they had unlocked an easy compromise on an issue that had ensnared American politicians for more than four decades. Richards saw something else: a political bribe that traded abortion for federal funds. It wasn't even a particularly politically astute one.

There was no way that House Republicans, who had spent years casting Planned Parenthood as a moral stain on the nation, would agree to Kushner's plan.

Top policy staff inside the White House who opposed abortion were dumbfounded when they heard from Ivanka about the plan. It seemed to them like she was on another planet, one where she didn't see how deeply the antiabortion movement had embedded their forces in the new government. The man who had led the charge against Planned Parenthood for nearly a decade wasn't just in the administration; he was now vice president.

In Bedminster, Richards plastered a smile on her face. Planned Parenthood could hardly undermine its central message—that services like abortion were fundamental to women's health—for an administration that represented everything they opposed.

"We really stand for the right of women to get the reproductive health care they need," Richards explained. "And we're not gonna trade that off for money." As they stood up to leave, Kushner offered another warning. The new administration planned to repeal Obama's health care law within weeks. If Richards wanted the deal, she'd better move fast.

As their car pulled out of the empty golf course, Richards told her husband that the whole experience—the golf club meeting, their proposal, even the headlines about Trump attacking judges blaring from the televisions above the bar—felt surreal. Obviously, no such "deal" was going to happen. But it sure seemed to Richards like the president's daughter, a New York socialite whose most recent job was running a fashion brand sold at Macy's, would be overseeing women's health for the nation. Ivanka and Jared were, thought Richards, "out of touch but obviously incredibly emboldened and feeling empowered." It was hard to wrap her mind around. Richards and her husband were quiet the rest of the way back into New York City.

Her dream of a Clinton administration that would not only defend but expand abortion rights had died. Yet it was hard for broad swaths of liberal America to see how quickly the politics of abortion had changed amid the chaos that overtook the country in those early months of the new administration. During the campaign, Trump had said—multiple times—that he planned to pick judges who would overturn Roe. He repeated that pledge after he was elected. But the nation didn't believe what it heard.

Many voters assumed that Trump's opposition to abortion rights was just part of the political game to win the White House. The new president was a celebrity, and America believed they knew his history. A Manhattan businessman who didn't know how to pronounce the books of the New Testament seemed unlikely to be the guy who eradicated abortion rights.

Even some voters who backed Trump didn't believe his administration posed a threat to abortion. "Participants tend to think Trump's position is malleable and he is not likely to prioritize abortion," wrote the National Institute for Reproductive Health in a report summarizing its findings from focus groups conducted in Ohio and North Carolina. Participants believe that he is "all rhetoric," the report said, and his inflammatory language was just to "shock people."

Another set of focus groups commissioned by Planned Parenthood found similar results. Voters who backed Trump said they would be frustrated and angry if he defunded the organization. "It's a deal-breaker," said a fifty-eight-year-old woman in Phoenix. "It will rob women of basic fundamental rights. I'm talking about female health care, which includes abortion. Which includes birth control. I think birth control is the greatest gift that they gave for womankind." If Trump attacked Planned Parenthood, added another woman, "I'd be pissed off as hell."

There was also little preparation for what was to come at the court. Nancy Northup, the head of the Center for Reproductive Rights, had felt so certain walking into Hillary Clinton's Election Night party with her husband at the Jacob K. Javits Convention Center in New York, ready to make history under that literal glass ceiling. Everyone was there. Little girls in sparkly shoes. Hipster moms in velvet pantsuits over THE FUTURE IS FEMALE T-shirts. Katy Perry, the pop star pumping out feminist anthems like "Roar." Chuck Schumer, who would soon be the Democratic Senate leader. Stephanie Schriock, the head of EMILYs List. Ilyse Hogue, the head of NARAL. And Richards.

Northup left around 9:30 p.m. when the results started to look a little weird and the night started to seem like a long one. When she walked in the door at home, her son told her it wasn't looking good. By 2:00 a.m., she was calling her sister, sobbing. Clinton's presidential campaign symbolized the dream of everything Northup had worked for her entire adult life, all the way back to college when she fought for the ratification of the Equal Rights Amendment.

On the subway into the office later that morning, Hillary Schneller, a senior lawyer at the Center for Reproductive Rights, frantically sent Leonard Leo's list of potential justices to Julie Rikelman, the head of litigation, with a note saying they'd better start digging into their records. The all-staff meeting that day was like a shiva—the grief, the quiet sobbing, and the sad platter of bagels—pausing to watch Clinton make her concession speech on all three televisions. All Northup could offer her team was a pep talk that sounded like a dirge. "We are built for this," she told her staff. Look at our wins in Bogotá, Colombia, and Nepal, she told them, citing places where the center had made strides to unwind total abortion bans. Protecting abortion rights at home during a Trump presidency would be hard, but not impossible, she said. As she spoke, one of her lawyers walked into the office with tears streaming down her face.

Now, a few months later, the center was waging that fight. But for many of its Democratic allies, the stakes—even at the court—weren't fully clear. Neil Gorsuch's confirmation had been an even swap: Antonin Scalia for another conservative. This was still the court that had struck down the Texas law. Even in some surprising places, the belief that the Supreme Court would save abortion continued. In Texas, NARAL dismissed the Republican trigger ban bill with a striking sense of confidence. "This constitutional amendment is a pretty unserious idea," said Blake Rocap, NARAL Texas's legislative counsel. "It would basically have no effect because, guess what? The Supreme Court already said you can't make abortion illegal."

For Planned Parenthood, the court was a second-order problem. The risk it faced in this new administration was immediate. Republicans had been trying to defund the organization for years, and the David Daleiden videos were still fresh. If they succeeded, it would result in hundreds of thousands of low-income women losing access to care and the likely closure of clinics across the country. In April, the administration undid an Obama administration rule preventing states from blocking funding for family-planning clinics that also provided abortions—essentially taking money away from Planned Parenthood. In Iowa alone, that move later resulted in the closure of four clinics, after the state's Republican governor approved a budget that removed Planned Parenthood's Medicaid funding.

Now, it seemed like Republicans would have the votes in Congress to go further than ever before. As Richards expected, the new administration quickly released another iteration of the efforts to repeal Obama's health care law and defund Planned Parenthood. This version would cut federal funding for one year, eliminating $550 million in Medicaid dollars, a temporary step that could open the door to more sustained cuts in the future. This was an "existential crisis," she said. With Trump in office, there was no longer a presidential veto to protect them, Richards knew. Saving their federal funding—not the more distant threat to Roe—had to be their top priority in this new era. Their best hope rested on whether they could channel all the frustration and energy of the Women's March into this new fight, she believed.

Richards used the new surge of donations to fund an advertising campaign and organize supporters to push back, dispatching them to flood Capitol Hill and question their representatives at raucous town hall meetings. When Pence posted a photo of negotiations over the bill in the White House, showing the vice president sitting at a long conference table surrounded by twenty-five white men, Planned Parenthood deployed its "pink army" to launch online attacks. Even Anna Wintour, *Vogue*'s editor in chief, wore a hot-pink Planned Parenthood button—magnetic, to avoid puncturing her clothes—as she watched the shows at New York Fashion Week.

Still, the legislation passed the House and seemed headed for success in the Senate. After rallying her troops in a protest on Capitol Hill, Richards returned to her hotel room to anxiously watch the live stream of the Senate vote. Then the unthinkable happened. John McCain bucked his party's leadership, voting against the legislation with a dramatic thumbs-down. Republicans didn't have the votes. The bill was officially dead. To Richards, it was another sign that their protesting and organizing succeeded. "I know Ann is laughing her ass off," Richards's husband texted her. "This day belongs to you and your folks. Here's to having many more like it."

In some ways, the failure of the defund legislation had less to do with Planned Parenthood and more with the popularity of the health care bill. Americans had grown accustomed to the benefits of the law, provisions like free contraception, allowing young adults to remain on their parents' health care plans, and mandatory coverage for preexisting conditions. By linking Planned Parenthood to that law, Republicans had unwittingly managed to protect the organization.

That fall, there was a second victory when Senate Republicans dropped plans to repeal the health care bill entirely, effectively admitting defeat by switching their focus to Trump's tax plans. And then, a third when Trump pressured Tom Price, the head of Health and Human Services and a longtime opponent of Planned Parenthood, to resign after reports that he spent $400,000 flying on private jets.

Richards had started talking to her board about stepping down before the 2016 election, but she stayed to steer the organization through the threats of the first year of the Trump administration. After nearly a dozen years, she had accomplished her mission of transforming Planned Parenthood into a political powerhouse. It wasn't just the lobbying efforts and flood of donations for Democratic campaigns. The protests that she helped organize in Texas with Davis created a new generation of abortion-rights activists, some of whom eventually came to work at Planned Parenthood. And now, after Clinton's defeat, there were millions of women who were "pissed off and ready for action," she said, and that power wouldn't get undone, no matter what the Trump administration did. "I knew that our work was far from over, but the tally was Women—3, Trumpcare—0," Richards later recounted. "The lasting legacy of this moment will be the generations of women it has inspired and energized." On her last day, supporters gave her a social media salute, firing off a flood of tweets with the hashtag #ThankYouCecile. Hopefully, Richards thought, their collective power could save abortion rights—and the Democratic Party—from Trump.

18

Purging "Pro-Life" from the Party

But the problems for the abortion-rights movement in this new era went far beyond Planned Parenthood. The world had turned upside down, and Democrats were nowhere near ready for the dangerous stakes of this new fight.

Ilyse Hogue, the head of NARAL, had no illusions about the new administration's broader goals. After all, Trump had made them very clear. He would select judges who would overturn Roe. She also had no illusions about the state of the court. While she wished Justices Ruth Bader Ginsburg, eighty-four, Anthony Kennedy, eighty, and Stephen Breyer, seventy-eight, long lives, she understood the reality. They were old, meaning Trump would likely get a second nominee. When he did, the balance of the court would flip to conservative control. And if the court changed, Hogue believed, Roe wouldn't survive.

Ten days after Trump won, Hogue gathered her leadership team in an upstairs room at Cork, a trendy Washington wine bar, to strategize. There was no way they would be able to stop Trump's first pick to the court. Democrats, particularly moderates, would see it as an even trade—one conservative for another to fill Scalia's old seat.

But effective opposition campaigns didn't manifest overnight, Hogue knew. They needed to build the structure now for the second battle, when Roe would truly be on the line.

"It's going to be pretty thankless," she told them. They all, she said, should be "eyes wide open about this."

Already their small resistance was vastly outmatched by the power of the incoming administration, though even Hogue did not know the full extent. As she spoke to her team in November 2016, just blocks away, Misha Tseytlin and his Alliance Defending Freedom connection mingled with the throngs of conservative lawyers celebrating in the gilded Mayflower Hotel—and brainstormed exactly how strict an abortion ban would force the Supreme Court to take up Roe. Two hundred miles north, in Trump Tower, Mike Pence and his team were vetting résumés and putting their movement into position.

Hogue didn't know about those secret operations. But it was clear to her that the administration planned to push a full-scale assault on abortion rights. To her, just like to the antiabortion movement, Trump's personal views were almost immaterial. Given his history of denigrating women and multiple accusations of sexual misconduct, Hogue assumed he would hardly stand in the antiabortion movement's way, regardless of whether he was a true believer in their cause. "We know that misogyny would rule in a Trump White House and that never bodes well for reproductive health care or advancing women's equality," she predicted, back in the spring of 2016, when even Marjorie Dannenfelser and others doubted his commitment to eradicating abortion rights. During the campaign, her staff had tracked the ties between Trump's world and the antiabortion movement, documenting the links between his campaign and groups like SBA and ADF. Now, with Trump in office, Hogue was frustrated that so many Democrats failed to see what was coming.

Her party couldn't even agree on a message about abortion. Some Democrats were in denial that Roe was at stake. Others, in an echo of the Republican autopsy in 2012, wanted to create a "big tent" that would embrace Democrats who opposed abortion rights if it would add to their numbers in Congress. Hogue saw an existential moment for abortion rights, one that left no room for any kind of political compromise. These differing strategies made Democrats weak and ill equipped to confront the incoming attacks.

That wasn't how it worked for Republicans, Hogue knew. Dannenfelser and her movement forced them to be a unified bloc on abortion, threatening primary challenges and to rally the base against any Republican who supported abortion rights. By 2016, anecdotal evidence suggested that not a single Republican state legislator identified as "pro-choice." That unity gave them power. Democrats needed to become the same kind of unbreakable force, she told her staff. Their voters were already there: a whopping 85 percent of Democratic women now thought abortion should be legal in all or most cases, up eighteen points from March 2016, before Trump claimed his party's nomination. Yet support for abortion rights, even after the shock of Trump's victory, was not enshrined as an inviolable litmus test among the highest ranks of the party.

If Roe could be saved—and to keep fighting, Hogue had to believe it could be—Democrats needed to rally behind defending it. Hogue thought they needed a version of the strategy Dannenfelser pursued after the Republican autopsy: make the abortion-rights movement a force Democrats wouldn't dare cross. "In order to have a hope of winning at the court, winning elections, we needed the Democrats to be able to effectively, and with integrity, model that they weren't going to yield on this issue," Hogue said.

It wasn't a cause that was getting much attention at the time. New liberal organizations, groups like Indivisible and spin-offs of the Women's March, sprang up after Trump won, quickly building chapters across the country. But their resistance movement was decentralized and diffuse, lacking a singular leader and splintered into multiple fronts. None of those groups were focused exclusively on combating Trump's push to pack the court or the risk that could pose to Roe. Other threats—from saving Obama's health care law to stopping Trump's immigration ban—felt far more immediate than what a bunch of judges, or even Supreme Court justices, Trump was likely to appoint could do years from now in the courts.

Plus, even after the Republican Senate refused to give Merrick Garland a hearing while Obama was still president, some Democratic senators believed the gravity of the town, norms like regular process in the Senate, would hold. When it came time to fight Neil Gorsuch, three Democratic senators from Republican states voted to confirm him, arguing that the Senate should defer to the new president. "Would he be the judge I'd pick? No, never," said Senator Heidi Heitkamp of North Dakota, one of the three. "But he is the judge that the duly elected president picked." And then there was the issue of the small fraternity of a half dozen Democrats, all men, in Congress who opposed abortion rights and more who were uncomfortable talking about the issue.

Democrats needed to be on war footing all across Washington, Hogue believed. And they weren't. They didn't see how fragile abortion rights were or that the battle over abortion was part of a bigger fight by conservative Christians to change the country. It was a sense of denial that Hogue understood. After all, she had once been that way herself.

When NARAL offered Hogue the job of president in 2013, she largely viewed abortion as the musty old battle of their mothers—an all-but-settled issue. She knew about the laws being passed in conservative states. She was from Texas and had watched the waves of restrictions pass through her home state. But those laws didn't seem like the most pressing political issue. "You're not going to take it, are you?" asked one of her mentors when she asked for his thoughts on the new opportunity. "You don't have to work on women's issues—you've proven you can work on issues that affect everyone. Why would you move backward, where women only go if they can't make it in the men's world?"

Hogue had different doubts about the job. Her own abortion during graduate school had sparked some soul-searching but little internal conflict. She had had the support of her parents, her boyfriend, and even her Catholic best friend. It was a notable moment but not one that defined her life's work, which was focused on pushing the Democratic Party establishment from the left. During her years in Washington, she had moved through the ranks of environmental and progressive organizations before becoming political director for MoveOn.org, the powerful liberal activist group. "Do I really want to be the 'Abortion Lady'?" she asked herself as she considered the offer from NARAL. "I've done so much in my career, and if I am the Abortion Lady—will I always be the Abortion Lady?"

What she saw in NARAL was a political opportunity, a chance to run her own organization in a town where women still struggled to gain control of campaign spending. Hogue believed she could use abortion rights and NARAL's $10 million budget to back candidates who would push the party to the left—on abortion, but other issues too.

Yet soon after taking the job, her understanding of the abortion battle began to change. Hogue watched as abortion-rights supporters cast the Hobby Lobby case as an issue of health care, while conservatives argued it was one of broader religious freedom. Average people didn't see birth control as health care, akin to a root canal or heart surgery, she realized. And besides, in America, a country built on a myth of rugged individualism, appeals to freedom would beat health care every time. Abortion rights were losing the narrative, she she came to believe.

Hogue drew another conclusion from Hobby Lobby, as well. The antiabortion forces weren't just fighting against abortion—they wanted to restrict contraception too. Abortion rights, she thought, weren't just about terminating pregnancies but unwinding the entire sexual revolution to a time when women had fewer rights and far less control over their bodies. They were the "foundational issue upon which everything else is built."

Through it all, Hogue was trying to get pregnant herself. Her infertility and miscarriages filled her with a profound sense of failure. Hogue began to realize that her sense of shame came "from the same place as the stigma about abortion, which is the singular vision of what women are put on Earth to do—to get pregnant."

Finally, at forty-five, she got pregnant with twins. At a hearing on Capitol Hill, an antiabortion advocate dared to ask of her belly, "Is that real?" Hogue took it in stride: "As though I actually had strapped on a prosthetic baby bump to wear to a hearing for some reason," she said. "It's like, 'What don't you get about choice meaning choice?'" Pregnancy and motherhood were the backdrop to women's lives, Hogue came to see, the source of so much pressure and political policing.

Her babies had just turned one when she told her abortion story from the stage at the Democratic National Convention in 2016. In private meetings, she offered another, more ominous warning of what might come should Trump win. The election was a broader clash of "fundamentally different ways" of looking at the role of women in American life, she told the Texas delegation at a breakfast gathering. "You have men like Donald Trump, Mike Pence, Rick Perry, and Greg Abbott who believe that women have one place—in the home, having as many children as possible," she said. "So that men can keep control and impose their worldview on us."

Now, those men were in charge. And Democrats, Hogue saw, weren't ready.

That became abundantly clear to Hogue in April 2017, when a pair of Democratic leaders made a point of going all the way to Omaha to endorse a mayoral candidate with an antiabortion record as part of a nine-state "unity tour." Heath Mello was a Catholic Democrat from the city's working-class south side, who had backed a series of abortion restrictions, including cosponsoring a twenty-week ban on the procedure.

The leaders were not focused on abortion. Senator Bernie Sanders saw Mello as the kind of working-class Democrat who could win in a conservative state like Nebraska. Tom Perez, the head of the Democratic National Committee, saw a "big tent" party that could build back from the losses of the Obama years by welcoming a diversity of views. "If you demand fealty on every single issue," Perez said, "then it's a challenge. The Democratic Party platform acknowledges that we're pro-choice, but there are communities, like some in Kansas, where people have a different position." (Perez was referencing a defeat for Democrats in a recent Kansas special election that had been closer than party strategists had expected.)

Hogue saw a betrayal. There were certainly communities in Kansas where voters had a different view of the health care law, immigration, and even Trump, but Democrats didn't accept those stances. Why should the party treat abortion differently? From her father's study in Dallas, where she was visiting her parents for Passover, Hogue fired off a statement blasting both Perez and Sanders as "not only disappointing" but "politically stupid."

"It tells your most active political base that we're just negotiable political property," she said.

Hogue wondered why party leaders were so willing to jettison abortion rights and cross the movement's leaders. Maybe it was the old political calculation that abortion rights energized the forces of opposition more than the Democrats who supported the issue. Maybe it was that the abortion rights groups were always with the party, so there was no cost for bucking them. Or maybe it was just misogyny, the idea that abortion was a "women's issue"—not a mainstream topic like taxes or foreign policy. Whatever it was, it had been the political reality for Democrats for decades. But in this new political moment, Hogue wasn't going to accept that anymore.

Her pushback complicated the dynamic for Cecile Richards, who was scheduled to appear with Sanders and Perez in Las Vegas a few days later. Perez quickly engaged in some quiet diplomacy, calling Richards and Hogue. He blamed Sanders for not fully vetting Mello. By the following afternoon, he had released a far more strongly worded statement. "Every Democrat, like every American, should support a woman's right to make her own choices about her body and her health," he wrote. "That is not negotiable and should not change city by city or state by state. At a time when women's rights are under assault from the White House, the Republican Congress, and in states across the country, we must speak up for this principle as loudly as ever and with one voice."

Still, even Nancy Pelosi, the highest-ranking woman in the party and a staunch supporter of abortion rights, publicly fretted about the party expelling those who felt uncomfortable with the procedure. "I grew up Nancy D'Alesandro, in Baltimore, Maryland; in Little Italy; in a very devout Catholic family; fiercely patriotic; proud of our town and heritage, and staunchly Democratic," she told *The Washington Post* a few weeks later, in May 2017. "Most of those people—my family, extended family—are not pro-choice. You think I'm kicking them out of the Democratic Party?"

The chairman of the Democrats' House campaign arm, Representative Ben Ray Luján from New Mexico, agreed and decided he would still give funds to candidates who opposed abortion rights in the coming 2018 midterms. "We have to be a big family in order to win the House back," he said.

Hogue knew she would have to take a more aggressive approach. She launched a direct strike on another Democrat, mobilizing a primary campaign against Dan Lipinski, one of the party's last self-identified "pro-life" Democrats. A seven-term Catholic congressman from Illinois who replaced his father in Congress, Lipinski voted at the start of Trump's term for a bill that would prohibit qualified health care plans from including abortion coverage and, later, a twenty-week abortion ban. Hogue convinced progressive organizations to sign a letter endorsing a liberal Democratic challenger, Marie Newman, boosting her from relative obscurity to a progressive cause. "This isn't some deep-red district. This district is solid blue," Hogue told NARAL donors as the intraparty fight heated up in early 2018. "The seat has been held by a Democrat for fifty-eight out of the last sixty years. Yet Lipinski votes more like a right-wing Republican." She embedded five staffers in Newman's campaign and eventually ran ads attacking Lipinski for voting to defund Planned Parenthood and voting fifty-two times against abortion.

The primary race split the Democrats. Pelosi backed Lipinski, while some of her liberal colleagues from Illinois supported Newman. Lipinski, a longtime favorite of SBA, likened Hogue's attack to the scorched-earth politics of Republicans. "This is part of the reason Donald Trump won," he said. "Democrats have chased people out of the party."

Hogue's efforts enraged leaders at the Democrats' House campaign arm, which had a policy of backing incumbents. When Luján, the chairman, called to make peace, Hogue told him there was an easy solution: stop endorsing anti–abortion rights candidates.

In the final days of the race, Dannenfelser, too, got involved in the Democratic primary to support Lipinski, a rare time SBA worked to help a Democrat win. She sent seventy canvassers to his district to door-knock at seventeen thousand homes of antiabortion Democrats. Lipinski narrowly staved off the challenge, beating Newman by about two thousand votes in March 2018. (Two years later, Newman would defeat Lipinski by two percentage points in a primary rematch.)

Still, Hogue's efforts had always been more about changing the party's message than quelling fierce internal divisions. By the time Newman lost, the partisan sorting of Congress over abortion rights was all but complete. To be a Republican was to oppose abortion rights, and to be a Democrat was to support them. It was a generational shift. When Obama took office in 2009, self-identified antiabortion Democrats held thirty-six seats in the House, comprising 15 percent of their caucus. By the Trump administration, their numbers had dwindled to three members of the House and three in the Senate. All six were men, and all but one were Catholic. The era of the self-proclaimed "pro-life" Democrat was over.

A corresponding shift happened on the Republican side. In 1992, when Republican-appointed Supreme Court justices protected abortion rights in Casey, there were around a dozen Republican supporters of abortion rights in the Senate. By 2017, there were only two—Susan Collins of Maine and Lisa Murkowski of Alaska.

The decisions by Representatives Charlie Dent and Rodney Frelinghuysen in 2017 and 2018, respectively, to retire marked the official extinction of the abortion-rights Republican in the House. Republican Majority for Choice, a three-decade-old advocacy group that sought to expand support for abortion rights in the Republican Party, began shutting down its operations. "We have to face reality," the founders wrote in *The New York Times* in June 2018. "The big tent has collapsed for good."

Now, the new Trump administration—led by Pence's handpicked army of allies—would demonstrate just how far the party had shifted on abortion.

19

Jane Doe

The girl traveled for months, from Central America up through Mexico, and into the United States. Just seventeen, petite with tan skin and long, dark hair, she was poor and wanted to build a life that would make her proud. She hoped to learn English, study and work, and maybe—"*Si Dios lo permite*," she told *Vice News*, "if God allows me"—become a doctor someday.

It was when she arrived at the shelter in Brownsville, a border town on the southernmost tip of Texas, with all the other teenagers and children—"unaccompanied minors," as they were known—that she discovered she was pregnant. She was about eleven weeks along. Back home, she had watched her parents beat her unmarried older sister with firewood and cables until she miscarried. Abortion was banned there. But here, she had another option. She told the authorities that she wanted an abortion, and as soon as possible. "I don't feel capable of being a mature woman or being strong or old enough to be able to take care of it," she said.

It wasn't a particularly unusual request. Throughout the Bush and Obama administrations, immigrants in the custody of the United States could generally procure abortions, so long as the government didn't pay for them. But this girl wouldn't have the same options as the unaccompanied migrant girls who had made the long trek to the border before she had. In the Trump administration, the request made the girl not just one of the tens of thousands of migrant children coming into the country that year, but a priority for the head of the Office of Refugee Resettlement—Scott Lloyd, the Catholic lawyer who was closely tracking the pregnancies of girls crossing the border. She wasn't the only girl in this situation. Over the course of Trump's administration, Lloyd's agency kept a spreadsheet documenting hundreds of similar girls, with columns listing their ages, the type of sex—consensual or assault—the likely gestational age of the fetus, and where they were being held. Many were sixteen or seventeen years old, a few were fourteen. At least one was eleven.

The notes offered a window into what the journey had been like for the girls. "Kidnapped in Mexico x 18 months; raped/forced into sex trade–pregnancy as a result to unknown male," read the notes for one sixteen year old, who was six months pregnant and being held in Texas. "With 49 year old male," read the entry for a fourteen year old girl, who was seven months pregnant in California. "Assaulted in home country and along journey by unknown assailants," read the entry for another fourteen year old girl, who was less than a month pregnant, in Illinois. The row for a seventeen year old in Illinois who was five months pregnant noted "Pregnancy with 40 yo husband" and "HIV positive due to Rape by stepfather." In at least two cases, the notes listed their LMP—or last menstrual period—as a way of trying to date their pregnancy. Lloyd argued that the deeply personal data captured by the federal government was necessary to track the girls' medical care and identify trends among the children coming into the United States.

Whether these girls requested an abortion was also listed in a column on the spreadsheet. Lloyd's policy was that those requests had to be approved by him in writing. And, he said, under his watch the government would not spend taxpayer funds on abortions. "If they were asking us to take them for an abortion, I mean, that would be something that we would have to necessarily expend resources to do," he said, explaining how a shelter staffer would have to travel with the girl. "And we weren't willing to do that." Lloyd was, however, willing to spend resources implementing a new policy that sent pregnant girls to a "life-affirming" pregnancy center, he said.

So the girl went. The staff prayed over her and forced her to look at a sonogram of her fetus, she said. But her decision was made, she said, and it was between her and her God—not them.

The battle between the girl and the Trump administration revealed how the antiabortion movement was turning dusty corners of the federal government into platforms for its crusade. It was a big goal built in small ways, through Excel spreadsheets, emailed orders, and new regulations crafted by armies of bureaucrats. It was expanded by lawyers, writing statutes in statehouses that they could push forward through the lower courts. And it was secured by the judges who were installed to seats on high courts.

That afternoon, the girl met Rochelle Garza, an attorney from the Rio Grande Valley in private practice who was frequently appointed by the court to represent girls seeking abortions. The rule in Texas was that minors needed approval from a judge to end a pregnancy, if they could not get consent from their parents.

But this time, when Garza got to the court with the girl and a lawyer from a nonprofit that offered legal aid to pregnant minors in Texas, something unusual happened. The federal field specialist for the resettlement agency was standing outside demanding to enter the confidential hearing in the judge's chambers. Strict rules were supposed to keep these proceedings secret because they dealt with children. The Trump administration official shouldn't have even known that they were in court that day. Inside the room, with the Trump official barred from entering, the judge cleared the way for the girl to get her abortion on September 29, after the counseling session mandated by Texas law. Private funds would pay for the procedure, and her lawyers would take her to her appointment. The only role of the shelter staff—and the federal government—would be to open the doors and permit the girl to leave for a few hours. Still, Garza had the sinking feeling that it might not be that easy.

She was right. The staff refused to allow the girl to be taken to her appointment. She would not get her abortion that day. Or for weeks that followed. Instead of the clinic, she was headed back to court. Garza knew that they needed help for a case that was quickly moving beyond Texas. To get the girl released from the shelter, they would need to sue Lloyd and the Office of Refugee Resettlement.

They connected with Brigitte Amiri, the deputy director of the ACLU's Reproductive Freedom Project. To her, the problem was bigger than just this girl. She had uncovered emails appearing to show that the agency, under Lloyd's leadership, attempted to stop another abortion already in progress, sending another migrant girl to the hospital to try to save the fetus after she took the first pill in the two-dose medication abortion process. It was an "abortion reversal"—a procedure pushed by antiabortion doctors that had been deemed "dangerous" and "unethical" by the American College of Obstetricians and Gynecologists. In other messages later revealed in a public records request by a liberal group, he mandated that staff tell a pregnant girl's parents about her abortion decisions against her wishes, violating her right to privacy.

To Amiri, it all seemed shockingly "brazen." During the Bush administration, the antiabortion forces were largely outside activists pushing their own agenda with some help from government officials. This, with Lloyd, was something new. The most radical activists were no longer outside pushing the administration. They were the administration. "There were always these entities, Catholic hospitals or charities, trying to say they didn't have to follow the law because of their religious beliefs," she said. "Now, the government had stepped into their shoes."

Still, when the girl's case came to Amiri, she thought it would be easy. The government could not ban abortion, a federal right under Roe that was protected by Casey. On October 16, Amiri filed an emergency petition in a federal court in Washington. Like the woman whose case established the federal right to an abortion, Jane Roe, this girl would also be nameless.

"I do not want to be forced to carry a pregnancy to term against my will," the girl said in her court declaration, before signing her alias in block letters: JANE DOE.

Every day mattered. The longer the girl waited, the more medically and logistically complicated her procedure would become. She had to be seen for counseling at least twenty-four hours before the procedure, in two separate appointments with the same doctor. If she reached seventeen weeks and six days, Amiri had told the court, the girl would have to travel several hundred miles north to a different facility; the mandatory counseling meant she would have to make the round trip twice. And because of the 2013 Texas law, the one that Wendy Davis filibustered but that passed anyway, abortion was now illegal after twenty weeks.

At the Department of Health and Human Services, Matthew Bowman, the former Alliance Defending Freedom lawyer, was advising Lloyd as deputy general counsel for the department. But now, to deal with the litigation, the administration put a fleet of eighteen lawyers on the case, including Scott Stewart, the newly appointed deputy assistant attorney general for the department's civil division. The girl, he argued, could either return home—to a country where abortion was banned—or find a sponsor who would help her get the procedure. The judge asked whether Stewart believed that Roe was still the "law of the land." Stewart didn't dispute the legality of Roe but signaled that undocumented minors had "minimal" constitutional rights to an abortion in federal custody, unless it was for a medical emergency.

"Despite the fact that she is in this country illegally and is in a detained shelter, or whatever it is called, she still has constitutional rights," the judge, Tanya Chutkan, said. "Do you agree with me there?"

Stewart refused to cede the point. "I'm not going to give you a concession on that, Your Honor," he said.

Judge Chutkan laughed, an exasperated chuckle. "This is remarkable," she said. She granted an order later that day, allowing the girl to leave the shelter on either October 20 or 21.

The government appealed Judge Chutkan's order. As the case was pending, the shelter staff didn't allow the girl to leave, to go to the clinic or anywhere else. Instead, they isolated her, wouldn't permit her to do Zumba with the other kids or go on trips outside of the shelter. The staff followed her every move, "*de día y de noche*," she told VICE News in an interview, caseworkers even tracking her into the bathroom. They asked what she would name the baby. She felt so alone.

People from this country that she was just beginning to know stood with her, Garza told her, writing and calling to show their support. "*Eres muy fuerte. Tienes un carácter muy fuerte*," Garza said. "You are very strong. You have a very strong character."

In all their conversations, Garza never told the girl that she might not get her abortion. Watching her struggle, Garza couldn't bear to say the words. Instead, Garza, Amiri, and their teams prepared for the next legal battle. When the hearing was announced for October 20, the date that Judge Chutkan had said the girl could have her abortion, Amiri raced straight from her office in New York to Washington, grabbing shoes from under her desk and stopping at Union Station to buy a change of underwear. By then, the girl was more than fourteen weeks into her pregnancy.

In oral arguments before the three-judge federal appeals panel, Amiri argued that the girl simply wanted the guarantees enshrined in Roe. Weeks earlier, the state judge in Texas had granted her the power to make her own decision. Lloyd and his team were substituting their judgment for the girl's own, effectively exercising veto power over her decision—and her constitutional right, she said.

"Since 1973, the Supreme Court has held that the government may not ban abortion," Amiri told the judges. "We're not asking for a sweeping constitutional ruling; we're asking for [something] basic, the validation of what the Supreme Court has already said for forty-some odd years, and that is the government may not block abortion for anyone."

The Trump administration pushed back. Their lawyers did not contest whether she had a right to an abortion, just that the government was not required to facilitate access to the procedure. She could, they said, return to her home country for the procedure. Their argument put the girl in an impossible position, given that she was not allowed to leave the shelter on her own, never mind the futility of making the treacherous, monthslong trek back to a place where abortion was illegal.

Amiri turned to one of the judges, a fit, middle-aged white man with side-swept brown hair graying at the temples. Based on his detailed questioning of the Trump administration lawyer, she could tell that he had done his research and read all the legal papers. His questions were tough but measured. He quizzed the lawyers on how far the right to an abortion established in Roe extended. "An adult woman who is pregnant in immigration detention unlawfully here, does she under current Supreme Court precedent have a right to obtain an abortion?" he asked. He wondered why the girl couldn't find a sponsor to act as her guardian and take her to the appointment. "Did she have names of people and phone numbers and addresses with her when she arrived in the United States?" he asked.

Amiri explained why that had proven impossible. The government had been seeking a sponsor for weeks already and had been unable to find anyone who would qualify. The process—background checks, home visits, and the rest of the vetting—would simply take too long now and would likely put the girl outside of the window for getting a legal abortion, she explained. The restrictions passed by the Texas legislature over the years had made scheduling an abortion difficult. And that wasn't even accounting for the "irreparable harm" to the girl's mental and physical health from being forced to remain pregnant. The delay so far, Amiri argued, was an "undue burden"—the kind that had been deemed unconstitutional by the Supreme Court in Casey.

When the hearing was over, the stakes felt even bigger than the girl. "If we lose this case, I don't know what Roe means," Amiri reflected. "The Trump administration would do to all of us what they have done to Jane Doe."

The ruling came by the time Amiri disembarked from her train home to New York. She stood on the sidewalk outside her daughter's pre-K classroom and sobbed. The girl should wait eleven more days, the court ruled, as the state tried to find a sponsor. If one was not found by October 31, the litigation could start again. But Amiri knew that by Halloween, the girl would be over seventeen weeks pregnant and they'd have to start all over with the district court. That process could easily take more than three weeks, meaning the girl would miss the twenty-week Texas deadline. It was, thought Amiri, a dishonest political punt. A way for the two Republican-appointed judges on the panel to please conservatives while dodging the big constitutional question the case posed to Roe.

Amiri rushed to file an appeal, asking the court to rehear the case en banc—meaning the larger full court would review the decision by the three-judge panel. Two days later, the circuit court voted to reverse the ruling and allow the girl to end her pregnancy by a 6–3 margin.

The Trump administration effort had failed. The girl was granted her abortion.

Amiri flipped through the pages of the ruling to see what the three judges who dissented had said. The same judge who questioned her about the girl's sponsor had written that he opposed the majority ruling. His words were not as aggressive as another judge's, a woman who wrote bluntly that Jane Doe had no constitutional right to an abortion. He stopped short of that kind of direct hit at Roe, writing that giving the girl what Garza and Amiri saw as her constitutional right represented "a radical extension" of abortion law.

The final decision was "based on a constitutional principle as novel as it is wrong," he argued, "a new right for unlawful immigrant minors in US government detention to obtain immediate abortion on demand." It was an argument that threaded together a judicial question—what rights an undocumented girl could receive—with the political language of the antiabortion movement, "abortion on demand."

The judge had given no indication of such views during oral arguments, when he asked civil questions. "It's like he got angry, and then it came out," said Amiri.

When the girl finally entered the clinic in the early morning, it was under cover of darkness. She wanted support, so Garza went into the room with her. Garza held her hand and rubbed her hair, and felt sad and tired and frustrated. In Washington, antiabortion activists were outraged. "We unequivocally reject abortion advocates' narrative that justice has been done in this case," Marjorie Dannenfelser said. "Instead the extreme agenda of the abortion lobby and the ACLU has claimed two victims and made a cruel mockery of the 'American dream.'"

But Garza had watched her struggle and saw her suffer as she was unable to control her own destiny. In the end, the girl was required to stay pregnant for a month longer than she wanted. It was amazing how divorced legal proceedings and politics could be from people's actual lives and decisions, how little the judicial system took into account human pain, Garza thought.

The episode showed the increasingly precarious state of abortion rights. The antiabortion movement had people like Lloyd positioned to originate policy. They had lawyers like Stewart and Bowman ready to defend it. They fell short in just one part of the system—the court, where they did not have a majority of judges. But they were working on that.

The story of Jane Doe was a sort of parable, a precursor to what America without abortion could look like if the antiabortion movement could put all the pieces into place. In many ways, the case was a trial run for a larger strategy, the antiabortion movement's revision of Jane Roe years earlier.

The court's ruling in the case didn't stop Lloyd, who continued to deny abortions to other pregnant undocumented girls on his agency's spreadsheet, including one who said she had been raped and threatened to harm herself. Even more unusually, the Justice Department soon turned its full force against Amiri, Garza, and even Garza's brother, who was her law partner, asking the Supreme Court to sanction the lawyers for alleged "material misrepresentations and omissions" in the case. To some observers, the action looked like retaliation against advocates by the federal government. The appeal was "a flagrant effort to intimidate the ACLU, one of the Trump administration's fiercest legal foes," wrote one legal analyst. The high court declined the request and the ACLU's case ballooned into a class action lawsuit on behalf of all the pregnant teens in custody. Eventually, three years after the litigation began, the government ended the policy banning the young migrants from getting abortions. Lloyd left the office in 2018, after the controversy over a Trump policy forcibly separating thousands of migrant children from their families consumed the country, for a new role at HHS focused on outreach to faith-based partners. Eventually, three years after the litigation began, the Trump administration acquiesced and issued a new policy in the fall of 2020, prohibiting obstruction or interference with access to abortion for unaccompanied minors who requested one.

After Jane Doe had her abortion, Garza, like Amiri, kept thinking about the judge who had written the dissent, arguing the girl shouldn't be allowed to have it. He couldn't see the trauma written on her face, thought Garza, but still he wanted to take away her rights. She did not know him, but she knew he had never seen the girl.

At the top of his dissent, the court had printed the judge's name in capital letters. "KAVANAUGH."

PART III

THE CHESSBOARD

JUNE 2022

Sioux Falls, South Dakota

Dr. Sarah Traxler put on her blue scrubs as soon as she arrived from the airport. Fifteen patients were waiting. It was the most they could fit in one day.

She had flown from Minneapolis to Sioux Falls, where Planned Parenthood ran the last remaining clinic that provided abortions in South Dakota. There was no doctor in the state who provided abortions, except for the rare medical emergencies in hospitals. So twice a week, once a month, for seven years, Planned Parenthood paid for Dr. Traxler to make the trip.

Her journey was particularly tense that morning, with rumors swirling and protesters already assembled at the Supreme Court. She was waiting on the jet bridge when the court announced its fifth and final case for the day, and it wasn't about Roe. Settled in seat 4B, her regular spot, she exhaled as her plane flew west, between two layers of gray clouds into the thin, pinkish-yellow light.

Planned Parenthood had already told her that after this week's round of patients, it would stop offering abortion at the clinic until the case was decided. If Roe were overturned, South Dakota had a law in place to automatically outlaw nearly all abortions. No one knew when the ruling would come down, so no one knew, exactly, what the legal liability would be if a doctor were in the middle of a procedure when it did.

Inside the clinic, Misty Parrow, the center's manager, lined up all the patient charts. A delivery came—a vase of sunflowers, a gift of encouragement for the staff from their regional Planned Parenthood affiliates. Parrow set them on a table in the back.

The black-and-white ad from the national Planned Parenthood headquarters, framed above Parrow's desk, felt particularly prophetic that morning. "The Supreme Court—aided and abetted by the White House—has opened the door for antiabortion extremists to impose limits on abortion in each state," it warned. "If they succeed, access to reproductive health care for a woman will depend on geography. Or her bank account."

"To take this battle to fifty state legislatures, your active support is needed," it said. "The fight to keep safe, legal abortion is entering its most crucial phase."

It was signed by Faye Wattleton, the first Black woman to lead Planned Parenthood—and dated 1990. That was more than thirty years ago, after the Supreme Court ruled in the Webster case that states could pass their own restrictions on abortion access, even with Roe. Parrow's job each day was a reminder that South Dakota had long done just that.

Over the seven years they had worked together, Dr. Traxler and Parrow had choreographed their routine to the minute so that Dr. Traxler could get through the long list of state-mandated questions and paperwork for each patient.

The first patient that day was twenty-nine, a veterinarian for large animals. Just recently, she had performed an ultrasound for a cow.

Dr. Traxler took her through the checklist. Did she want to see the ultrasound? Yes. Did she want to take home an image? Yes. Did she want to hear the heartbeat if it was detectable? Yes. She wanted it all, all the information, she said—she and her partner were both scientists, after all.

She was seven weeks and two days pregnant. One of the state-mandated forms asked her to circle on a scale of one to ten how sure she was she wanted to have an abortion. She circled a three.

She had grown up in a Catholic family. Everyone supported her to make her own decision, she said. But one moment she would be decided, then a few hours later, she would change her mind. She had worked so hard to get to this point in her career, she said, and while she and her partner had great jobs, they were not married, and they were not sure if they were ready to have kids. He supported her no matter what, she said, but that also left the weight of the decision entirely up to her.

She had a tattoo on her arm: a verse from the New Testament. She had gotten it seven years earlier, after she was sexually assaulted in a field when she was out with the cows. She remembered telling her father what happened. Her voice grew quiet.

"I said, 'Give me something that will make me want to live through this,'" she said.

He wrote her a letter, quoting this verse. It was about the power of love. She inked it into her body.

She had driven more than two hundred miles to get here, one way. Three more trips to go.

In South Dakota, abortion was a two-step process. First, patients had to attend a mandatory counseling session. Then, after a seventy-two-hour waiting period, they could return for their abortion. Those laws, passed in 2011, meant women seeking abortions in the large, rural state often had to travel hundreds of miles for the procedure, even as Roe remained standing. Recently, Republican governor Kristi Noem had signed legislation adding a third mandatory visit for women seeking medication abortions.

The laws were burdensome for abortion providers too. There had not been an abortion doctor living in the state since around

1997, so Planned Parenthood paid to fly in providers. Dr. Traxler flew in twice each week when it was her turn, first on Monday for the counseling and intake, then on Thursday for the procedure. On a wall in her office, Parrow had a giant calendar for the whole year, tracking the rotation of which doctors would fly in on which day to provide abortions. She had mapped it out through September, in case the clinic could stay open.

Everything had become so complicated, but the women's reasons for coming never changed, Parrow said, just the requirements that they had to meet. That was the point of the laws. Roe did not need to be reversed to effectively end abortion. Abortion just needed to be made functionally impossible.

In South Dakota, it was working. In 2008, there were 848 abortions in the state. By 2021, there were only 192.

Those numbers could get even smaller at any moment. If the court overturned Roe, the decision would trigger a 2005 state law prohibiting all abortion except to save the life of the pregnant woman.

In another room that morning, a patient wiggled her hip bones down on the ultrasound table. She chose not to see the images or hear a heartbeat. But when Dr. Traxler asked if she wanted to take home the images, she said yes. Moments later, she changed her mind.

It was not her first choice, being here. When she had thought about being pregnant for the first time, she had imagined being happy. Now, when she read posts on Facebook groups for moms, she just felt anxious. She and her partner had just moved into a new apartment, and they needed to get a new car. It felt like they were struggling to survive, she said. She was twenty-one. Really, she said, she was not ready.

"I'm just a lowly waitress," she said. "I really don't make a lot of money."

Adoption did not feel like an option either. There were so many kids in the system right now who were going to foster care, and she could not do that to another child, she said.

"I don't want my kid going into the system and then thinking that I didn't want them, because it's not that I don't want them," she said. "It's just that I don't want to have them be struggling with me."

Her voice grew tight and shaky. The abortion would cost her about $400, and combined with the cost of the first appointment, it was more than she made in a month of tips, she said. She had to come up with the money by Thursday. But the abortion would be much cheaper than raising a child, she thought.

She worried she was not making the right choice. The father was worried about how stressed she was, she said. She was trying to manage several illnesses, including borderline personality disorder, depression, and anxiety, and she had felt terrible since she stopped taking her medications while pregnant.

"It's so hard taking care of myself as it is," she said.

During the ultrasound, she did not look at the screen. The fetus measured at twelve weeks and two days. She sat back up and wiped off the gel.

Like most of her friends and family, she was "pro-choice," she said. But she felt weird about getting an abortion almost into her second trimester. She knew in South Dakota, it was legal to get an abortion through the twelfth week of pregnancy at a clinic and through the twenty-second week at a hospital.

"I don't know, that feels a little long to me," she said. "But if it's legal, I mean, I can't say anything against it, I suppose."

Before she left, she asked if they could do the abortion on Friday instead of Thursday. It would still be after the seventy-two-hour waiting period, she said, and she had to work at the restaurant on Thursday and did not want to lose her shift.

No, Dr. Traxler explained. The law required that the procedure be done by the same doctor who conducted the counseling, and she could only fly in on Thursday.

"All right," the patient said. "I'll just tell them that my doctors say that my pregnancy is nonviable and they're going to remove it on Thursday. I'll tell my grandma that, and then she'll take my shift."

Dr. Traxler asked if she wanted to talk through her feelings. "We're here for you no matter what you decide," she said before walking to her next appointment.

Dr. Traxler remembered when her daughter was about ten, and they went on a mother-daughter date to the ballet. Her daughter started telling a story she had heard about her friend's cousin, who was nine years old and pregnant. Dr. Traxler stopped. She talked with her daughter about appropriate touch and consent. When they finished, her daughter had a wish for her friend's cousin: "I wish there was a way she could become un-pregnant," she told her mom.

Dr. Traxler was relieved to be able to tell her that there was. "I said, 'It's called abortion; it's what I do for a living. I make people not pregnant anymore who don't want to be pregnant,'" Dr. Traxler remembered telling her. "She looked up, and she said, 'Oh, she should totally do that.'"

Dr. Traxler was young, too, when she first heard about abortion in the foyer of her Southern Baptist church in Louisiana, and opposed the procedure. But then in college, one of her friends had one. Listening to her wrestle through the decision, Dr. Traxler changed her mind. Eventually, she left the church.

Now, her daughter was almost twenty and very angry about what was happening, Dr. Traxler said. Everywhere, women's roles were increasingly being confined, by the lack of childcare, by the pandemic, by the pending decision from the court, she said. Everything felt backward.

Dr. Traxler worked her way through the next dozen patients. Julia, twenty-eight, said she was against abortion like her Christian family. But she was also a single mom, with three-year-old twins and a five-year-old, who were living in Honduras with her mother. She sent back $2,000 monthly to support them. She couldn't afford another child. "I wouldn't be able to provide them the lifestyle I am providing them," she said. "It's not a big lifestyle. But it's a decent one. I'm preparing them for the future."

Another woman brought her daughter, who played with her Barbie car in the exam room, as her mother explained that she was not there because of finances but because caring for a child was so much more than that—it was time, emotion, physical labor. Some patients that day did not speak English. Another was a transgender man.

Then Dr. Traxler came to the last name on her list. The final patient, waiting across the hall.

Amber sat in the chair, small and pale and swallowed up in a huge red hockey sweatshirt. Her orange-blond hair was limp around her cheeks.

Her best friend tucked her feet up on Amber's chair. She was pregnant, too, due on Christmas Eve. When she found out she was pregnant, she called Amber—"You'll be next!" she said. And she was. They were twenty-one and twenty. But things had changed. "She's having her kid, and I'm not having mine," Amber said.

The two women listened to Dr. Traxler's voice on an audio recording.

> *South Dakota law requires that I tell you that you have the right to review all of the material and information described*

in South Dakota Codified Laws Section 34–23A-1. Section 34–23A-1.2 34–23A-1.7 inclusive. Section 34–23A 10.1 and section 34–23A-10.3. Section 34–23A-1 contains the definitions and terms used in South Dakota laws regarding performance of abortions.

The tape stretched on for five long minutes, describing the things the state had determined Amber needed to hear before she had the procedure. It told her she might be able to get some assistance for childcare or neonatal care. That the father of the child would be legally required to pay child support, even if he was the one who said he would pay for the abortion. It told her the name and number of a nearby antiabortion pregnancy health center. Amber had to listen and then report back what numbers she heard at the end, to prove she had listened all the way through.

She didn't need any of that. She had circled a ten. She asked for a surgical abortion to be sure it was completely over.

Parrow went through her health history. Amber said she was diagnosed with bipolar I, borderline personality disorder, and gastroparesis, but had not found lasting treatment that helped her. She vaped, but had stopped drinking six months ago. She used marijuana for her nausea. Parrow asked her questions, questions she had asked hundreds of patients over the years.

Are you in a monogamous relationship?

Have you been hit, slapped, kicked, or otherwise physically abused by anybody?

Have you ever been forced to participate in a sexual activity that made you feel uncomfortable?

Has your partner tampered with your birth control, refused to wear condoms, or pressured you to become pregnant?

Are you afraid your partner will hurt you if you say you have an STI and your partner needs to receive treatment?

You're aware of all the other options that are available and you're confident in your decision to continue the abortion?

Amber answered each one. "I've been asked like five times by everybody today. They're like, 'Are you sure?' And I'm like, 'I'm 110 percent,'" she said.

She felt safe now, living back home and six minutes from her best friend. She told her ex's parents she planned to get the abortion, and they supported her, she said.

The young women rolled their eyes at the mention of Amber's ex and railed against his misdeeds. In the breakup, he tried to take furniture she had bought with money she got from OnlyFans, Amber said. They remembered becoming friends, when Amber had just a trash bag with four outfits and a pair of boots.

Amber said she would do the STI test another time, once she checked if insurance would pay. Her paperwork was time stamped 3:34 p.m.

Three days later, just after 3:34 p.m., she returned.

She had the last abortion legal under Roe in the state of South Dakota.

Days later, after the Supreme Court decision, she posted on social media. "If I wasn't able to get my abortion, I wouldn't be here right now," she said. "I would have unalived myself.

"My abortion saved me."

2018–2020

20

Exactly Fifteen Weeks

In the summer of 2017, a few weeks before Jane Doe crossed the southern border into the United States, the Alliance Defending Freedom convened hundreds of top conservative leaders to the luxurious Ritz-Carlton, Laguna Niguel, in California for a private four-day summit. The stated goal was to discuss religious freedom. But the deeper ambition was to develop their agenda for the new Trump era. Their guest list included ten state attorneys general and solicitors general, a collection of the most powerful Christian lawyers in the country, and Jeff Sessions, President Trump's new attorney general and a key ally who had described Roe as "one of the worst, colossally erroneous Supreme Court decisions of all time." Sessions initially kept his remarks, and the promise he made to the group, a secret from the public.

"Under this administration, religious Americans will be treated neither as an afterthought nor as a problem to be managed," Sessions said in a closed-door evening address.

When reporters discovered the details of Sessions's speech, public outcry centered on the fact that America's top law enforcement official addressed a group known most prominently at the time for its opposition to gay rights. But ADF's work was growing, largely under the radar as it sought to become a mainstream Christian rival to the ACLU. No one on the outside knew just how extensive ADF's ambitions were, or that ADF was laying groundwork to challenge Roe.

ADF had invited another delegation that sought to keep its participation off the official record: a team from the Wisconsin attorney general's office, including Misha Tseytlin, the solicitor general who just eight months earlier was brainstorming about abortion law at the Federalist Society cocktail hour. When a reporter from the USA Today Network-Wisconsin later unearthed that delegation's participation, a state spokesperson simply said that Tseytlin had co-led a session at the conference. No one disclosed what it was about. Tseytlin's remarks that day remained unknown to the public.

But Tseytlin, a man most Americans had never heard of, was there to present a very specific strategy: a legal path to end Roe.

Lawyers had a moral duty to act, Tseytlin told the group. He proposed the idea for an abortion ban that set a limit just a few weeks earlier than twenty weeks. States like Texas, his own state of Wisconsin, and fifteen others had enacted bans at about twenty weeks, which ended abortion rights earlier than the viability line required by Roe and Casey. And yet Roe still stood as the law of the land. They needed to undercut the decision more openly, he argued, with bans that started earlier.

His session was well-attended by lawyers in the antiabortion movement and some staff from the offices of state attorneys general, but not packed. While abortion remained a focus for the true believers, issues like religious liberty and speech captured far more attention at the gathering.

Even to those in the room with Tseytlin, it was far from clear that the plan that was hatching would, just five years later, lead to the most consequential Supreme Court ruling on abortion rights in half a century. The early years of the Trump administration had been good for ADF. The group now had some three thousand allied lawyers in its network, brought in more revenue than the ACLU, and was growing rapidly. Its march on the Supreme Court continued, and ADF lawyers were about to defend the baker in Colorado who refused to make a cake for a same-sex couple's wedding. Part of ADF's power was built from events like this one, bringing together state attorneys general and solicitors general, along with allied attorneys from across the country to strategize on priorities. Some of those guests were reimbursed for travel expenses. For this summit, the group paid part of Tseytlin's travel costs. The organization asked guests to maintain the secrecy of their discussions, as it did for most of its events, according to participants. ADF did not disclose its list of allies and encouraged lawyers involved with its efforts not to even acknowledge attending its events, according to attendees.

Like the Federalist Society, ADF aimed to connect lawyers and legal allies to further its goals. But ADF was also profoundly different. It was an explicitly conservative Christian legal advocacy project, designed to leverage lawyers, elected officials, and activists to achieve policy goals in line with their religious mission. ADF had a new president, Michael Farris, who had initially opposed Trump's election—Trump's views on abortion "appear to have been written on an Etch A Sketch," he once said—but the group saw new opportunity and was now intensifying its efforts at cultural transformation.

Similar to Trump, ADF was building a public identity around the idea of Christians being under siege, especially as American values on sexuality, marriage, and family expanded in the wake of the Obergefell decision making same-sex marriage legal. ADF's own religious commitments became stricter. The group added more specific belief requirements to its statement of faith, including that "rejecting one's biological sex rejects the created image of God," that "God intends sexual intimacy to only occur between a man and a woman joined in marriage," and that life "must be respected and protected from conception to natural death."

In Tseytlin's closed-door session, the idea of moving up limits from twenty weeks faced resistance from some antiabortion activists. Even with Trump in office, the movement remained divided over the best legal path to end abortion rights. The national movement had been focused on abortion bans at twenty weeks, or twenty-two weeks, depending on how they counted the weeks of pregnancy, and groups like the Susan B. Anthony List thought the strongest argument would be to convince the public that a fetus could feel pain at that time. Some worried that an earlier limit would be too aggressive for the justices. If their test case got to the Supreme Court and lost, it could set their movement back years.

But another flank of the movement wanted to take advantage of this moment of power and move more aggressively to pass laws that flouted Roe's viability requirement. They wanted to try all kinds of bans, from six-week cutoffs to laws banning abortion based on fetal selection for race, sex, or disability to see what kind of a proposal could, eventually, entice the Supreme Court to weigh in on the issue.

ADF believed the most effective strategy would be to find the magic number of weeks that would force the court to reconsider Roe. The limit had to be not so early as to be immediately struck down by lower courts but still below the viability line to undercut Roe. Arkansas had already passed a twelve-week law, and it was blocked by the courts, so that seemed too low. ADF lawyers decided to get a state to ban abortion at fifteen weeks. The spark of Tseytlin's cocktail hour conversation became a flame.

Their goal would be to remove Roe's viability line without directly asking the court to take the more drastic—and likely more politically inflammatory—step of directly overturning the decision. It could be a first step in a longer strategy to end legal abortion entirely.

For centuries, people have debated the question of when life begins, when a human life has civil rights, and when the responsibility for it begins and ends. ADF's fifteen-week plan did not emerge from biological discussions about when an organism becomes an organism, or philosophical ones about the relationship between body and soul. Nor was the policy grounded in the medical realities of modern-day pregnancy for American women. The fifteen-week mark was before a fetus could live outside the womb and was several weeks before doctors generally conducted the first significant fetal anatomy scan. It was simply a test case, designed to push the legal limit, to put Roe in check, or if they were successful, checkmate.

ADF's mission was to craft the legislation that would start the process of trying to reach the Supreme Court, and its leaders knew exactly whom to hire to write it. Denise Burke had worked at Americans United for Life for almost two decades, writing model legislation on various abortion restrictions and advising state legislators and state attorneys general on how to pass it. She was one of the movement's top authors on antiabortion measures. The legislation would need to be airtight to survive the journey through conservative statehouses and the inevitable legal challenges in the lower courts in order to eventually arrive at the Supreme Court.

ADF lawyers identified states where they believed the bills had the best chance. They looked for favorable governors, attorneys general, and state legislatures. Three states stood out: Mississippi, Arkansas, and Utah. Each was in a different circuit court region. The thinking was that if the laws were debated in different circuit courts, and the courts issued conflicting rulings, the Supreme Court would be more likely to take up one of the cases and arbitrate among them. It was those kinds of conflicts—what lawyers called *circuit splits*—that often attracted the interest of the justices, who saw part of their mandate as ensuring that the law was applied consistently across the country.

"A circuit split would mean there had to be a resolution," said Dannenfelser, who was on ADF's board.

While ADF tried to reverse engineer its way to the Supreme Court, antiabortion activists on the state level were also trying to advance tighter abortion bans. ADF tracked them all. Every legislative session was another opportunity to move forward, and abortion opponents on the ground, like the ADF lawyers, were driven by a sense of spiritual mission. The most religiously devout states overlapped with the legislatures pushing for abortion restrictions.

Mississippi topped the list, with 59 percent of adults identifying as "very religious," according to Gallup.

Since 2004, there had been only one clinic in Mississippi where women could get an abortion—Jackson Women's Health Organization, with its unmistakable bubble-gum-pink walls. The Pink House, as everyone called it, was just a seven-minute drive from the capitol building, where lawmakers tried to find ways to shut it down with bill after bill. And again and again, the Pink House and its lawyers at the Center for Reproductive Rights pushed back in the courts, arguing the laws violated the standards set in Roe and Casey. Through it all, the Pink House survived.

In the fall of 2017, a few months after Tseytlin went to the Ritz for the ADF summit, a conservative Christian lobbyist named Jameson Taylor started what he called his annual "intelligence gathering" on what antiabortion legislation he wanted to push next session and how the antiabortion forces could, once again, take another shot at the Pink House. He made the rounds to various Christian groups and called different policy experts, including Kellie Fiedorek, a young lawyer who worked for ADF. Her job was to build out the ADF network in the states, to push their model legislation through the statehouses, and create an army of allied local lawyers who could defend it.

Soon Taylor was listening as ADF lawyers made their case that the Supreme Court might uphold a law that banned abortion before Roe's standard of viability—and that Mississippi was an ideal testing ground. Burke at ADF explained how the legislation she was writing would work. To end the federal right to an abortion, activists needed a law that could actually reach the Supreme Court without first getting struck down for obviously violating Roe. Passing a ban that was too aggressive would be categorically struck down in the lower courts. That was the entire reason to try something in the gray zone, not perhaps as early in pregnancy as they would ideally like, but before twenty weeks. ADF was crafting the legislation with Justice Anthony Kennedy in mind—Tseytlin's old boss—in hopes he might be a swing vote to uphold a law that crept restrictions forward and, in the process, eradicate the viability standard that was the underpinning of Roe.

As a law, it was "very, very imperfect," Taylor reflected. He knew a fifteen-week ban would only criminalize about 3 percent of the 2,550 abortions in Mississippi each year. But stopping procedures was not really the point. ADF's primary goal was to write bills as a litigation strategy, not craft laws that would be the strongest public policy or end the greatest number of abortions. The Mississippi bill was a legal tool to provoke a Supreme Court challenge to Roe. It could set a bigger plan in motion to eventually achieve their ultimate goal of ending all abortion in America.

"ADF made a very good case," Taylor said. "There was a chance that the court might look at the viability line and see it is really a bit of a moving target."

Some lawmakers in Mississippi worried they would be sued if it passed and did not want to be saddled with the exorbitant cost such litigation could bring. The Whole Woman's Health case had cost Texas nearly $1.1 million to argue and another $2.5 million in attorneys' fees after a federal court ordered the state to cover costs for the Center for Reproductive Rights. But ADF had a plan for that, too, offering to have its lawyers defend the law at no cost to the state. This free legal counsel was a selling point for Taylor when he lobbied the legislators to take up the bill.

Plus, Taylor had an important ally in the statehouse who he knew would push an antiabortion bill—Representative Becky Currie, a nurse, devout Christian, and three-term legislator who was one of the state's most ardent advocates for their cause.

CURRIE WAS AN exception in Mississippi, the rare female Republican lawmaker. "I've been pro-life since I was eighteen and pregnant," she said.

For Currie, the practice of regularly introducing abortion bans was simply part of being spiritually faithful, even if they would be struck down. She was baptized in the Southern Baptist Church at nine and grew up in McComb, Mississippi, a town smaller than some evangelical megachurches. She always wanted to be a nurse and the first in her family to graduate from college. When she found out she was pregnant just after finishing high school in 1975, her older sister came to see her right away to talk through options. But Currie felt she had no choice—abortion was legal under Roe, but the culture in rural Mississippi was not as liberal as in the big city of New Orleans, where her sister worked, and she felt a lot of shame—so she married the father as she finished her first trimester. They soon divorced, and she moved back in with her parents, who babysat so she could go to nursing school.

She worked in the ER, and labor and delivery, but when she felt God prompting her to run for political office, she did. She'd felt drawn to politics ever since a friend's mother, a lawyer unlike her own stay-at-home mom, had invited her as a teenager to a meeting of the local Republican club. The job would be part time, like it is for many state legislators in America, and paid a modest amount. In 2008, she entered the house chamber, which had been controlled by Democrats since the Reconstruction era after the Civil War. Three years later, Republicans took control as part of the Tea Party wave, and antiabortion activists suddenly had more support for their agenda.

Currie's experience as a nurse shaped her political views. She often told the story of an incident in the ER as a young nurse when a pregnant woman came in and delivered far too early. The details varied some in her telling—sometimes the premature infant was a girl, sometimes it was a boy, sometimes it was fifteen weeks, others fourteen weeks. But what Currie remembered most was that she waited until the heart stopped so she could put the remains in a plastic container to send to the lab. What Currie understood about what happened was that the fetus "wanted to live."

"I just never got over that," she remembered.

So decades later, when she met with Taylor about a new antiabortion bill, fifteen weeks seemed to Currie like a good marker. She introduced the bill, called the Gestational Age Act, in early 2018. "The more we worked on the bill, it just felt anointed," she said. "You just know when it was right."

Such legislation, with Currie as the public face, was the ultimate realization of the strategy that Dannenfelser and Kellyanne Conway had lectured the men about all those years ago. She was exactly the kind of woman Dannenfelser envisioned having power when she started SBA. A single mother, Currie had decided against having an abortion but still fulfilled her dream of becoming a nurse and then a politician. She could speak personally and authentically about the subject and her faith in a way that required none of their hotel conference room trainings.

Currie was far from alone. At this critical juncture, women had become the face of the antiabortion movement. Antiabortion activists had honed their strategy of relying on women to champion their policies. Across the country, Republican women made up less than 10 percent of state legislators from 2008 to 2017, but they were significantly overrepresented as sponsors of antiabortion bills, according to an analysis of the period. Of the more than 1,600 antiabortion bills that were introduced during that stretch in state legislatures, nearly half had a female Republican cosponsor, and a third had a female Republican as the primary sponsor. It became more complicated for Democrats to paint abortion opponents as anti-woman, when women were leading the charge.

But as Currie proudly championed the bill, she did not know the full story. She thought her vision for fifteen weeks, rooted in her foundational story of the beating fetal heart, had generated the plan. No one had told her that the Alliance Defending Freedom had coordinated its strategy with Taylor before their meeting, or that fifteen weeks was part of its specific legal plan to undermine Roe, she said. Or that Misha Tseytlin, the former solicitor general of Wisconsin, had brainstormed this possibility at Leonard Leo's

Federalist Society cocktail hour and advanced it at a posh California resort alongside high-profile Republican leaders and attorneys. To her, the bill simply made sense based on her experience as a nurse watching a premature delivery.

"I really thought we came up with fifteen weeks," Currie said later. "But when talking to other groups, it was kind of like the decided number. But also maybe that is just how they talk to legislators, let them think it was their idea."

The legislation, steered by Burke, was written in a way that suggested it was rooted primarily in medical reasoning. But in reality, it featured specific legal language for ADF's longer-term argument to undercut Roe. Roe had called the developing embryo and fetus "potential human life." This bill described it as "an unborn human being" and highlighted specific details of prenatal development as evidence. Between five and six weeks' gestation, "an unborn human being's heart begins beating," the bill claimed. said. At eight weeks, "an unborn human being begins to move about in the womb." At nine weeks, "teeth and eyes are present, as well as external genitalia." At ten weeks, "vital organs begin to function." The legislation stated that the United States was one of seven countries in the world to allow for abortion after twenty weeks of pregnancy, laying the groundwork to argue that the country was an outlier among developed nations.

The bill picked quotes from the decisions in Roe and Casey that acknowledged that states had an interest in protecting "the potentiality of human life" and "the life of the unborn." ADF's idea was to design the legislation to draw out what it saw as an inherent conflict in those two rulings—both allowed abortion before viability but also said that states had an interest in preserving potential life. The bill itself would argue that Mississippi was doing what the Supreme Court allowed, acting in the interest of potential life, and force the court to reconcile the difference.

Currie didn't pick up on the bigger legal strategy embedded in the legislation, a bill she believed she had crafted with Taylor and

Representative Andy Gipson, a lawyer and Baptist minister who had sponsored the state's religious freedom bill, which established "biological sex as objectively determined by anatomy" and forbid state government from punishing people who refused to provide services, medical care, or housing because of a religious opposition to same-sex marriage and transgender rights. Yet before she introduced the legislation on the house floor, Currie said she received emails from ADF, a group she said she didn't recognize. The lawyers encouraged her to frame the law as about the mother, not about the baby, and to focus on the medical harms to women from abortion after fifteen weeks, she said. The argument reflected their strategy to make the ban more palatable to the general public as it moved through the courts and into the national spotlight. But Currie did not see why that kind of marketing campaign was necessary. Mississippi had an antiabortion supermajority, and they would pass the law, which was her goal.

The same week Currie introduced the bill in Mississippi in January 2018, ADF leaders in Washington, DC, unveiled their plan to a group of grassroots allies the morning after the March for Life. They outlined their steps at the Evangelicals for Life conference, hosted by the public policy arm of the Southern Baptist Convention, in another closed-door gathering. Even those who were paying attention to what was happening in Mississippi saw just another abortion ban, but slowly and quietly, ADF was bringing larger swaths of its network into its mission.

"We have a plan to make Roe irrelevant or completely reverse it," Kevin Theriot, vice president of ADF's Center for Life, said as they explained how Mississippi had just introduced a bill banning abortion at fifteen weeks, which had never before been done.

The court would not be able to ignore a ban that limited abortion just to the first trimester, Burke told them. "We're kind of basically baiting them, 'Come on, fight us on turf that we have already set up and established,'" she said. Mississippi would be the first of several states to pass their fifteen-week bills, she said.

"Once we get these first-trimester limitations in place," Burke said, "we're going to go for a complete ban on abortion, except to save the life of the mother."

Back in Mississippi, Democrats, as expected, protested when it was time to debate the bill on the house floor. The bill "does nothing to help the mother who has the unwanted pregnancy. You're not putting any money into social programs that will help her out," said Representative Adrienne Wooten, a Democrat from Jackson. "What is this body going to do when these children get here? Is this body going to take this baby into their own house?"

The legislation amounted to a public health experiment with immense consequences: What would happen if such a poor state, one already among the worst for maternal mortality, further restricted abortion? Already, Mississippi was one of the most dangerous places in the country to give birth. The state had the nation's highest fetal mortality rate, highest infant mortality rate, highest preterm birth rate, highest miscarriage rate and low birthweight rate. Those public health realities didn't impact the bill's chances of passage. The challenge Currie faced wasn't whether her law was too restrictive—it was whether it went far enough. Some local antiabortion activists pushed for a so-called heartbeat ban instead that would make abortion illegal at about six weeks of pregnancy.

Republican leaders rallied their forces behind the fifteen-week plan. Christian groups like the Mississippi District United Pentecostal Church convinced hundreds of pastors to sign a letter to assuage reluctant lawmakers that they had the support of churches if they moved forward. The American Family Association, which was started in Mississippi and whose founder also helped start ADF, blasted supporters with emails urging them to call legislators.

As the bill made its way through the legislative process, Taylor began taking regular prayer walks around the capitol. As he circled the senators' reserved parking spots, the leafy trees, and the landmark bronze monument honoring the Women of the Confederacy—"Our Mothers, Our Daughters, Our Sisters, Our Wives"—he prayed. A lifelong Catholic, a distinct minority in the largely evangelical state, Taylor felt like he was doing the work God had called him to do.

Currie, too, began to feel like the bill had a special divine purpose. "I feel like I've done my job, and I hope the Lord does," she reflected.

When Governor Phil Bryant signed the bill into law, with Currie smiling next to him, it became the tightest restriction on abortion in the nation. It made no exceptions for rape or incest, just a narrow provision to preserve the physical life of the woman or in cases of "severe" fetal abnormality. "We'll probably be sued in about half an hour," Bryant said to chuckles from supporters in the room.

His estimate wasn't far off: it was less than an hour before Jackson Women's Health Organization—the Pink House—filed the lawsuit through their attorneys at the Center for Reproductive Rights. The district court issued a temporary restraining order the next day, putting the law on hold while litigation progressed. In its brief, the center pointed out the limited impact such a law would have on the actual abortions happening in the state. The Pink House performed abortions only until sixteen weeks of pregnancy, the center's lawyers wrote, and had done just seventy-eight abortions when the fetus was identified as being fifteen weeks or older in 2017.

Going after that small fraction, of course, was exactly the plan. Not too early in pregnancy and not too late, but exactly the time that might compel the Supreme Court to wade back into abortion jurisprudence. "We were seeking to be incremental and strategic," Taylor said. Christian activists were learning to control their "moral passion," to accomplish their long-term goal, he said.

To the outside observer, the law looked like just another dead-on-arrival right-wing effort to outlaw abortion, not meaningfully different from the hundreds of such laws passed in recent years. But to those on the inside, this law set in motion a carefully calculated experiment, with a new hypothesis designed to reach a new conclusion. "The abortion clinic in Mississippi took the bait, so to speak, and immediately filed suit," John Bursch, an ADF lawyer, said.

There were still so many unknowns. For the law to serve its intended purpose, antiabortion activists needed a majority on the Supreme Court. ADF attorneys and their allies like Tseytlin had designed the legislation to target Justice Kennedy, but he was still a relative wild card.

"As a Christian, sometimes you don't know God's plan, and he kind of makes things happen," Currie said.

21

The Pick

The White House was already making things happen. The administration's behind-the-scenes charm offensive to push Justice Anthony Kennedy into retirement—and give Donald Trump a second Supreme Court pick—had finally succeeded in late June 2018, just months after Mississippi and ADF passed the fifteen-week abortion ban. The pressure campaign over who should get the nomination began almost immediately.

Senator Heidi Heitkamp, the Catholic Democrat from North Dakota, was called to the White House for a meeting with the president and his top aides. The whole enterprise was more than a little awkward, she thought. In the twenty-four hours since Kennedy delivered his resignation letter to Trump at a lunchtime White House meeting, the president had traveled to an arena in Heitkamp's home state, where he urged thousands of cheering fans to vote her out in the coming midterms—and then turned around to ask for her support for his next Supreme Court justice.

Sitting in the Oval Office, she listened patiently as Trump ticked off the names on the list. What did she think of this judge? What about that one?

It was clear to Heitkamp that the president hadn't yet decided on his pick and was trying to suss out who she preferred. Trump saw her as a gettable vote, a Democrat running for reelection in a deeply conservative state. Plus, she had backed Neil Gorsuch, his first nominee to the court. But this nomination was different, she thought, as Trump kept talking. Kennedy was a swing vote, and he'd backed abortion rights in the past. Awarding Trump a second justice from his list would create a new conservative majority, empowering the court to reshape American life on a whole swath of cultural issues, including abortion, affirmative action, and same-sex marriage.

As Trump rolled through the names from his list, Heitkamp, who supported abortion rights, kept her views to herself. Wedged between Trump aides Don McGahn and Marc Short, she told the president that she had to do her own due diligence. She didn't know any of these people, and she could hardly promise to support some name without finding out more about the individual judge.

She stood up to leave and turned back to the men. "If your court reverses *Roe v. Wade*, the Republicans might be a minority party for a generation," she said. The White House shrugged off her warning. There was no evidence to suggest it might be true. In election after election, abortion simply didn't motivate Democratic voters.

Inside the White House, another political pressure campaign was underway too. But this one was aimed at the president. More than a year before Kennedy announced his resignation, he had encouraged Trump to add a new judge to his list. The name he suggested was the same man McGahn was now pushing: Brett Kavanaugh, a former Kennedy clerk with a long record in Republican politics. He was added to the third iteration of the list in November 2017.

As a lawyer in the George W. Bush White House, Kavanaugh worked closely with Leonard Leo, his emails from that time show, including on Samuel Alito's confirmation and other judicial appointments. McGahn, a longtime Federalist Society member, saw Kavanaugh as a model for the kind of judges conservatives should put on the court. He even used Kavanaugh's decisions as a benchmark to evaluate potential lower-court nominees.

McGahn had an early record of success on judges, delivering the Gorsuch nomination and dozens of lower-court judges by the summer of 2018. He told Trump that Kavanaugh offered the easiest win in the Senate.

But some antiabortion movement leaders had their doubts. Not only was Kavanaugh a creature of the Washington "swamp"—a reason Leo intentionally kept his name off the first two iterations of the list—he also seemed a bit squishy when it came to social issues, particularly abortion. Until his ruling in the Jane Doe case, Kavanaugh had never addressed the right to an abortion in any of his writing as a judge. In public editorials and private conversations, antiabortion activists made clear that they saw his dissent in the Jane Doe case as unconvincing, because of his implication that he would allow the abortion if the girl found a proper sponsor.

Pence's staff and allies in the White House had been moving a different option into position: Amy Coney Barrett, a former Antonin Scalia clerk, beloved University of Notre Dame law professor, and Catholic mother of seven. She was a new member of the Seventh Circuit Court of Appeals, tapped by a lawyer in Mike Pence's office to be one of the first judges Trump appointed when he got elected—getting her on the bench and burnishing her credentials for a future opening on the Supreme Court. The seat she took had been held open by Senate Republicans for more than a year, after they refused to give a hearing to President Obama's candidate, Myra Selby, the first woman and African American to serve on the Indiana Supreme Court.

Barrett had become a conservative heroine during her confirmation hearing, when Dianne Feinstein, the top Democratic senator on the Judiciary Committee, raised concerns about whether her Catholicism would prevent her from being impartial: "The dogma lives loudly within you," Feinstein said. Conservatives saw Feinstein's criticism as an unfair religious test, emblazoning the slogan on coffee mugs and shirts in pride.

Unlike Kavanaugh and Gorsuch, who rose through the ranks of presidential administrations and white-shoe law firms, Barrett embodied a more grassroots form of conservatism. Her roots were in New Orleans and the Midwest, and unlike every other current Supreme Court justice at the time, she did not go to law school at Harvard or Yale. "I'm a Catholic, and I always grew up loving Notre Dame," Barrett said. "I wanted to be in a place where I felt like I would be developed and inspired as a whole person." She was a star, top in her class, just a few years younger than Marjorie Dannenfelser and the conservative sisterhood taking root in the early 1990s in Washington. One of her professors, John Garvey, who became the president of the Catholic University of America, recommended her to Scalia for a clerkship with just one line: "Amy Coney is the best student I ever had."

She returned to Notre Dame to spend her career teaching, while raising her seven children, including two adopted from Haiti and her youngest with Down syndrome. She was a member of the People of Praise, an especially insular religious community that had about 1,650 adult members, including her parents, and drew on the ecstatic traditions of charismatic Christianity. Her advice to students was simple: Pray before accepting a new job. Tithe 10 percent of your income to church and those in need. Commit yourself to a parish and build a life and community there.

She represented an ideal of conservative womanhood, where one could be both a superstar mother, part of a tight-knit religious community, and a brilliant and ambitious career woman. Unlike Kavanaugh, Barrett was not really involved in politics, aside from some Federalist Society events and speaking at an ADF fellowship program for law students. But in her research and writing, she devoted herself to originalism and textualism, and her work drew the attention of the conservative legal establishment. On the appeals court, Barrett soon built a largely conservative record and registered concern over striking down abortion restrictions.

Most important to the antiabortion movement, she had made her personal views opposing abortion very clear. Barrett believed life began at conception and opposed Obama's contraception mandate. She was known for her deep sense of calling to family, faith, and her work. She had the biography that Dannenfelser and her allies of conservative antiabortion women could only have hoped for back in 1993, when Ruth Bader Ginsburg became a justice.

If Trump selected Barrett, then Senators Susan Collins or Lisa Murkowski, the two Republicans left in the caucus who supported abortion rights, might be unwilling to vote to confirm her given her record on abortion rights. But Short believed there was an opportunity to pick up Democratic support instead. Senator Joe Manchin, who backed Barrett for the appeals court, had signaled to Short that he could support an antiabortion judge, as long as that judge left Obama's Affordable Care Act—which provided crucial healthcare coverage for many in his poor home state of West Virginia—untouched. Senator Joe Donnelly, a fellow Catholic from her home state of Indiana, was another gettable vote, Short believed. Like Heitkamp, the two Democrats were up for reelection in conservative states.

Still, Barrett had been a judge for less than a year. If she were ever to be on the Supreme Court, she needed more judicial experience.

If there was any disappointment when Trump picked Kavanaugh, antiabortion movement leaders did not show it publicly. They released statements praising the pick and got to work. Leo's forces were ready. Within hours of Kavanaugh's formal announcement, the Judicial Crisis Network announced plans to spend millions boosting Kavanaugh's image as an impartial jurist. Kavanaugh might not have seemed as sure of a bet for the antiabortion movement as Barrett. But he was a Federalist Society man who had attended their annual conference for twenty-five years, and by Leo's own estimation, a very large number of their members believed Roe was wrongly decided.

Besides, the president had his own plans for Barrett, he told a number of people. "I'm saving her for Ginsburg."

ROCHELLE GARZA, ONE of Jane Doe's lawyers, practically gasped when she heard the news. "This guy?" she thought. "Are you kidding me?"

For Garza, the story of the girl's case suddenly had even greater significance. Now the administration was doing more than targeting a migrant girl in detention, she thought. They wanted to do to America what they had tried and failed to do to Jane Doe. Trump had picked, for the biggest promotion of all, the judge who wrote the dissent that would have functionally revoked the girl's right to an abortion. "He's going to take away everyone's reproductive rights," Garza thought.

Whether Kavanaugh would reach the court hinged on just a handful of senators. The group included Heitkamp; Manchin and Donnelly, the two other red-state Democrats; and Collins and Murkowski, the two Republican women who supported abortion rights.

Collins interviewed Kavanaugh for two hours in her office in August. In their conversation, he assured her that he understood the importance of Roe in American life. "Roe is forty-five years old, it has been reaffirmed many times, lots of people care about it a great deal, and I've tried to demonstrate I understand real-world consequences," he told her, according to private notes later reported by *The New York Times*. "I am a don't-rock-the-boat kind of judge. I believe in stability and in the Team of Nine." Collins emerged from the meeting offering a largely positive review, sending an early signal that she would likely support his confirmation. He had convinced her that he believed Roe was settled law.

Democrats, meanwhile, struggled to unite behind an opposition strategy. The idea that Kavanaugh—a White House lawyer for the Bush administration and a suburban dad from the liberal bastion of Bethesda, Maryland—would overthrow nearly a half century of established law seemed hard to swallow. Some Democrats believed he was more like John Roberts, an institutionalist who generally took an incremental approach to changing the law, than Clarence Thomas or Samuel Alito.

Ilyse Hogue at NARAL argued for a clear assault: a straight, targeted message that Kavanaugh would destroy Roe. But Senator Chuck Schumer, the minority leader of the Senate, worried that mounting an aggressive anti-Kavanaugh campaign could hamper their efforts to win control of the body in the coming midterms. In meetings with Hogue and liberal activists, he worried that asking donors to fund a focused anti-Kavanaugh effort would make it harder to raise money for their broader electoral efforts in the fall. This was a fight Democrats would likely lose, he reasoned. Better to take the defeat fast and leave time to focus on winning back control of the Senate—a victory that would likely make Schumer into the new majority leader.

As the date of the confirmation hearing drew near, abortion-rights advocates continued to push back. The Center for Reproductive Rights, which never endorsed Supreme Court nominees because its lawyers argued before the court, broke its decades-old policy to oppose Kavanaugh. "His judicial philosophy is fundamentally hostile to the protection of reproductive rights under the U.S. Constitution," the group warned.

Garza prepared to testify before the committee that Kavanaugh placed an "unjustifiable" hurdle to abortion rights in Jane Doe's case. Brigitte Amiri of the ACLU met with Democratic Senate staffers and reporters, trying to raise alarms by noting that in Kavanaugh's dissent to the Jane Doe case, he referred to Roe as "existing precedent," the implication being that such a ruling could be overturned. Amid its leadership transition away from Cecile Richards, Planned Parenthood and other abortion rights groups organized hundreds of protesters to descend on Washington, gathering on the steps of the court, shouting chants in the middle of the Senate cafeteria, and climbing the stairs to drop leaflets with the rallying cry "#StopKavanaugh" into the atrium in the Hart Senate Office Building.

Still, even as they fought, some in the abortion-rights movement began making the earliest preparations for the ultimate defeat. Hogue began shifting resources into state and local races, hoping to win back governors' mansions and break Republican supermajorities—the only way to stop passage of the state restrictions that she thought would eventually reach the court. That process was far from an immediate solution. It could take years, she realized, as it had taken their opponents.

The morning of Kavanaugh's confirmation hearing, red-cloaked women stood silent sentry outside room 216 of the Hart Senate Office Building, their white bonnets and floor-length scarlet robes inspired by *The Handmaid's Tale*, Margaret Atwood's dystopian story about a world where women had no rights. Inside, Republican women filled many seats, their presence sending the opposite message that Kavanaugh was an ally.

Through it all, Kavanaugh sat expressionless, hands folded on the table in front of him, a stoic witness to the chaos. His mission was simple: survive unscathed.

KAVANAUGH WOULD NOT achieve that goal. His hearing would go down as one of the most contentious in history, remembered for a woman's emotional testimony of sexual assault, his outraged denial, and America's inflamed response. Christine Blasey Ford, a research psychologist from California, alleged to *The Washington Post* that Kavanaugh had pinned her down at a party when they were teenagers in the early 1980s and groped her. Kavanaugh denied the incident completely. America was ripped apart over questions of belief, power, and women's bodies.

Since Trump won the White House, outrage over sexual mistreatment of women in American life had birthed a new movement—#MeToo—that brought down 201 powerful men the year before

Kavanaugh was nominated. Now, Blasey Ford v. Kavanaugh became the ultimate clash of gender and politics, in the pitched political area of a Supreme Court confirmation hearing that already had enormous implications for women. In the media and in the hearings, the debate over women and their bodies moved from abortion to a new, but related, fight over the power of men and women in society.

But earlier that month, Kavanaugh had another series of exchanges—ones that were far less memorable once the storm of sexual assault allegations came. Before Kavanaugh and Blasey Ford testified, there was a first set of hearings that followed the more typical pattern for potential Supreme Court justices, where senators on the Judiciary Committee questioned the nominee on his or her legal record.

In those hearings, Feinstein, the highest-ranking Democratic member on the committee, led her party's line of attack. Peering down at Kavanaugh, her objective was to show the country that Kavanaugh was unfit because of a range of issues—including Roe.

At age eighty-five, Feinstein had been through eight Supreme Court confirmation hearings. Her first was for Ginsburg back in 1993, shortly after she was elected to the Senate in the Year of the Woman, as part of the wave of women outraged by the treatment of Anita Hill during Thomas's confirmation hearing. She had been a tough San Francisco mayor who survived threats and an assassination attempt in the tumult of the 1970s, and ran for office as a feminist. "They don't get it yet in Washington, but they will once we get there," she said then. During Thomas's hearing, the Judiciary Committee had been all men. Now Feinstein was one of four women, all Democrats, on the committee, and one of twenty-one women in the Senate.

Yet, after so many years in the Senate, Feinstein had become deeply vested in the bipartisan traditions of polite comity and respect that once governed the chamber. She quizzed Kavanaugh on his views about Roe, just as senators in her position had done in every hearing since she'd been in Washington. And Kavanaugh, citing judicial propriety as candidates always did, largely declined to answer.

Feinstein pulled up an email he had written in 2003, when he was a lawyer in the Bush White House. The court, he had written then, "can always overrule its precedent." She wanted to know if Kavanaugh stood by that assessment. Did he consider Roe to be "settled law," as he reportedly had told Collins in his meeting with her?

Roe, Kavanaugh replied, was "settled as a precedent of the Supreme Court" and should be "entitled the respect under principles of stare decisis," the legal doctrine that says precedents should not be overturned without a very compelling reason.

"One of the important things to keep in mind about *Roe v. Wade* is that it has been reaffirmed many times over the past forty-five years, as you know," he said.

Feinstein interrupted him. In all her Supreme Court confirmation hearings, she said, the answer on Roe was always the same. "When the subject comes up, the person says, 'I will follow stare decisis,' and they get confirmed, and then, of course, they do not," she said. "So I think knowing going into it how you make a judgment on these issues is really important to our vote as whether to support you or not."

As Kavanaugh replied, McGahn sat directly behind him, jotting notes on a legal pad.

"I understand how passionate and how deeply people feel about this issue. I understand the importance of the issue. I understand the importance that people attach to the *Roe v. Wade* decision, to the *Planned Parenthood v. Casey* decision," Kavanaugh said. "I do not live in a bubble. I understand. I live in the real world."

Feinstein pressed again. Did he believe Roe was settled law? Yes or no?

Kavanaugh, again, returned to the answer given by so many in his position so many times. Roe was precedent. Even more, the decision in Casey that followed nearly two decades later made it "a precedent on precedent," he said. Feinstein moved on to her next issue.

That kind of polite evasion was largely how discussions of precedent always went for both Republican and Democratic nominees. In 2005, John Roberts called Roe "settled as a precedent of the court." In 2006, Samuel Alito called it "a precedent that has now been on the books for several decades." Sonia Sotomayor, three years later, said Roe was "the precedent of the court, so it is settled law." In 2010, Feinstein had a similar exchange over Roe with Elena Kagan, who referenced "the continuing holding" of the decision. And in 2017, Neil Gorsuch said that "a good judge" would consider Roe "as precedent of the U.S. Supreme Court worthy as treatment of precedent like any other."

But now, this crucial moment for federal abortion rights revealed how those traditional back-and-forths obscured the true stakes to the public. The legal jargon was difficult to understand. The questioning did not explain the judicial philosophy that drove a judge's interpretation of the law. An everyday viewer could walk away from watching the discussion without understanding that Roe was actually on the line.

Truthfully, there was little reason to even imagine that a culture-altering decision like Roe could ever be overturned. Precedent almost always stands. Republicans had vowed to overturn Roe for decades, but it never happened. To the public, Roe seemed indestructible, an indelible part of American life for two generations.

But in fact, the Kavanaugh moment was different. In a way, Trump had already betrayed the judicial impartiality Kavanaugh was trying to project. The antiabortion movement—through Trump—had a specific legal target and Trump had joined its mission. He said all the judges on the list had been selected because they were "pro-life." And when asked, in the third presidential debate, whether he wanted to see Roe reversed by the justices he had picked, Trump said it would happen "automatically."

In that old 2003 email, Kavanaugh, like Trump, pointed out another basic legal reality: precedents can change. The sense of their infallibility is based on legal traditions, not actual law. The principle of stare decisis is just that—a principle, not a mandate. And when precedents do change, they redefine the course of American history. *Brown v. Board of Education* in 1954 overturned Supreme Court precedent in *Plessy v. Ferguson*, ending the "separate but equal" doctrine behind Jim Crow laws and racial segregation in public schools. A precedent in 1918 allowed child labor, and the court overturned that decision during World War II.

Later in the questioning, Senator Richard Blumenthal, Democrat from Connecticut, returned to the question of Roe, but this time through the Jane Doe case. He told Kavanaugh that his dissent was a "signal" to the Trump White House, delivered in the language of the antiabortion movement, that he was "prepared" to overturn Roe. Kavanaugh denied that his use of "abortion on demand" was a code word, noting it was a term also used by legal scholars.

Blumenthal then asked the central question one more time, even more directly than Feinstein. "Can you commit, sitting here today, that you would never overturn *Roe v. Wade*?"

Once again, Kavanaugh dodged. "So. Senator, each of the eight justices currently on the Supreme Court, when they were in this seat, declined to answer that question," he said.

When the first round of hearings ended, even some of Kavanaugh's champions in the antiabortion movement still weren't sure if he would be with them on Roe or how far he would go. That was the whole point of citing precedent for Kavanaugh and the decades of judicial nominees who preceded him. It revealed nothing. And because the infallibility of precedent was a myth, it meant nothing either.

22

The War over Wen

When Heidi Heitkamp finally rose from her desk in the Senate chamber to cast her vote on the Kavanaugh nomination, she felt a deep sense of history. So much of what the Senate did was routine, passing the federal budget or statements of support for one cause or another. But for Heitkamp, this was a vote that could change the country for generations to come. Above her, in the gallery, female protesters screamed and chanted "Shame on you" at her Republican colleagues. Mike Pence, who was presiding from the dais, banged his gavel again and again, repeatedly asking the sergeant at arms to restore order. Heitkamp voted no, knowing the decision would cost her reelection. Susan Collins believed Brett Kavanaugh's promises of precedent and voted to put him on the court, along with one Democrat, Joe Manchin, who crossed party lines.

Kavanaugh was confirmed. He was the most unpopular nominee in thirty years, put on the court by a 50–48 vote, one of the slimmest margins in American history.

With Kavanaugh on the bench, the court was now more conservative than at any other point in modern history—by one scholar's estimate, since before World War II. Antiabortion activists had moved a pivotal piece of their strategy into place. There was a distinct conservative majority of five justices, and a liberal minority of four, without the confusion of a swing justice like Anthony Kennedy.

Still, only 39 percent of Americans believed Kavanaugh would vote to overturn Roe. An even smaller number of Republicans—a little more than a quarter—believed he would, according to polling.

Ilyse Hogue and Marjorie Dannenfelser and their allies on both sides had been preparing for this battle for years, starting before Donald Trump was inaugurated. They spent millions of dollars on Kavanaugh's confirmation, releasing a deluge of ads and protests, calls to Congress, and knocks on doors trying to sway public opinion to their side. Roe was mentioned more than 280 times in the hearings and in the testimonies and letters submitted to the committee from both sides.

But the drama over Christine Blasey Ford's explosive accusations pushed the issue to the back burner of the public conversation. Sexual assault became the dominant conversation, one that lingered into the elections. "I don't want to call it a distraction, because that sounds like it wasn't equally important," Hogue told *The New Yorker* days before voters headed to the polls. "But I think that, because of the power of that story, it eclipsed the other concerns."

Many antiabortion activists believed that Ford was persuaded to testify by Democrats who were afraid of losing Roe. But Ford didn't see herself as protecting Roe, according to Ricki Seidman, one of her advisers. She believed the Senate would confirm a conservative and simply wanted one without a history of sexual assault allegations. "I never had a conversation with her about Roe," said Seidman. Just as with Wendy Davis and her Texas filibuster, liberal America had grabbed headlines for protesting Kavanaugh's nomination. But now, Hogue saw how little that mattered. "People rose up in record numbers, and Republicans didn't even pretend to care," she said.

Kavanaugh was a capstone to female rage during Trump's first two years in office, and Americans responded weeks later in the midterm election with a Year of the Woman reminiscent of 1992. Democrats took power in the House, which soon had a female speaker when Nancy Pelosi reclaimed the gavel. A record total of thirty-six new women won House seats—all but one were Democrats. Their ranks included a litany of historic female firsts, including the first Muslim women in Congress and the first Native American women in Congress. There were four female military veterans. There were old political hands—like Donna Shalala, a member of Bill Clinton's cabinet—and new faces, like Alexandria Ocasio-Cortez, the twenty-nine-year-old who won an upset victory in New York City against a longtime party leader. Some, like Ocasio-Cortez's new "squad," were progressives. Others were moderates. But they all supported abortion rights.

It wasn't all good news for Democrats: Republicans expanded control over state governorships and rode a conservative backlash to the outcry over the charges of sexual assault to strengthen their control in the Senate, flipping four seats, including Heitkamp's in North Dakota. She might have lost even if she voted to confirm Kavanaugh, she realized. But there was little question that, politically, it would have been better for her to trust his promises of precedent, like Collins had, and vote to confirm him. Though it was hard to see at the time, with their wins in the Senate and governors' mansions, Republicans had increased the power of their antiabortion majorities in the places that mattered most in their longer-term fight against abortion rights.

Still, for the first time in the House, a majority of the representatives supported abortion rights. The last time Democrats controlled the House—before the 2010 Tea Party wave—there were still dozens of largely male antiabortion Democrats in their ranks, who along with antiabortion Republicans made it impossible to advance legislation protecting Roe. The effort pushed by Nancy Northup in 2013, titled the Women's Health Protection Act to be as broadly appealing as possible, never even reached a vote.

Representative Diana DeGette, a Democrat from Colorado who led the House Pro-Choice Caucus, saw new opportunities. Their best chance to codify Roe, to write it into national law instead of just relying on the 1973 court ruling, could come in as soon as two years—if Democrats held the House and gained control of the Senate and the White House. It was hardly impossible, she thought; Trump was so polarizing that Democrats just might be able to beat him in 2020. Still, a bill would be a heavy political lift, and there was no guarantee that any legislation wouldn't eventually be undercut by the court. But they could start getting ready now.

They needed to rally their troops, take advantage of the protests swelling on the outside to mobilize inside Congress. But their strongest ally, Planned Parenthood, was losing political traction. The brief, troubled tenure of Cecile Richards's successor, Dr. Leana Wen, would illustrate a central problem of the abortion-rights movement in the final years of Roe. At the height of the onslaught of the Trump administration, Planned Parenthood was at war with itself, arguing over tactics, strategy, and even the simple question of how to talk about abortion. While the antiabortion movement executed a multipronged attack to take down Roe, abortion-rights advocates couldn't seem to agree on the basics.

Wen, an emergency room physician, was the first doctor to run Planned Parenthood since the 1960s, and unlike Richards, she had limited political experience. She was an immigrant who worked her way from poverty to medical school—starting when she was just eighteen—then to a Rhodes Scholarship and, eventually, a position leading Baltimore's public health department.

Where Richards saw a political army in Planned Parenthood, Wen saw a medical powerhouse. "I want Planned Parenthood to be the doctor for American women," she told the board when she interviewed to replace Richards, according to a participant in the meeting. Planned Parenthood, under her leadership, could become an innovative health care system equal to Mayo Clinic. Its affiliates would be one-stop shops for health care, staffed with clinic workers prepared to address a range of problems from mental health disorders to substance abuse. It was a significant shift in vision, and Planned Parenthood's leadership was all in. She got the job with the board's unanimous support.

Not long after the 2018 "pink wave," Wen came in her hot pink blazer when Pelosi, the most powerful female politician in the country, invited her to be part of the resistance at Trump's State of the Union address. The Democratic women below her in the House chamber looked like beacons in their suffragist white blazers, standing out amid the seat of dark suits. And yet as Republicans thundered applause for Trump, Wen couldn't help but hear a very different message. One not of defiance, but of defeat. "Lawmakers in New York cheered with delight upon the passage of legislation that would allow a baby to be ripped from the mother's womb moments before birth," Trump said, devoting a section in one of his biggest speeches to target abortion rights. "These are living, feeling, beautiful babies who will never get the chance to share their love and dreams with the world. And then, we had the case of the governor of Virginia, where he basically stated he would execute a baby after birth."

"Execute a baby." The remark was a new twist on the graphic terms Trump used in the third presidential debate, this time drawing from a political controversy that had consumed Virginia and the nation in recent days. Democratic governor Ralph Northam, a pediatric neurologist, had stumbled into a political firestorm when he defended legislation that would lift some of the restrictions on third-trimester abortions in the state. Asked in a radio interview if the bill would allow an abortion even as a woman was in labor, he said no. Abortions late in pregnancy were rare and only done when the fetus faced "severe deformities." In cases where a woman goes into labor with a nonviable fetus in the third trimester, he continued, "the infant would be delivered, the infant would be kept comfortable, the infant would be resuscitated if that's what the mother and the family desired. And then a discussion would ensue between the physicians and the mother."

Northam thought he was describing a mother facing an impossible, unthinkable choice in a pregnancy gone terribly wrong. But to antiabortion activists, it was infanticide. Republicans from the

Virginia statehouse to Capitol Hill pounced on the remarks, depicting Democrats as monsters who would condone the murder of an infant.

The line had been a late addition to Trump's speech after Dannenfelser and a small set of conservative leaders came to the White House for a private preview of his remarks. Trump burst into the room, where they were meeting with Vice President Mike Pence and Kellyanne Conway. "Can you believe that crazy governor of Virginia?" he said, talking about the issue for five minutes, before switching to talk about expanding his wall across the southern border.

Over the weeks that followed, Trump embraced the infanticide message at rally after rally, turning the phrase *execute the baby* into a staple of his reelection events. During his first two years in office, Trump had rarely mentioned abortion in his public remarks. Now, in 2019, he mentioned the issue regularly, in inflammatory and inaccurate ways. "The baby is born," Trump said at a rally in Wisconsin. "The mother meets with the doctor. They take care of the baby. They wrap the baby beautifully, and then the doctor and the mother determine whether or not they will execute the baby."

Republican candidates across the country started following Trump's lead, making claims that Democrats promote "birth-day abortions" and were "the party of death." Coordinated campaigns by Dannenfelser and her allies targeted swing voters in battleground states with digital advertising repeating the claims. Again, it was an old message made new: the Willkes' 1971 handbook taught that abortion and infanticide were no different; both were forms of euthanasia, one prenatal, one postnatal. It was a core belief of the antiabortion movement, grounded in its fervently held belief that a single-cell zygote is a full human person deserving of civil rights.

The political conflation of murdering babies with abortion later in pregnancy was a misrepresentation of complicated medical procedures, a way to undercut all abortions by highlighting the small number of cases that surveys showed made Americans the most uncomfortable. Only about 1 percent of abortions happened after twenty-one weeks, just short of the viability line. Very limited data existed on the number after twenty-six weeks, though one older study estimated it was about 0.02 percent—a few hundred abortions. Providers who conducted these procedures described the devastating choices and circumstances that led to them. There were girls who were sexually abused before getting a period so they didn't realize they were pregnant. There were women who wanted a child but discovered late in their pregnancy that delivering could risk their life or future fertility. And then there were the women carrying fetuses with severe conditions who, if born, would suffer before dying shortly after birth. In those rare cases, the parents and doctors would have a discussion about end-of-life care after birth—not executions or infanticide.

Wen knew those medical realities didn't matter, at least not politically. As with the Daleiden videos, the antiabortion movement had defined the terms of this new debate, and abortion-rights advocates were struggling to catch up. A majority of Americans were aware of the "infanticide" claims, surveys by progressive groups found, showing that the message had reached into the political mainstream even if it was not true. Some Democrats argued against responding at all, saying that reacting to what they saw as clear misinformation would only amplify Trump's and the Republicans' claims. Wen disagreed. "Sometimes there is a temptation to let the absurdity stand on its own, but we have to recognize that this is a different time," Wen told *The New York Times*. "He's deliberately conflating infanticide with abortion late in pregnancy. And it's important that we as doctors and health care providers explain the extremely rare and devastating circumstances of abortion later in pregnancy."

For much of the Trump administration, Planned Parenthood had leaned into an unabashedly pro–abortion rights message, linking its mission to an array of liberal causes, including immigrant rights, racial justice, and even net neutrality. The night of Trump's

2018 State of the Union, Richards had cohosted an alternative event—the State of Our Union—organized to celebrate the power of women with a coalition of labor organizers, sexual assault survivors, and immigrants' rights advocates. Planned Parenthood was still a health care organization, with dozens of independent affiliates running hundreds of health care centers across the country. But now, it was also a leader of the Trump resistance, a potent, hot-pink symbol of liberal power in a country where all their values were under siege.

To Wen, the success of the campaign to rebrand abortion late in pregnancy as infanticide illustrated how deeply Planned Parenthood's strategy had failed. The hurricane had already struck, she thought; Roe was barely hanging on after the shift on the Supreme Court with Kavanaugh's confirmation. Their mission now was not only political advocacy but emergency management: how could resources be sent from places with trigger laws to places where abortion remained legal? Could they transport patients across state lines?

Planned Parenthood remained the top provider of abortions in America. But that was only one part of its medical practice, far smaller than services like testing for sexually transmitted infections and providing contraception. Some of its clinics offered family medicine, like treatment for rashes or gastroenteritis or conjunctivitis, pediatric care for low-income women, infertility services, or prenatal care. In thirty-one states, clinics offered transgender hormone therapy.

The only way to save Planned Parenthood's mission was to depoliticize it, Wen believed. If they could make clear that abortion was a part of health care, and only a small piece of Planned Parenthood's work, the attacks wouldn't carry as much power. "People aren't coming to Planned Parenthood to make a political statement," she told BuzzFeed News. "They're coming because they need their vaccinations. They need their well-woman exams. They're getting HIV tests."

The strategy marked a dramatic break from Richards, who required that all the organization's affiliates provide onsite abortions, a rule that prompted a few health centers to leave Planned Parenthood entirely. Instead of Richards's campaigns like "#Fight4Birth-Control" or "I Stand with PP," one of Wen's first efforts was called "This Is Health Care." She posted new sections on the group's website about chronic health conditions like diabetes, asthma, and the common cold—over objections from aides who worried it could expose the organization to attack, since they didn't provide care for those illnesses.

At a basic level, Wen believed she could do what would prove to be impossible: simply talk about abortion as a medical procedure. The new approach was a tactic Richards would have never considered and a line of thinking Ilyse Hogue at NARAL was actively trying to change among Democrats. And it would end shortly after it began. Just eight months after she started the job, Wen would be pushed out in an ugly public spat.

To many on her staff, Wen's vision of depoliticization seemed ridiculously naive, even dangerous. Wen, they thought, believed in a fantasy, a myth that abortion could be discussed solely as a clinical procedure. The antiabortion movement saw Planned Parenthood as a symbol of everything wrong with America. If it didn't defend itself, Planned Parenthood could lose what little ground it still had.

Tensions within the organization grew as the antiabortion forces in the White House advanced. Every month brought another blow. At the National Institutes of Health, the administration banned researchers from using fetal tissue in their work—the same kind of material Planned Parenthood officials discussed in the Daleiden videos. A new Health and Human Services rule required some insurers to issue a separate invoice for the amount of premium attributed to abortion services, a mandate insurers warned could result in the elimination of abortion coverage.

And at the United Nations, the antiabortion movement expanded its efforts to encompass not only the nation but the world.

US negotiators pushed to remove references to "universal access to sexual and reproductive health and rights" from an annual document about empowering women. In his address before the annual UN meeting later that year, Trump stressed his country's commitment to protecting "innocent life," as his administration unveiled a letter signed by the United States that there "is no international right to an abortion." The letter's other nineteen signatories were largely autocratic nations and those with poor records on women's rights, including Saudi Arabia, Yemen, Sudan, Libya, Russia, and Bahrain.

But the existential blow to Planned Parenthood came just weeks after Wen went to Trump's State of the Union address. The Trump administration announced it would ban any organization that performed or referred patients for abortions from receiving money through Title X—the federal program that pays for contraception and other reproductive health care for millions of low-income Americans. The policy change would eliminate as much as $60 million in annual funding from the program for Planned Parenthood clinics.

The change made antiabortion pregnancy centers, which were largely not medical facilities, and other community health organizations eligible to receive the grants, so long as they did not mention abortion as an option for their patients. In practice, the rule redirected tens of millions of dollars from Planned Parenthood to these centers. The Trump administration soon awarded $5.1 million in Title X funds to the Obria Group, an antiabortion organization that ran centers in six states. The group encouraged abstinence, marriage, and "natural family planning," and didn't offer hormonal birth control, including pills. At the time, Dannenfelser sat on its board.

It was a defunding, not by Congress, as Republicans had tried to do since Pence introduced the first bill more than a decade earlier, but by executive action. And this time, no senator could save them, like John McCain had in the early months of the administration.

Wen cast her opposition in clinical terms, accusing the Trump administration of violating medical ethics. "Imagine if the Trump administration prevented doctors from talking to our patients with diabetes about insulin. It would never happen. Reproductive health care should be no different," she told *The New York Times*. Planned Parenthood's lawyers prepared to sue the administration to block the policy as its policy experts contemplated whether the organization would need to withdraw from the program entirely—a once nearly unimaginable step.

Yet as she pushed back against the flood of outside attacks, Wen was fighting an internal uprising. Meetings with Planned Parenthood's state affiliates and national staffers exploded in recriminations after she publicly described abortions later in pregnancy as "extremely rare and devastating circumstances." To many of her staff, it felt like Wen was casting their movement back to Clinton's old language of "safe, legal, and rare." Wen wasn't just wrong, they thought, she was complicit in the stigma and shame that surrounded abortion in America.

Tensions between Wen and the liberal politics of many of her staffers consumed the organization. High-profile political aides quit. Damaging details about her brusque management style began seeping into the press, including a handbook that detailed best practices for working with her. Her rules included maxims like, "Make sure to frequently look up [from Twitter] and make eye contact with Dr. Wen to see if she is trying to communicate urgent information" and "Try not to look at emails more than once. Take care of it then."

Wen and her staff didn't just disagree. They didn't even speak the same language. Wen refused to use "trans-inclusive" language, reported BuzzFeed News, like pregnant "people" instead of pregnant "women." She argued that such terms would "isolate people in the Midwest," while her more progressive staff said the terms were more encompassing of all of Planned Parenthood's patients.

Wen was standing in a restroom stall when she overheard two people airing their frustrations: "I thought we'd get a rock star rabble-rouser, a congresswoman, or a senator," one said. "Instead, we got a doctor." Ten days later, Wen was fired in another unanimous board vote. She learned of her official ousting by reading about the news in *The New York Times*.

THE WAR OVER Wen laid bare a central tension of Planned Parenthood. The organization was both a health care provider and a political juggernaut. Amid the frenzied politics of the Trump era and the ever-growing restrictions in the states, balancing those two functions had become increasingly difficult. Planned Parenthood was a sprawling operation, a federation of fifty-three affiliated but separate state operations, with a nearly unmanageable financial structure, according to some board members. Each affiliate operated independently, with its own leaders and board, and fundraising apparatus to pay for staff, medical equipment, and services for uninsured patients. They paid dues to the national office, which focused more on campaigns, politics, and lobbying. And now, three years after they thought they would live in Hillary Clinton's America, every part of the operation was under attack.

A divided mission wasn't a challenge faced by Planned Parenthood's opponents, who had purely political groups, like the Susan B. Anthony List, and largely separate networks of crisis pregnancy centers. Planned Parenthood offered health care, with services that included breast cancer screening and vasectomies. The pregnancy crisis centers largely offered non-medical-grade sonograms, classes on baby care, free diapers, and other kinds of social support. They were not, nor did they aspire to become, the kind of world-class medical system that Wen had dreamed of making Planned Parenthood into.

As Planned Parenthood scrambled, longtime board member Alexis McGill Johnson took the reins as interim president. Almost immediately, she renounced Wen's efforts to minimize the organization's work providing abortions. "I think when we say, 'It's a small part of what we do,' what we're doing is actually stigmatizing it," she told *The Washington Post*. We are a proud abortion provider." One of McGill Johnson's first acts was to announce that Planned Parenthood was withdrawing from the Title X program due to Trump's new rule. That action only underscored the risks abortion rights faced in this changed national landscape. Republican governors were signing an unprecedented wave of abortion bans into law. And now, Kavanaugh was on the court, replacing Kennedy, who ruled in favor of federal abortion rights, with a justice who posed a potential threat to those rights. "A lot of us are awakening to the fact that if you are wealthy, if you live in the New York ZIP code or California ZIP code or Illinois ZIP code, your ability to access reproductive health care is not in jeopardy in the same way that it is in other states," McGill Johnson said.

Her early months were spent working to stabilize Planned Parenthood and rebuild trust within the organization after the infighting of Wen's tenure. Then McGill Johnson began to reimagine the organization entirely. Richards, a daughter of the Democratic Party, had focused on building political power. Wen, a public health expert, had emphasized its health care services. McGill Johnson, who built a career combating bias and discrimination, decided to prioritize racial equity.

Lori Alexis McGill was a self-described "movement baby," born five months before Roe, sandwiched between second-wave feminism and Black Power. Her mother worked her way up from a secretary at AT&T Bell Laboratories to the company's vice president of human resources, while paying her father's way through medical school. Her parents, she told *The Root*, were "race folks"—in dashikis and Afros, marching and organizing.

She went from Princeton to Yale, where she began going by her middle name, Alexis. After earning a graduate degree in political science, she taught courses on Black politics, race, and poverty at Yale and Wesleyan. She helped hip-hop icons like Russell Simmons and Sean "Puff Daddy" Combs form organizations, like the 2004 Vote or Die campaign, to turn out younger Black voters.

Her work with Planned Parenthood began in 2011, after a billboard in SoHo caught her eye. There, about a half mile from the Planned Parenthood clinic in Lower Manhattan, was a photo of an adorable Black girl in a pink sundress. The words printed above her read: "The Most Dangerous Place for an African American Is in the Womb." The ad was purchased by Life Always, a Texas antiabortion group, and part of a series of billboards posted by antiabortion organizations in urban areas that used photos of Black children to level charges of racism and genocide against abortion providers. It was a racist demonization of Black women's reproductive choices, McGill Johnson thought, something she associated with conservative states, not New York City. "I just was shocked, like, 'What is going on here?'" she remembered thinking.

A few weeks later, she found herself at a dinner party with Richards. At the time, she was leading the Perception Institute, the anti-discrimination think tank that she helped found to tackle racism and bias in school systems, police departments, health care providers, and corporations. She brought up the billboard. "This is horrible. You're the head of Planned Parenthood. You need to do something about this," McGill Johnson said. Richards shot back: "No, you need to do something about this." McGill Johnson joined the board soon after.

Now, with McGill Johnson as president, racial equity would become Planned Parenthood's new "North Star," she promised. In her Planned Parenthood, the staff would wake up every day and think about the experience of Black women, as patients and employees. She started programs to eradicate implicit bias in Planned Parenthood's care, from interactions with office staff to medical treatment to billing.

She wasn't Planned Parenthood's first Black president, a distinction that belonged to Faye Wattleton more than forty years earlier. But McGill Johnson believed that this was the time for her expertise to help correct historical wrongs and build an abortion-rights movement that better represented people who looked like her.

"What does it mean to show up unapologetically for your staff? To be able to say, 'We're going to talk about race, about intersectionality, about Margaret Sanger?'" she asked in an interview with *Elle*. "We are going to make a big bet on equity. It's our moonshot."

It was yet another vision for Planned Parenthood, a third shift in direction for the organization in as many years. Just three years earlier, in 2016, it had the power of the Obama White House and the protection of the Supreme Court. Hillary Clinton seemed ascendant, and they were preparing to expand abortion rights. Now, the organization was weakened, riven by infighting and boxed into refusing tens of millions in federal funds. It was perhaps the most vulnerable time in Planned Parenthood's more than one-hundred-year history, exactly as its opponents had hoped.

23

Gaming the Courts

Days after Brett Kavanaugh was confirmed in October 2018, Leonard Leo went on a media tour to boast about his new justice. His Federalist Society, he said, sitting down with PBS, had become much more powerful than just a "ragtag group of largely law students." Their ranks now included some of the country's most powerful people. Yet even as he won his decades-long dream of a conservative court, Leo urged caution. "If a vacancy occurs in 2020, the vacancy needs to remain open until a president is elected and inaugurated and can pick," he said. "That's my position, period."

Senate Republicans should not be hypocritical, he suggested. They should treat Trump as they did Obama with Antonin Scalia's seat, and deny the president the ability to get a justice on the court so close to the election. It was not a particularly hard vow to make. No president since Ronald Reagan had gotten three justices in a single term.

Leo believed the contentiousness of the confirmation process—how wronged Kavanaugh felt by it all—would work in his favor, making the new justice more uncompromisingly originalist and conservative in his views. "Brett Kavanaugh has seen how unforgiving the Left can be," he told *Time* magazine. "So Justice Kavanaugh has every incentive to basically do what he wants to do and ignore the Left."

But Kavanaugh was just one piece of the antiabortion leaders' plans, especially because they were not sure how far he would be willing to go. The entire machine they had been building to undermine abortion rights was starting to whir. They'd gotten the White House, expanded their margin in the Senate, and had justices they believed supported their cause on the court. In twenty-two states, Republicans now held complete control of state governments—both chambers of the legislature plus the governorship—giving them total power over abortion legislation. As Democrats celebrated their pink wave, the antiabortion movement looked to what it did control, which was significant. Power mattered, but to matter, it had to be in the right places at the right moment.

All those years of liberal protests—in the Texas State Capitol, on the National Mall for the Women's March, and on the steps of the Supreme Court during Kavanaugh's nomination—were proving to be no match for unified conservative control in statehouses. Republican states had now enacted 424 abortion restrictions since Tea Party Republicans took over state capitals in 2011. Eight years later, a new reality was rapidly becoming clear: in many parts of the United States, it was now more difficult to get an abortion than at any time since *Roe v. Wade* legalized the procedure nearly fifty years earlier. By early 2019, around twenty cases, with different legal strategies to gut Roe and Casey, were in litigation in lower courts, lined up to possibly reach the Supreme Court.

Activists in Mike Pence's home state were hoping Indiana's law banning abortion for race, gender, or disability preference might introduce new protections for the fetus. Alabama lawmakers hoped their strategy of banning the most common method of abortion would undercut Roe. In Ohio, the state Right to Life group reversed seven years of its incremental approach and backed a six-week "heartbeat" ban, which the governor soon signed into law. "Now is our time," Michael Gonidakis, president of the group, told *The New York Times*. "This is the best court we've had in my lifetime, in my parents' lifetime."

Antiabortion activists did not build just one plan. They built an ecosystem. So many people were working to dismantle Roe, in so many different ways, with so many different arguments, that eventually something was bound to work, they hoped. Even ADF was creating additional possible pathways to maximize its potential success. And suddenly, just after the 2018 midterm elections, they needed options.

A federal judge declared Mississippi's fifteen-week law unconstitutional and blocked it, permanently. The law "unequivocally" infringed on the due process rights of women guaranteed in the Fourteenth Amendment, ruled US District Court judge Carlton W. Reeves. He expressed frustration that Mississippi and other states insisted on passing these bans knowing they would be struck down, at a "tremendous" financial cost to the taxpayer.

"The Mississippi Legislature's professed interest in 'women's health' is pure gaslighting," he wrote in his decision. "The real reason we are here is simple. The State chose to pass a law it knew was unconstitutional to endorse a decades-long campaign, fueled by national interest groups, to ask the Supreme Court to overturn Roe v. Wade."

The fifteen-week law "is closer to the old Mississippi—the Mississippi bent on controlling women and minorities," Reeves, only the second Black judge appointed to a federal judgeship in the state, wrote in his opinion. "The Mississippi that, just a few decades ago, barred women from serving on juries 'so they may continue their service as mothers, wives, and homemakers.' The Mississippi that, in Fannie Lou Hamer's reporting, sterilized six out of ten black women in Sunflower County at the local hospital—against their will. And the Mississippi that, in the early 1980s, was the last State to ratify the 19th Amendment—the authority guaranteeing women the right to vote."

His opinion infuriated conservatives but did not stop ADF's plan to force a higher court challenge. Mississippi would, of course, appeal to the Fifth Circuit, and an ADF lawyer lined up to defend Governor Phil Bryant in his amicus brief, the "friend of the court" arguments that outside parties submit to support their position in a case.

But the ruling did complicate their strategy. Mississippi's law had been blocked so quickly. Some lawyers on ADF's team wondered if fifteen weeks was too early, and if they should try a number closer to twenty weeks. They started crafting another piece of model legislation that set the limit at eighteen weeks.

Like the fifteen-week mark, the eighteen-week mark had nothing to do with moral teachings about when a fetus becomes a person, the rights of a pregnant woman, medical realities, or the small number of abortions that occurred after that point in pregnancy. If the model legislation benefited women and children in that moment in that state, it was an ancillary outcome to the primary objective. This bill was again a litigation strategy and ADF was searching for that legal sweet spot. Their plan was still incremental: first to get rid of Roe's viability line, chipping away at the decision; and then, sometime in the future, ask the court directly to overturn Roe in a separate case.

Still, there was the problem that reaching the Supreme Court was a gamble in any situation. The court receives more than seven thousand requests for oral arguments each year but takes up only about eighty.

To increase their odds of getting picked, they needed a circuit split. If different federal circuit courts of appeals issued conflicting rulings about similar laws, the Supreme Court might feel compelled to resolve the legal dispute and set a new standard for the nation. Mississippi was never going to be enough. To provoke a Supreme Court challenge to Roe's viability rule, the strategy had to be much wider. They needed to find other states to pass their laws. ADF knew that any restriction would be contested in court by abortion-rights organizations, prompting another ruling. They would try to manufacture a split.

Attorneys reviewed the map. Mississippi was assigned to the Fifth Circuit Court of Appeals, increasingly known for its hard rightward turn under Trump, which might uphold the law. That would get them one ruling. Then they looked for states with favorable legislatures and governors who would be likely to pass an abortion-restriction bill. They trained their sights on two: Utah, in the Tenth Circuit, and Arkansas, in the Eighth. Both states had veto-proof Republican supermajorities in their legislatures, plus Republican governors.

ADF's strategy in state after state was to rely on the web of conservative Christian activists on the ground. Most every state had a policy group that promoted their values and an informal network of Christian lobbyists, legislators, local political activists, and church volunteers.

ADF invited these people to conferences, like the one Misha Tseytlin had attended, to organize them behind their shared goals of changing American culture through the law. Their closed-door legislative workshops, training, and networking sessions had a minimal online footprint, leaving little public trace of ADF's efforts to assess the nationwide state of play for their priorities and coordinate strategy.

ADF could trust these devoted activists to push their shared agenda, even if the grassroots didn't see the full legal chessboard. To strike at Roe, all it had to do was activate its allies and tap their local networks. ADF would stay two steps removed, ensuring the plan and its role as a master broker would remain in the background.

They already had a head start in Utah, where they had tried to create a split when they first pushed the Mississippi law in 2018. Gayle Ruzicka, president of the Utah Eagle Forum and a mother of twelve, had grown excited when she had first heard the pitch from a friend with the state attorney general's office who was volunteering with ADF. "'I've been working with them, there's this great bill, this fifteen-week bill, and they've written it in a way where we think we can get it through the courts,'" she remembered him saying. "The whole idea was, 'This is something that could overturn Roe.'"

Ruzicka needed no convincing. Like so many others in the movement, ending abortion was her life's ambition. For years, she had been a forceful presence inside the statehouse, peering down at lawmakers from the galleries, pressuring them to vote her way. She had worked with Phyllis Schlafly, the conservative anti-feminist activist, for decades, running a long-standing Christian policy center in the state. Decades earlier, she had organized the mothers in her community, the Church of Jesus Christ of Latter-day Saints, against issues like sex education and drugs.

They had to move quickly—the Utah legislative session was already in motion, and it was short. Ruzicka mobilized her allies, including Mary Taylor, who led Pro-Life Utah. She found a potential Republican sponsor, Senator Margaret Dayton, then the state's longest-serving female legislator, and gave her ADF's bill. Dayton had opposed abortion for years and had proposed legislation like banning abortion based on the sex of the fetus. But she did not want to support abortion up until fifteen weeks. Abortions later in pregnancy were like "child sacrifice," Dayton said, "like sacrificing children on the altar of convenience."

Like Becky Currie in Mississippi, Dayton said she didn't really know the ADF lawyers who came up with the bill. But she trusted Ruzicka to be her intermediary and just bring her the information, and agreed. "It wasn't my endgame, but it was better than nothing," she said. She also did not know details about Currie's bill in Mississippi or ADF's work to get that legislation moving. "We thought we were leading," she said, "and we were glad to do so."

From the outset, Dayton ran into trouble. The men in the Republican caucus seemed comfortable with the idea, she said, but some of the women did not want to take a stand either way. She ran out of time, and the bill stalled before she introduced it. Dayton decided to not seek reelection due to health issues. Ruzicka watched Mississippi's fifteen-week law move ahead alone.

When the time came for the 2019 session, Ruzicka set up a mission control center at long tables in the capitol cafeteria, organizing homeschool kids and retirees to rally lawmakers. She recruited a new Republican woman to sponsor the bill, Representative Cheryl Acton, a mother of four who ran for office to advance "freedom, civility, and the worth and dignity of every individual and family." But then, after the district court struck down Mississippi's law, Ruzicka heard from Acton and ADF lawyers: they wanted Utah to try eighteen weeks instead.

Kellie Fiedorek, the ADF lawyer who ran the network of state allies, went out to Utah to help direct the plan, Ruzicka said. Mary Taylor and Ruzicka were crushed. Banning abortion at fifteen weeks would stop more procedures and save more babies, they argued. But they listened to Fiedorek. The big-time lawyers were the experts, and if the fifteen-week law was truly never going to make it to the Supreme Court, they did not want to waste time. "We were so sad. There were tears," Taylor reflected later. "We were so heartbroken to have to give that ground."

Still, Ruzicka tried to focus on the ultimate prize: overturning Roe. "It's always strategy," she said. She pivoted to her next step: working to pass a trigger ban that would outlaw nearly all abortions in Utah if Roe were overturned.

As Ruzicka and Taylor worked in Utah, ADF ran a similar play in Arkansas, laying the groundwork in yet another circuit court. Just like in Mississippi and Utah, ADF got in touch with the person who ran a top Christian policy group in the state. In Little Rock, that was Jerry Cox, president of the Family Council. Around the time of Kavanaugh's confirmation, he was busy planning bills for the 2019 legislative session that aimed to advance biblical values in state law. His group was part of a network of dozens of similar groups in about forty states, affiliated with Focus on the Family, the evangelical group that shared a founder with ADF. Cox's policy group regularly attended ADF gatherings for lobbyists and policy allies like him to strategize legislative action.

It was a symbiotic relationship, reflecting ADF's outer network. "They don't have the boots on the ground like us," Cox said. "If they want to see a law passed in the state, they are dependent on us to walk into the capitol and find a sponsor, get people to vote for it."

ADF offered much in return. It helped smaller organizations like his, Cox explained. Local nonprofits often lack the financial resources to hire lawyers on their own to write legislation. ADF could deliver the bills to advance his values. "It's kind of like ordering up a hamburger," he said. ADF then tracked the legislation across the states to produce results on a larger scale.

Like Jameson Taylor in Mississippi, Cox had worked with ADF lawyers several years earlier to enact a religious freedom bill like Pence's in Indiana, as conservatives pushed back against gay marriage. And, like Ruzicka and Taylor, Cox had been working on antiabortion legislation in Arkansas for years, since Democratic governor Bill Clinton signed a parental consent law that he championed in 1989.

Cox initially wanted to try a fifteen-week bill after watching Mississippi. He knew the magic number of weeks could not be less than fifteen—Arkansas had tried a twelve-week law in 2013, and the courts struck it down. But an eighteen-week ban would not have much of an impact on stopping abortions. In 2017, only seventy-five abortions were performed in Arkansas after eighteen weeks, just 2 percent of all the abortions the state health department recorded.

But Fiedorek's strategy convinced him. The point was the litigation tactic, not really the policy itself. The process would repeat ADF's play in Mississippi, but with the new twist of eighteen weeks. ADF brought Cox into the fold, telling him about its work in Utah and explaining its broader legal strategy. "They said if both of these percolate up through the system, we might end up with a split between circuits with the Eighth Circuit holding ours, and the circuit that Utah is in, going the other way," Cox remembered. "And therefore we would get a case in front of the Supreme Court."

Cox deferred entirely to ADF's direction on the eighteen-week bill, just as Ruzicka had in Utah. He wanted to be certain that the bill would do "what we intend, which is to give the court an opportunity to either overturn Roe or chip away at it.

"We said, 'Write it the way you want to because this is going to go before the Supreme Court,'" he remembered telling ADF. "They wrote every bit of that bill. We totally relied on them."

The pipeline was extraordinarily powerful. It appeared to the public, and even some local activists, like a grassroots strategy, emerging organically from a groundswell of conservative pushback to abortion rights among activists and state legislators. But the inner maneuverings of ADF's shadow network revealed that the cultural change campaign was really coming from an elite group at the top. The local activists pushing these bills deferred to ADF lawyers and acted simply as vehicles to turn the group's ideas into actual policies—and lawsuits.

Cox asked Representative Robin Lundstrum, a lifelong Southern Baptist who was on his board, to sponsor the bill. Lundstrum was another ideal spokeswoman, representing the conservative womanhood her movement wanted to emphasize. She had a doctorate in health sciences and had started her career working for a rape hotline in Tulsa that connected victims calling 911 with an advocate who met them in the ER and helped them navigate everything from prosecution to pregnancy choices. She remembered being in her early twenties, sitting with a rape victim who decided to give birth and through the experience found some meaning in her trauma. That experience made Lundstrum oppose abortion even in cases of rape and incest—and more open to the death penalty for abusers.

"In my estimation, we don't punish the child; we don't abort a child for rape and incest. If we want to punish someone, it should be the perpetrator. We need to up the penalties," she explained.

Lundstrum decided to sponsor the most hard-line version of the bill. It would have no exceptions for rape and incest. It would change the way pregnancy is dated, to count weeks from a woman's last period instead of from fertilization. Arkansas's existing twenty-week ban dated weeks to fertilization, so this change effectively moved up the timeline by a month. The legislation was written as an eighteen-week ban. But in effect, it was closer to Mississippi's fifteen weeks.

Even though there was a Republican supermajority, the bill was "a slugfest" to get passed, Lundstrum said. Partway through the process, she heard that the governor, Republican Asa Hutchinson, was trying to kill the bill because it had no exceptions for rape and incest. She rushed to his office with Senator Jason Rapert, her co-sponsor in the Senate.

"Let me be frank, out of the four people in this room, only one of us has been pregnant, and I have been pregnant four times," she told him. "Unless you know something I don't, the cake is baked at eighteen weeks. You know you are pregnant." But, she remembered, "He said, 'Add back the rape exception, otherwise we will kill it.' . . . We did, much to my chagrin."

Hutchinson signed the bill on March 15. Much of the language was identical to Mississippi's, down to "unborn human being" and the fetal development at various weeks—except for the eighteen-week change. In Utah, Governor Gary Herbert signed his state's version a week later.

The same legislative session, Arkansas also passed a trigger ban that would outlaw nearly all abortions if Roe were overturned. The idea was to get all the pieces in place. That legislation was sponsored by Rapert, who later that year started the National Association of Christian Lawmakers, which organizes lawmakers around "clear Biblical principles." His group was the first to unite conservative Christian lawmakers, federal, state, and local, around their shared religious values, which could then be turned into legislation they could push in statehouses across the country. The group cited an Old Testament verse as a rallying cry: "Blessed is the nation whose God is the Lord." It was a step toward a long-term outcome of lowering the wall separating church from state.

Even with ADF's planning, many pieces had to fall into place for Roe to be overturned. In Mississippi alone, where the case was still waiting at the Fifth Circuit, there was also the matter of the attorney general, the law enforcement official who would be responsible for fighting for the law in court. Mississippi's attorney general, Jim Hood, an antiabortion Democrat, was running for governor. There would be an open race to replace him, in a state that backed Trump by double-digits just three years earlier. Now, ADF would likely get a Republican attorney general, but it could be one who wasn't known as a particular champion of its cause.

Lynn Fitch, the state's treasurer and most powerful female elected official, had jumped into the race. Unlike Currie, Fitch hadn't built her political career out of the antiabortion movement. She rarely talked about the issue, though she realized the next legal steps of the case would be waiting for her if she won. When Mississippi's fifteen-week ban passed, the Democratic woman who would run against her in the general election—Jennifer Riley Collins, the executive director of the American Civil Liberties Union of Mississippi—warned that it would "seriously harm low-income women, women of color, and young women." If elected, Collins would be the first African American to win a statewide office in more than a century, when a handful were elected during Reconstruction. But the fifteen-week ban wasn't a major issue in the Republican primary. So Fitch, then state treasurer, largely kept quiet on the law, focusing her early campaign on crime, human trafficking, and protecting gun rights.

The Supreme Court had also handed the antiabortion movement a setback in February 2019, blocking a Louisiana law that required doctors performing abortions at clinics to have admitting privileges at local hospitals. The law would have left the state with only one doctor in a single clinic authorized to provide abortions. John Roberts joined the liberal justices to keep the clinics open. The short order gave no reasons for the decision. Only Kavanaugh published a dissent, saying he would have let the law go into effect to see if additional doctors could obtain admitting privileges. The case did not end the law, just put it on hold pending an appeal, meaning it was likely headed back to the court to be argued on the merits during the next term. If that happened, those arguments could end up becoming the first true test of what the antiabortion movement hoped would be its powerful new majority.

For now, abortion-rights supporters heralded their victory. "The Supreme Court has stepped in under the wire to protect the rights of Louisiana women," said Nancy Northup, the president of the Center for Reproductive Rights. "This should be an easy case—all that's needed is a straightforward application of the court's own precedent."

Senator Susan Collins of Maine, who voted for Kavanaugh, dismissed his dissent as any kind of sign that he would take a more forceful strike against abortion rights in the future. "To say that this case, this most recent case, in which he wrote a very careful dissent, tells you that he's going to repeal *Roe v. Wade*, I think, is absurd," she told CNN. "There is a deliberate misreading of what he actually wrote, or people have just assumed and not read the decision."

But leaders of the antiabortion movement saw Kavanaugh's dissent as a signal that he could be with them. Their network kept working, pushing an unprecedented rush of abortion bans through conservative statehouses in 2019. Those laws gave ADF and other antiabortion lawyers options as they looked toward the Supreme Court. The laws were being lined up "like airplanes on the runway," Cox said. Mississippi's—or ADF's—fifteen-week law was already "airborne," he said, preparing for its case at the Fifth Circuit. And behind it, the taxiway was filling.

24

The Thread

Ilyse Hogue of NARAL worried as she tracked the numbers. It was the spring of 2019, the Democratic presidential primary campaign was already underway, and twenty-three candidates were vying to combat Donald Trump in the coming general election. Abortion-rights advocates desperately needed a champion for their cause. The situation seemed to grow more dire by the week, as state after state passed abortion bans. In May, Alabama surpassed Mississippi for approving the most restrictive abortion law in the country, a near total ban, including in cases of rape and incest, with limited exceptions for the health of the mother.

Most of the Democratic primary candidates responded with force. Senator Elizabeth Warren warned of "back-alley butchers" and "desperate women." Senator Kamala Harris solicited donations for abortion funds. Senator Kirsten Gillibrand called for Americans to "fight like hell" against the new bans.

But the front-runner was more like the kind of Democrat Hogue had tried to purge the party of the year before than his rivals were. Like Trump, who Marjorie Dannenfelser once worried wouldn't support the antiabortion cause, Joe Biden wasn't known as a stalwart champion of Hogue's movement. He released one comment about Alabama's new near-total ban, using language about "choice" that abortion-rights supporters had long ago disavowed. "Roe v. Wade is settled law and should not be overturned," Biden wrote on social media. "This choice should remain between a woman and her doctor."

That kind of restraint didn't cut it for Hogue. She didn't know about ADF's specific plans. But she saw an ecosystem of antiabortion activists pushing toward the Supreme Court. "All of these state legislators are acknowledging that these bills are designed to actually gut Roe and criminalize abortion—and they're doing that now because they don't know if they'll have the White House in 2020, and they need to move fast," she said in an interview with *The Riveter*, the online publication of a women's professional network.

Democrats needed a more aggressive approach, and it couldn't wait. The next president had to be the fiercest defender of abortion rights. And for Hogue and other abortion rights activists, that wasn't Biden. He refused to meet with their movement. He wouldn't talk about the issue publicly. And he continued to support the Hyde Amendment, which barred the use of Medicaid funding for most abortions, despite the party rejecting the policy in its 2016 platform. Hogue knew his record—and she didn't like it. Biden, she and others in her movement believed, represented a generation of Democrats who were squishy on abortion rights and whose era had passed.

Unlike Trump, Biden held strong beliefs about abortion. He was raised in the Catholic church in the post–World War II era. As a child, Biden learned that life began at conception and abortion was murder. But as a Democratic politician, he championed the liberal pluralism that he saw as central to American values. Torn between allegiance to his faith and his politics, Biden would spend nearly a half century struggling to square his two belief systems.

He entered the Senate at age thirty in 1973, just weeks before Roe was decided, as he sought comfort in his faith following the deaths of his wife and infant daughter in a car crash in Delaware. In an interview with the celebrity biographer Kitty Kelley the next year, when Americans were divided over issues of drugs and young people who had avoided the draft, he made his opposition to the procedure clear. "When it comes to issues like abortion, amnesty, and acid, I'm about as liberal as your grandmother," he said. "I don't like the Supreme Court decision on abortion. I think it went too far. I don't think that a woman has the sole right to say what should happen to her body."

In his early years in the Senate, Biden was an antiabortion Democrat who backed a constitutional amendment allowing states to overturn Roe. Over the four decades that followed, his position evolved. Biden still backed policies limiting abortion access, like the so-called partial-birth abortion ban championed by the Bush administration and the Hyde Amendment. He believed taxpayer funds should not pay for abortion procedures. But in later interviews, he defended Roe as correctly decided.

By the time he ran for president in 2007, against Obama and Clinton, Biden had come to a decision: Roe was the best means in a "heterogeneous society" to find some "general accommodation on what is a religiously charged and a publicly charged debate," he said on *Meet the Press* that year. He drew a firm line between his policy choices and his faith, taking the opposite view from conservative Catholics like Leonard Leo and Marjorie Dannenfelser. "I'm prepared to accept that at the moment of conception there's human life and being, but I'm not prepared to say that to other God-fearing, non-God-fearing people that have a different view," he told the Catholic magazine *America* in 2015.

Biden's position was clear: personally antiabortion; politically pro–abortion rights. It was a view that made him like so many Americans with their own, idiosyncratic views on the topic. For decades, public opinion surveys struggled to capture those complexities, making polling about the specifics of abortion policies notoriously unreliable. So much depended on how the questions were phrased. Were the words *pro-life* and *pro-choice* used? Politicized terms like *partial-birth abortion* or clinical ones? Different surveys would deliver results that seemed contradictory, such as a majority of voters saying they wanted abortion to be legal in "all or most cases," but large shares also backing various restrictions, like fifteen-week bans or parental notification.

But a few policies had clear and broad support. A majority of Americans backed some form of federal abortion rights. A majority of Americans supported Roe. A majority believed abortion should be legal in cases of rape or incest, or if the mother's health was at risk. Americans became more uncomfortable with abortion as pregnancy progressed, though they disagreed on precisely when the limit should be set. And many Americans believed taxpayer dollars shouldn't pay for abortions.

And so, in 2020, as the other Democrats running for their party's nomination offered uncompromising defenses of the procedure, Biden rarely spoke about the issue publicly. When he did, it was always in euphemisms, never uttering the word *abortion*. Privately, he worried that the uncompromising pro–abortion rights rhetoric of his rivals could alienate the moderates his party would need to win a general election against Trump. And despite a pressure campaign from abortion-rights activists, he refused to budge on his support for the Hyde Amendment.

To the activists, Biden's candidacy felt like moving backward to a time when abortion was kept in the shadows. As they saw it, Hyde was an issue of reproductive rights but also racial justice and health care. The policy meant that more than 7.9 million low-income Americans—overwhelmingly women of color—were denied coverage for an abortion, making them more likely to end up carrying a pregnancy to term if they couldn't find the money to pay for the procedure. As Republican states ratcheted up their efforts to pass restrictive abortion laws, Biden's position signified to some liberal voters that he was out of date and out of touch with the stakes of this new fight, campaign aides warned. Just as Trump's Make America Great Again movement pushed the Republican Party further to the right, the response to Trump's administration had emboldened the liberal flank of the Democratic Party. Positions once considered radical, like expanding the Supreme Court, abolishing Immigration and Customs Enforcement, and eliminating the Hyde Amendment, had become mainstream, championed by top candidates in the party's primary.

Most of his primary opponents had adopted the party's position in their platform. Several now highlighted their opposition to the policy to cast Biden as out of touch. "No woman's access to reproductive health care should be based on how much money she has. We must repeal the Hyde Amendment," Senator Kamala Harris of California wrote on social media.

Celebrity allies, powerful Black female Democrats, and abortion-rights activists pushed Biden to change his position on Hyde. "You can't tell me that this vice president who has been a champion for women would want to continue a discriminatory policy that is so detrimental to poor women, to women of color, to low-income women," Representative Barbara Lee, a Democrat from California and progressive champion, told *The New York Times* of Biden's position. Under pressure, Biden came to realize that the times had changed from when he first supported Hyde all those decades ago. It wasn't just the Democrats who had shifted: Republicans had become more uniform in their opposition to abortion since the early 1990s, when Biden was being lobbied as a swing vote on the issue in the Senate. They'd embraced state abortion bans, which, Biden thought, had forced a discussion about racial and economic equity. That, too, was a core tenet of Catholic social teaching, which stressed helping the poor and vulnerable.

In early June, Biden headed to Atlanta to address a DNC fundraising dinner. The Georgia legislature had passed a six-week abortion ban just weeks earlier. Reading the additional pages aides inserted into his speech for the event, he made peace with changing his thirty-year-old position. "I signed up to do this to win," he said. "That has to be part of the equation." When he took the stage, his stance was clear. "If I believe health care is a right, as

I do, I can no longer support an amendment that makes that right dependent on someone's ZIP code," he said.

Still, even after his announcement, Biden wrestled with how the rapid escalation of abortion bans and the radicalization of the antiabortion movement during the Trump administration had made his support for Hyde, a policy he long viewed as a compromise position between his faith and his politics, rapidly untenable. "What hit me was we're in a situation where when the assault was going on in Georgia, what's going on in Alabama, Missouri, it's just outrageous," Biden said, campaigning in Iowa. "How do you say, 'Well, guess what, it's gone, it's gone'? So that's the reason why I made that decision."

Yet, while Hogue and her allies won over Biden in the primary, they did not maintain their grip as the race moved toward the general election. As Warren, Harris, and others embraced policies like requiring private insurers to cover abortion and making abortion pills available over the counter, Biden stayed mum. His campaign didn't release an abortion policy plan and declined to respond to a *New York Times* survey on the candidates' views. There was little evidence from 2012 or 2016 that the issue energized large swaths of Democratic voters, his aides argued, so why force Biden to highlight an issue that he struggled to discuss publicly?

The Democratic Party followed his lead. At its national convention in August 2020, the word *abortion* was never uttered. On the rare occasion the issue was raised, it was through the language of racial justice, with more oblique references, like when Harris, the vice-presidential nominee, spoke about inequities in "reproductive and maternal health care."

The silence frustrated Hogue. Biden was their nominee. He would be challenging the most antiabortion president in history. And he didn't seem to want to talk about abortion at all. In strategy memos and presentations to politicians and aides, she urged Democrats to talk more about the issue. Yet, even the abortion-rights movement could not agree on what to say. With the general election looming, each of the three major national abortion-rights political organizations took a slightly different approach to the issue. Under Alexis McGill Johnson's leadership, Planned Parenthood cast the race as a battle for reproductive health care, embracing another new slogan—"Bans Off Our Bodies"—as the number of restrictions ballooned in Republican states. EMILYs List ran only one notable general election ad about abortion, attacking incumbent Senator Susan Collins for backing Brett Kavanaugh as she ran for reelection in Maine. And at NARAL, after investing in a yearslong research project to figure out the best messaging for the movement, Hogue was trying to rally Democrats around the idea of framing abortion as a personal freedom—a classic American value. In presentations detailing their new approach, which was based on intensive polling and focus groups, NARAL strategists advised Democrats to play offense by describing the full scale of state restrictions and promising to create a country where "people respect other people's personal decisions around parenthood and pregnancy." Much of their research showed that "freedom to decide" was a more powerful argument for Americans than Planned Parenthood's messages about health care and women's rights.

To local abortion-rights activists in states that had passed restrictive abortion laws, the whole discussion about messaging felt entirely out of touch. As Democrats debated whether to talk about abortion and movement activists fought over how to discuss it, abortion providers were struggling with the most basic function of all: providing it.

While Planned Parenthood remained the biggest abortion provider in the country in 2019, it wasn't performing the majority of abortions in America. About 60 percent of abortions happened in small, unaffiliated independent clinics, which performed most of the controversial procedures later in pregnancy.

The flood of state restrictions had forced more than a third of those clinics to close their doors. In 2012, when Obama was president, there were 510 independent abortion clinics, according to the

Abortion Care Network, the national association of independent clinics. By 2019, their numbers were down to 344.

Those clinics had little lobbying power and none of the fund-raising prowess or brand recognition of Planned Parenthood. "We don't have the infrastructure," said Tammi Kromenaker, the straight-shooting feminist activist who ran Red River Women's Clinic, the only remaining abortion clinic in North Dakota. "You need an advocacy person? That's me. You need a legal person? That's me. Someone to plunge the toilet? That's me."

Many of these providers felt dismissed and powerless. Some of them blamed Planned Parenthood for dominating the debate, sucking up financial resources to bolster its own operation while ignoring the clinics struggling to provide services in the most hostile areas. "When people are up in arms and angry and upset about the bans, their instinct is to give to Planned Parenthood," said Kwajelyn Jackson, the executive director of the Feminist Women's Health Center in Atlanta, an independent clinic. "People want to do what's easy. Planned Parenthood is easy to think about."

Alabama provided a striking example of the disconnect. In the weeks after its near-total ban was passed, celebrities and liberal donors poured money into Planned Parenthood. Musicians, from Lizzo to Carole King to John Legend, promoted the group's #BansOffMyBody campaign. Ariana Grande donated the proceeds from her concert sales, and the founder of Tumblr pledged $1 million.

But Planned Parenthood didn't actually perform abortions in the state. Its two Alabama clinics hadn't offered abortion services since March 2017, according to data from the state department of health, though they advertised the service. Meanwhile, Gloria Gray, the head of the independent West Alabama Women's Center in Tuscaloosa, was having trouble paying her bills. Her clinic performed more than 3,300 abortions in 2018, more than half of all the procedures in Alabama. Yet she couldn't afford a $20,000 fence to keep the protesters off the property. While Planned Parenthood collected millions, her crowdfunding effort produced about $4,000. "We saw an outpouring of love and support throughout the whole country, to which we're very grateful," said Gray. "But we as independent providers have not necessarily seen a lot of benefit from that."

Even within Planned Parenthood, disparities persisted between the national office, which raised hundreds of millions to be spent on lobbying and campaigns, and its independent affiliates, which paid dues to the national office to operate their clinics under the organization's brand. Some of their health centers in conservative states struggled financially, constantly racing to keep up with laws requiring they meet standards that made it expensive and burdensome to operate.

There had been no movement-wide strategy to prepare for the multipronged legal assault from the antiabortion forces. "They are pulling us in fifty million different directions. You can't just go to the US Congress. It is this legislature, that one. This one meets this month. This one meets every other year. It's Whac-A-Mole," said Kromenaker, in North Dakota. "I don't think anybody ever thought it would get to where it is right now."

Kromenaker grew up Catholic and opposed abortion. She broadcast her views, even pasting a GOD IS PRO-LIFE bumper sticker in her dorm room at Minnesota State University. Then a friend had an unwanted pregnancy, and her views changed. It was "an immediate flip of the switch," she said. After graduation, Kromenaker got a job as a part-time patient advocate at the clinic in North Dakota. Eventually, she became the owner of the small brick building in Fargo. The clinic didn't see a ton of patients. Maybe twenty or twenty-five on Wednesdays, when staffers performed abortions. But many of those patients traveled hours to reach the state's only abortion provider. After more than two decades, the lavender walls of the intake rooms, the rituals of patients and procedures, even the hate mail had become the rhythm of Kromenaker's daily life.

Kromenaker echoed a version of Leana Wen's philosophy. Planned Parenthood's focus on progressive politics had not helped her in North Dakota—or preserved the political career of Heidi Heitkamp, their former senator—and in the fall of 2019, it felt like very little could. The attacks were coming too fast and too frequently. "I don't think anyone ever foresaw that we would need a movement strategy," she said at the time. "We've had Roe." If abortion-rights activists could do it all again, Kromenaker thought, they wouldn't have stopped at the Supreme Court back in 1973. They would have worked to enshrine abortion rights state by state, town by town, to protect Roe from conservative state legislators.

But, of course, that wasn't what happened. And now there was no broader plan—or even a unified national message—to fight back in this crucial moment. If Roe fell, a trigger law would ban abortion in her state within thirty days. Similar laws were on the books in a dozen other states. They would essentially make the procedure illegal across broad swaths of the South and Midwest.

To Kromenaker, it was clear that the fate of Roe now rested on the frail shoulders of Ruth Bader Ginsburg, the now-elderly Supreme Court justice whose picture was displayed on a banner in Kromenaker's office. Roe itself felt like it was dangling, too, she thought.

"I can only be hopeful that we don't get to the place where it is all taken away for us to realize what is going on," she said. "It feels like it is hanging by a Ginsburg thread."

25

Mississippi Womanhood

In Jackson, Lynn Fitch, now the Republican attorney general of Mississippi, had unpacked all her boxes, hired new staff, and dragged an old, heavy desk into her new office. It was the desk of her mentor, Evelyn Gandy, the first woman elected to a statewide constitutional office in Mississippi. Like Gandy, Fitch was making history: the single mother of three was the first female attorney general in the state.

That turbulent summer of 2020, thousands of protesters from Black Lives Matter Mississippi marched below her office on the twelfth floor of the Walter Sillers State Office Building, a Brutalist tower named for a famed segregationist politician. They knelt in silence for eight minutes and forty-six seconds, as long as the white officer in Minneapolis had pressed his knee into George Floyd's neck. Days after Floyd's murder, Fitch had decided to drop the prosecution of a white police officer who had shot and killed a Black man during a traffic stop in 2015. She said that the officer's actions were "necessary self-defense." Her decision had helped fuel the largest demonstration in Jackson since the Freedom Summer of 1964, the height of the civil rights movement. Half a century later, families and activists were demanding change in a state that remained one of the most segregated in America.

"When Mississippi changes, America changes," an organizer declared at the podium. And in the midst of the coronavirus pandemic and a racial reckoning, Mississippi was changing. Just not the way the protesters might have thought. History was turning in far quieter corners.

Up above the protests, the legal fate of the fifteen-week abortion ban was sitting on Gandy's old desk. Like Judge Carlton W. Reeves in the district court, the Fifth Circuit Appeals Court had also rejected the law, with all three judges on the panel agreeing that it should be struck down. The lower court's decision would stand unless the state of Mississippi appealed. For the Supreme Court to take the case, Fitch would have to ask. That was the role of the state attorney general. She could file for *cert*—formally known as a petition for *writ of certiorari*—the legal request for the high court to review the lower-court decision.

Within the Fifth Circuit's rejection was a notable concurring opinion, written by Judge James Ho, a former clerk for Clarence Thomas and leader in the Federalist Society who was appointed by Donald Trump during his first year in office. Republicans in Texas had blocked Barack Obama from filling his seat on the court for three years, running out the clock until the end of Obama's term. Thomas swore Ho into office at the Harlan Crow Library in Dallas, a private collection of the billionaire donor who was close to both Thomas and Leonard Leo.

Ho agreed with the Fifth Circuit's ruling to strike down the law, saying the court was required to follow the precedent of Roe. But functionally, his opinion was a dissent wrapped in the packaging of agreement, one that laid the legal groundwork for the new conservative majority on the Supreme Court to take an interest in the case. If Fitch and her team decided to appeal to the court, Ho's writing offered guidance for the kind of reasoning that might compel the justices to take up the case.

In his opinion, Ho offered an extensive originalist explanation for why the precedent of Roe was not supported by the text of the Constitution or its original meaning. He cited issues like Reeves's decision to decline testimony from an SBA scholar who argued that a fetus could feel pain as early as ten weeks, suggesting that the Supreme Court should consider the fetal pain argument. Ho drew a line from this case to when lower courts allowed controversial testimony in *Brown v. Board of Education*, which overturned Supreme Court precedents and ended racial segregation in public schools.

He also slammed Reeves for suggesting the fifteen-week law was sexist and racist. "I find it deeply disquieting that a federal court would disparage the millions of Americans who believe in the sanctity of life as nothing more than 'bent on controlling women and minorities,'" he said. Instead, he pointed to a rising "pro-life feminism," citing a group of female scholars who had spent years arguing that legalized abortion doesn't liberate women—but oppresses them.

As a politician, Fitch had rarely focused on abortion. Few in the antiabortion movement even knew her. But she subscribed to Ho's broader concept of conservative feminism, a philosophy that purported to empower women but was not rooted in the liberal movement of the 1970s.

Fitch's personal story and ambitions represented a strain of femininity that ran deep in Republican states like hers, one that tried to square women's professional achievements with more traditional ideals of womanhood. Their vision was grounded in traditional Christian femininity. And it was closely tied to the cultural mission of antiabortion activists like Marjorie Dannenfelser and Kellyanne Conway and the rising class of conservative women—elected officials and judges like Amy Coney Barrett in the Seventh Circuit Court of Appeals—who were becoming the new faces of their cause.

The thinking amounted to an attempt to reappropriate the feminist movement that had transformed the country since Roe. In some ways, Fitch's rise mirrored that of Ann Richards, another divorced mother who had started her career as state treasurer. But the two women symbolized very different ideals of American womanhood. Richards was an icon of the liberal feminism of the boomer generation, a movement intertwined with the battle for abortion rights and Roe. Fitch symbolized the conservative backlash to that movement.

Fitch entered government in 1984, after becoming one of just fourteen women to take the bar in Mississippi that year—so few that they could all sit at one table. Gandy, her mentor, hosted Fitch and the other female lawyers for regular meetings to plot ways to expand their role in state politics. When Gandy suggested the idea of a women's professional committee at the state bar, she asked Fitch, then a lawyer for the state legislature, to present the proposal to the all-male commissioners. "Can you get all those woman things done in a year?" they asked. Fitch bit her tongue and said she'd "certainly try." Eventually, she got a seat as a commissioner herself, serving as she developed her private practice as a bond lawyer.

Along the way, Fitch had three children, and then divorced. Wanda Lynn Fitch Mitchell, wife and mother, became Lynn Fitch, single mom. School tuition and medical expenses, gas and phone bills, a fraternity pledge trainer for her son and sorority dues for a daughter: Fitch and her husband battled over it all for years in court filings, down to the $196.88 to replace the windshield on her son's car. A second marriage to a former Secret Service agent for Ronald Reagan ended in divorce after two years, just as her campaign for state treasurer heated up. But with her tight-knit group of girlfriends and color-coded calendars and babysitters, she made it all work, ignoring when her male colleagues disparaged her for sneaking out for school plays or to help her father.

As state treasurer, her passion was women's economic advancement, a focus that fit neatly into the purview of her role. "As women, we're doing better, we're earning more, but we still have old-school concepts about budgeting, about not looking at the big picture," she told female business leaders at the Tupelo Country Club. She threw her support behind an equal-pay law, named after Gandy. It failed to move out of the legislature for years—a loss Fitch attributed in part to the fact that the state had fewer female legislators than most of America—something Becky Currie knew well too.

When Trump was nominated, Fitch was a committee member for the Republican Party platform and successfully added a clause mandating that fathers were responsible for their babies from birth through adulthood. "It was an opportunity to put some language in there for states to pass legislation in regard to women's inequality," she told *The Daily Mississippian*.

Fitch was rarely asked to prove her antiabortion bona fides. In Mississippi, opposition to abortion was a given in politics, even among Democrats. Nationally, just 12 percent of Americans thought abortion should be illegal in all cases. In Mississippi, 59 percent of adults thought abortion should be illegal in all or most cases. In the rare instances that the fifteen-week law came up during her race for attorney general, Fitch promised to do "everything she could" to move the case along if she won.

And as soon as she got into office, Fitch made good on that promise. She began preparing to ask the Supreme Court to review the Fifth Circuit's decision to strike down the law. The chances that this abortion case would be accepted by the court seemed low, especially given the Fifth Circuit's reputation for a conservative bent. The two other abortion laws challenged by Center for Reproductive Rights at the Supreme Court since 2016—the Texas law that Wendy Davis had filibustered and a Louisiana restriction—were both upheld by that lower court.

By this point, the lawsuit bore the name of Dr. Thomas E. Dobbs III, the leader of the state's health department, who notably had no role in the litigation. When the Pink House and the center initially sued to stop the law, it listed the state's top health official as a defendant because the health department oversaw abortion regulation in the state. That official was his predecessor and when she retired, the name of the suit changed to his. Dobbs, an epidemiologist and expert on infectious disease, was focused on combating the pandemic and wanted nothing to do with the litigation. "We want to just keep on doing our good work and stay out of the crosshairs," he later said.

For Fitch, too, the abortion law was something that just landed in her lap. If the court took up the case, it could be the biggest abortion ruling since Casey in 1992. And she would be the face of it. If Mississippi wanted to be able to handle a case as big as Dobbs, Fitch needed a top-notch litigator. For the first time in the history of the state, Fitch hired a solicitor general to handle appellate strategy. Kristi Johnson, the US assistant attorney general who got the job, started the cert petition in March 2020 as hospitals filled with COVID patients.

As promised, the Alliance Defending Freedom had helped defend the law in the lower courts. John Bursch, an ADF lawyer who represented the governor to support the law at the Fifth Circuit, said he reviewed a draft of Johnson's cert petition. He boasted of a high rate of acceptance for cert petitions at the court and aimed to hone Mississippi's argument. His goal was to buttress Ho's argument from the Fifth Circuit and again highlight all the legislative findings in the law that were originally included for exactly this moment.

ADF lawyers also knew John Roberts was likely the swing justice, so Mississippi wrote the cert petition with him in mind. As ADF had long planned, the intent was to chip away at Roe—not foremost to overturn the decision altogether.

"The goal was to get the court to write an opinion that he would join, that would wipe out the illogical, unconstitutionally tethered viability line," Bursch said.

In June, days after the racial justice protests below her office and after months of preparation, Fitch's team filed their petition to the Supreme Court. It was two weeks after law enforcement officers fired tear gas and rubber pellets into a crowd of peaceful protesters in Lafayette Square across from the White House, moments before Trump marched through the plaza to St. John's Episcopal Church—where he held up a Bible in a declaration of Christian power and values.

Fitch's team took a broad approach in its petition. Mississippi asked three main questions to give the justices room to decide which to answer: 1) Were all pre-viability prohibitions on elective abortions unconstitutional? 2) Which standard should be used to evaluate the validity of a pre-viability law, the one established in Casey, which was evaluating the "undue burden" a law might create for a woman, or the one in the 2016 Texas case, which was about balancing the interests of the state in promoting health of the woman and her fetus and the burdens on the woman? 3) Could abortion providers sue on behalf of a woman against a state's law against abortions after the first trimester?

The word Roe itself was mentioned in the court filing only in passing, with brief name-checks of the historic case. The idea that Roe could be overturned through this case was only referenced by implication in a footnote. "To be clear, the questions presented in this petition do not require the Court to overturn Roe or Casey," the petition said. "They merely asks the Court to reconcile a conflict in its own precedents."

At the time, few people were paying attention to Fitch's petition or what was happening with the fate of the state's fifteen-week abortion law. Or really with any abortion law or pending court case. With the pandemic sweeping the nation, schools shuttered, the economy teetering, and the presidential election underway, there was plenty else to focus on.

The social issue that dominated political discourse in 2020 was race, not abortion or women's rights. As protests inflamed the country, Democrats seized on the growing awareness of racial injustice, making the issue central to their election campaigns. Republicans tried to ride a conservative backlash, stoking fears about crime and looting. They also attempted to re-create the spark of their 2016 campaign, rallying social conservatives with pleas to reelect the "most pro-life president we have ever had" and continue the work of his administration. Trump even attended the March for Life in late January, at the start of the election year.

He showed up on the Mall triumphant, the first president to attend in person. His appearance was a powerful signal of how important conservative Christian voters were to his coalition and his new Republican Party. Still, abortion stayed far under the radar for most independent and liberal voters, a distant second to the moment of racial reckoning.

But even though many voters didn't see it at the time, the issues of race and abortion were very much intertwined. Black women were disproportionately likely to have abortions: Black women of reproductive age made up 14 percent of women in the United States but received 42 percent of abortions nationally, according to data from the Kaiser Family Foundation, which tracks health statistics.

Almost nowhere were the reproductive health discrepancies more obvious than in Mississippi, a state where Black women of reproductive age were nearly 43 percent of the population and received 80 percent of abortions. Black women in Mississippi were more than three times as likely to die of pregnancy complications as white women. Black babies were twice as likely to die as white babies during their first year of life.

Abortion-rights activists saw those numbers and argued that abortion bans like the fifteen-week one in Mississippi were racist policies that hurt the health, financial standing, and autonomy of Black women. Restricting abortion, they believed, was a way to maintain control over Black women's bodies and economic futures by prioritizing a fetus over the women's lives. Already, access to abortion for poor Black women had been limited for generations by Hyde. The new bans—many in Southern states with high percentages of Black women—would limit their access to abortion even further.

Reproductive justice activists saw a deep connection between racism and limits on reproductive rights. For the first 250 years of the American experiment, Black women who were enslaved had no legal control or bodily autonomy over their reproductive lives. The ability of enslaved women to reproduce was central to the income of slave owners and the perpetuation of the institution. Mothers were separated from their future children at the moment of conception, with their wombs considered the prenatal property of slave owners. To many in the reproductive justice movement, state control over women's reproductive choices furthered this racist legacy.

As the Black Lives Matter movement grew, the abortion-rights movement made common cause with their efforts. "Ever since we were brought here against our will, this country has been a hostile birthing environment for Black women, and a dangerous place to raise Black children," wrote SisterSong, the reproductive justice organization run by Monica Raye Simpson, in a formal statement of solidarity between the two movements released in 2016. "We offer to the Movement for Black Lives our commitment to hold gender justice as dear as racial justice, with reproductive justice as the core of both these aspirations."

Antiabortion leaders also saw fresh evidence in the Black Lives Matter movement for their case that ending abortion was a civil rights cause. It was an old argument, reaching back to John C. Willke, but one they believed had new resonance when much of America was suddenly outraged about the continued police shootings of Black people. "This remarkable moment in American history fails to recognize a grave injustice similar to the one that it seeks to remedy," wrote James L. Sherley, a Black scholar at the Charlotte Lozier Institute, the research arm of SBA. "Among the many shouts demanding freedom and equal protection for Black Americans, silence excludes the millions of targeted preborn Black children who also deserve justice and humility."

The comparison was enormously controversial, just as the Holocaust comparisons were, equating fetuses with enslaved people and victims of police brutality. The antiabortion movement argued that abortion providers—most centrally Planned Parenthood—were targeting Black women for a campaign of "genocide" against Black babies by locating in areas with large Black populations. Those claims made implicit and racially charged assumptions about the agency of those women, argued abortion-rights advocates. Just because a clinic was located in a Black neighborhood didn't mean their doctors were forcing patients to abort their pregnancies.

Still, that turbulent summer, the post-Roe generation of millennial and Gen Z antiabortion activists seized the rallying cries of racial justice activists as their own. After the Democratic mayor of Washington, DC, painted "Black Lives Matter" in giant yellow letters on the street across from the White House, antiabortion activists lifted the effort for their own purposes. Students for Life activists painted "Black Preborn Lives Matter" on murals across the country. Kristan Hawkins, their leader, organized a coalition with Black-led organizations that installed six billboards featuring the slogan and a clenched baby fist pumped to the sky. Trump's reelection campaign spun up limited-edition "Baby Lives Matter" onesies, mimicking the BLM logo.

The campaign looked like a stunt from young conservative activists— yet another effort to "own the libs"—but it reflected an ideology about civil rights that permeated their movement up to the highest ranks. Two days before Trump's speech at the March for Life, Betsy DeVos, his education secretary, compared the antiabortion cause to abolition and, implicitly, enslaved Black people to helpless fetuses.

This moment in the antiabortion struggle, DeVos said in her speech at Washington's Museum of the Bible, reminded her of President Abraham Lincoln. "He, too, contended with the 'pro-choice' arguments of his day," she said. "They suggested that a state's 'choice' to be slave or to be free had no moral question in it." In DeVos's telling, Lincoln reminded "those pro-choicers" that slavery was a vast moral evil. "Lincoln was right about the slavery 'choice' then, and he would be right about the life 'choice' today," she said. "Because as it's been said: Freedom is not about doing what we want. Freedom is about having the right to do what we ought." Her comments were another attempt to claim the heritage of civil rights for the antiabortion movement. Democrats quickly cast them as a willful, racist perversion of American history.

The antiabortion movement's racial arguments were most extensive when it came to Planned Parenthood and its founder, Margaret Sanger. Activists frequently highlighted Sanger's relationships with racists and eugenicists, proponents of a discredited pseudoscience that promoted the genetic fitness of white people. Historical records showed that Sanger courted members of those types of people. In 1926, she addressed a women's auxiliary branch of a Ku Klux Klan chapter in New Jersey, an appearance she later described in her memoir as "one of the weirdest experiences."

Antiabortion activists circulated quotes from Sanger's extensive body of writing that portrayed her as supporting racist ideology. The most damning quote, one often circulated on antiabortion websites and social media, was from a December 10, 1939, letter. "We do not want word to go out that we want to exterminate the Negro population," they would quote, often pairing the remark with comments from Hillary Clinton or Barack Obama praising Sanger.

The full context of the letter actually undercut the very point the antiabortion movement was trying to make. Her letter was an attempt to dispel the misinformation of her day. Sanger was writing to a program director, arguing that they needed Black doctors and the support of Black ministers to help counter inaccurate suspicions that Planned Parenthood was running a racial sterilization effort by providing birth control.

"The minister's work is also important and he should be trained, perhaps by the Federation as to our ideals and the goal that we hope to reach," wrote Sanger. "We do not want word to go out that we want to exterminate the Negro population and the minister is the man who can straighten out that idea if it ever occurs to any of their more rebellious members."

While Sanger's early work focused on immigrant women, later in her career, she founded what she called the "Negro Project" with leaders including W. E. B. Du Bois, Mary McLeod Bethune, and Rev. Adam Clayton Powell, and worked to provide birth control in Southern Black communities. In 1966, the year Sanger died, Martin Luther King Jr. praised her work as having "a striking kinship" with the civil rights struggle.

Still, the criticisms of Sanger promulgated by the antiabortion movement reached to the highest court. In a 2019 case over two Indiana abortion laws, Thomas argued that the court was "duty-bound" to address provisions of the law, which prohibited abortion based on race, sex, and disability. In his opinion, Thomas offered his extensive version of the history of eugenics. He noted that Sanger "distinguished between birth control and abortion," but, he said, "Sanger recognized the eugenic potential of her cause." He added: "Abortion is an act rife with the potential for eugenic manipulation." A series of historians described his analysis as "historically incoherent," saying that top eugenicists largely opposed birth control and abortion. The court declined to address that part of the law, effectively leaving in place the lower-court decision striking it down.

Loretta Ross, a founder of the reproductive justice movement who had spent years researching Sanger, believed that Thomas and the antiabortion movement were intentionally weaponizing Sanger's legacy. "I don't believe she was fundamentally a racist when judged against the norms of her day," she wrote in the *Huffington Post* in 2018. "She was no more prejudiced than all white people were and are." But, Ross argued, Planned Parenthood's refusal to directly confront Sanger's legacy had provided a "golden opportunity" for opponents of abortion to undercut the cause of abortion rights. The dynamic left Black feminists like Ross in the difficult position of defending the historically white-led organization against an antiabortion movement that they saw as far more racist. "Our allies often fail to validate black women's leadership, while our opponents paint us as brainwashed traitors to our race," she wrote.

McGill Johnson, the first Black president of the organization in more than a quarter century, believed that Planned Parenthood could not move forward in this new era of racial justice without confronting Sanger's legacy. She had her own 2020 analogy for Sanger's 1920 set of beliefs, one that used a term for a privileged and racially insensitive white woman. "'First came Margaret, then came Karen," she told her team. "Margaret is Karen's godmother, basically."

To McGill Johnson, Baby Lives Matter felt like an updated version of the old billboard she saw a decade ago, the one that declared, "The Most Dangerous Place for an African American Is in the Womb" and that sparked her interest in joining Planned Parenthood's board. The higher abortion rate of Black women was not because of a nefarious plot by abortion providers. It was due, McGill Johnson argued, to structural racism and a raft of socioeconomic factors that made Black women disproportionately at risk for unintended pregnancy. Studies showed that Black women were less likely to receive sex education, more likely to live in "contraception deserts," and uninsured at roughly twice the rate of white women and girls—making it difficult to obtain contraception. Unintended pregnancies that led to unintended births would not only deny Black women their reproductive freedom and risk their health, they could trap them in cycles of economic disadvantage. Some research showed that banning abortion nationwide could lead to a 33 percent increase in deaths among Black women, compared with rates for 2017, because carrying a pregnancy to term was more medically dangerous than having an abortion.

McGill Johnson saw links between the decline of abortion rights and racial inequality. Like Ilyse Hogue, she saw how antiabortion activists were passing abortion restrictions and bans through conservative statehouses with the goal of striking at Roe, though she didn't know which law would eventually reach the Supreme Court. At Planned Parenthood's June meeting, she opened her remarks with a provocative question: "Who are we going to be when we're no longer defending Roe?" Her goal was to prepare her donors, activists, and organization for the emotion of losing Roe, so when it happened they could be in the mindset of reimagination and reconstruction, not just mourning and loss.

Rights had been lost before in America, McGill Johnson reminded the audience. Reconstruction expanded constitutional rights for formerly enslaved Black Americans. Then, the court and Congress, as a way of settling the disputed election of 1876, struck down those laws prohibiting racial discrimination. Rights can get lost in a multitude of ways, she warned.

FITCH'S UPBRINGING TOLD a different story of Mississippi's racial legacy. Wanda Lynn Fitch came from Holly Springs, a place described on the historic town marker as an antebellum cotton town that was home to thirteen generals of the Confederacy. Fitch's father, W. O. Fitch—or Bill, as he was known—had moved the family back to his rural hometown near the Tennessee border after making his fortune in finance. He had inherited a prime parcel of an old plantation and enrolled his daughters in Marshall Academy, a private school founded as a segregation academy—one of thousands of such schools started by white parents across the South after the *Brown v. Board* decision required racial integration in public schools. He opened his own consumer lending company and started buying parcels of land, growing his property to eight thousand acres. Along with Lynn's mother, Clydean, he restored the antebellum buildings on the Galena Plantation. The couple relocated the original log cabin of Nathan Bedford Forrest, a Confederate general and the first grand wizard of the Ku Klux Klan, onto their property and rebuilt the house as their residence.

On weekends, the Fitch family would saddle up the horses and ride through the open prairie fields and clusters of pine and hardwood thickets. Lynn, a fourth-generation hunter, shot quail like her father and grandfather did. But life in Holly Springs wasn't enough to hold her. She left for Ole Miss, where she flew through college and law school in five years. By twenty-three, she was a practicing lawyer, working in the attorney general's office and married to a law school classmate from the Mississippi River Delta.

Twenty-seven years later, when she launched her campaign for state treasurer, her father was the largest donor to her political operation. His fields and historic lodging attracted powerful guests—the state's governors and professional athletes—who traveled from across the country to hunt the twenty-five thousand quail that roamed the property, with guides and bird dogs. Justice Antonin Scalia, an avid hunter, made annual pilgrimages. Fitch had always felt the strong pull of her roots and admired the conservative justices. Now, with the decision to petition the Supreme Court to hear her case, she was continuing Scalia's legacy.

Just two weeks after Fitch filed her petition, the Supreme Court ruled on *June Medical Services v. Russo*, its first major abortion case since Trump shifted the balance of power to the right. The decision was a setback for the antiabortion movement. A five-justice majority struck down the Louisiana abortion restriction, which would have left the state with one abortion clinic, when it returned to the court. The Louisiana law was essentially identical to the one in Texas that Wendy Davis had filibustered and that had been rejected by the Supreme Court in 2016. The antiabortion movement leaders had been worried about Brett Kavanaugh's commitment to their cause. But he ruled for them, joining the minority in favor of upholding the Louisiana law.

Still, they did not have enough votes to win. For a second time, Roberts, who had also ruled in their favor in the Texas law, flipped to join the court's four-member liberal wing and strike down the Louisiana restriction. "I joined the dissent in Whole Woman's Health," he wrote, "and continue to believe that the case was wrongly decided. The question today, however, is not whether Whole Woman's Health was right or wrong, but whether to adhere to it in deciding the present case."

His commitment to precedent put ADF's strategy into doubt. The fifteen-week plan, and the eighteen-week one after it, asked the court to approve something much more comprehensive that would strike at a far more established precedent: a ban that would remove Roe's viability standard. Kavanaugh wasn't enough to secure an antiabortion majority. "This decision demonstrates how difficult it is to drain the DC swamp and how important it is that President Trump gets reelected so that he may be able to appoint more pro-life justices," said James Bopp Jr., general counsel for National Right to Life. That seemed unlikely: there were no public signs that any of the four liberal justices planned to retire, even Ginsburg, who was the oldest on the bench.

Still, Fitch had done her part in making the ask. Allies of the movement did what they always did, taking the next step, even if it ended in failure. They rallied behind her effort, filing amicus briefs to the court asking the justices to take up the case, some at ADF's encouragement. The Roman Catholic Dioceses of Jackson and Biloxi were the first to submit one to the court, asking the justices to consider "religious authorities to shed light on issues of morality that come before the Court," they wrote. They explained what they saw that morality to be, citing a verse from the Bible when God said to the prophet Jeremiah: "Before I formed you in the womb I knew you."

The case was distributed to the Supreme Court justices for consideration on September 2. And everyone waited.

26

The Days of Awe

"My God," Justice Stephen Breyer thought.

The member of the court's liberal wing heard the phone ring midway through the Mourner's Kaddish prayer. The sun had set on the East Coast, and the melodies and rhythms, the nigunim of Rosh Hashanah, washed through the early autumn evening of September 18. He was at home due to the pandemic, watching services on Zoom with his daughter and grandchildren. He told his wife he would answer the call later. This was one of the holiest days of the Jewish year, remembering the day God created the world. The final hours of the old year had passed. A new year was coming. The Days of Awe, the ten-day period of repentance and renewal when the gates of prayer are open, had begun.

Then the other line rang, and he couldn't ignore that call too. It was the Supreme Court marshal's office. His heart sank. Ruth Bader Ginsburg, feminist icon, had suffered complications due to metastatic pancreatic cancer.

At eighty-seven, she was gone.

Jewish tradition says that only the most righteous die during the Days of Awe, that God waits until as long as possible, until the final moments of the year, to take them. His friend Ruth, only five years older than Breyer himself, had waited until then to go too. The call came as Breyer was reciting the Kaddish, words so ancient that they are not Hebrew but Aramaic. It became a prayer of mourning in the Middle Ages, as Christian crusaders killed Jews across the Rhineland.

> *Y'hei shlama raba min-sh'maya v'chayim aleinu v'al-kol-yisrael, v'im'ru: amen.* May there be abundant peace from heaven, and life, for us and for all Israel; and say, Amen.

Breyer took a moment to write down his thoughts. "A great justice, a woman of valor, a rock of righteousness, and my good, good friend," he wrote.

Ginsburg would have known the complications of the reference, "woman of valor" or *eshet chayil*, from a biblical poem in Proverbs 31 about how to be a good woman. Her mother kept a list of such role models, and Ginsburg memorized their stories. She had also learned early that too often, because of her gender, she didn't count. When her beloved mother died of cancer, one day before her high school graduation, young Ruthie skipped the ceremony to stay home with her father and mourn, only to be told she could not pray the Kaddish because she was a girl. "The house was filled with women, but only men could participate in the minyan," she said, referencing the quorum of ten Jewish adults required to recite the prayer.

As an adult, Ginsburg largely abandoned traditional religious observance but felt deeply called by Judaism's commitment to justice. It was a value that guided her determination to fight sexism and discrimination all the way to the Supreme Court. It inspired her to push the court to respect non-Christian religions—changing policies like ending the requirement that Supreme Court bar certificates be stamped with the date "in the year of our Lord," referring to the Christian calendar, and pushing the court to not sit on the Jewish High Holy Days, even when she was told that no one complained that the court gathered on Good Friday. In her Supreme

Court chambers, she hung a framed lithograph of the Hebrew command from Deuteronomy: "*Tzedek tzedek tirdof*—Justice, justice shall you pursue."

The same spirit infused her dissents, such as her opinion in *Gonzales v. Carhart*, the 2007 abortion case that upheld the so-called partial-birth abortion ban, which stressed how a woman's power to fulfill her potential was tied to her ability to control her reproductive life. Widespread across Jewish tradition is the belief that the fetus is not considered a person. If the mother's life is at risk, the fetus is considered a *rodef*, or pursuer, and rabbinic tradition requires prioritizing her life over the fetus.

For a generation of progressives, Ginsburg had seemed like the picture of strength and fortitude, a larger-than-life icon who vanquished the forces of sexism. Now, physical realities had overtaken her. Her famous black bejeweled "dissent collar," which she wore on the days she pointedly disagreed with the court's majority opinion, would be donated to the Smithsonian's National Museum of American History, along with her black leather briefcase, inscribed with her famous initials, RBG.

On the steps of the Supreme Court later that night, hundreds gathered with flowers, candles, and homemade signs. A woman chanted Kaddish through a bullhorn to the crowd.

When Ilyse Hogue of NARAL heard the news, she was sitting down to Rosh Hashanah dinner. She had promised her twins that she would take the weekend off. Her phone rang and she ignored it. It rang again. Then her husband's phone started pinging with notifications. "You need to get your phone," he told her after checking his text messages.

Suddenly, it mattered less whether Brett Kavanaugh would rule with them or not. The antiabortion wing of the court could get another member. Hogue's views and the abortion-rights movement would almost certainly be a minority at the court for a generation. Everything had unraveled so fast these past few years. This was the final fight.

The timing was terrible. The Senate was in recess. The country was still in the midst of a pandemic. And early voting was underway in four states. Within hours of Ginsburg's death, Senate majority leader Mitch McConnell pledged that whomever Donald Trump picked to replace her would receive a confirmation vote. He had the votes, with a majority of fifty-three thanks to Republican gains in the Senate in the 2018 midterms. Republicans could lose Senators Susan Collins and Lisa Murkowski, the two Republicans who supported abortion rights, and still win the seat. The Democrats knew that was the only reality that truly mattered.

There were forty-six days until the presidential election, far fewer than the nine months between when Scalia died and Election Day. Yet, Leonard Leo's pledge that Republicans would not confirm a Supreme Court justice in an election year was forgotten. No president since Ronald Reagan had confirmed three justices to the court. Trump could be the one to do it, and it looked like he would. Ginsburg's death meant that conservatives could capture a new majority. The kind of supermajority that could take down Roe.

Democrats would fight. And it would be a battle, Hogue knew, they would lose.

MARJORIE DANNENFELSER WAS having a small picnic under the trees at the Supreme Court that night, eating crackers and cheese with some of her kids, when one of her staff members called with the news. The situation felt "sublime," she said. It had all come to this moment, a brief pause that would decide the direction of abortion law in America. The fall of Roe was not immediate, but it was now in sight, she thought.

"It's what we've been working for all these years," Dannenfelser said that evening. "What is most important is what happens to our court and Constitution. You don't get a shot that often."

Opposing abortion was, she continued to believe, good politics for the Republican Party. Dannenfelser argued that the suburban women who formed Joe Biden's base were not monolithic; more would be on the Republican side than the left might anticipate. A third justice would help bring those moderates back home to Trump, she calculated, overcoming the chaos of his administration and his low marks on handling the pandemic. Her sense of the politics would prove misplaced, but it revealed how deeply she believed her movement had changed minds and converted America to the morality of their cause.

Yet, for Roe, the outcome of the election no longer mattered. Nor did the composition of Congress. The die could be cast with this court seat. This confirmation battle.

In her office, Dannenfelser had a detailed map drawn on a wall-size whiteboard. From a distance, it looked like the kind used by political campaigns to track polling and turnout, swing districts, and congressional votes. But this one was color-coded by unified Republican control of state legislatures and governors' mansions, and partitioned by court of appeals jurisdiction. A red triangle meant the state had passed a "heartbeat bill," generally a ban started around six weeks; a green square signified a "pain-capable" abortion law, typically a twenty-week ban. Red stars showed the courts of appeal where Republican-nominated judges outnumbered Democratic ones—of the eleven, they controlled seven. It was a map of how all the laws were moving up toward the ultimate court that mattered.

With Ginsburg's death, the final piece of the puzzle map was snapping into place. There were still questions, of course. Which of the twenty or so abortion cases lining up at the lower courts might reach the Supreme Court next? Would it be Dobbs? If it was not Mississippi, could it be Utah or Arkansas? How far would Kavanaugh go on Roe? The antiabortion movement just needed to ensure that, with days to go, it got the nominee it wanted and that the Senate confirmed him—or her.

Ginsburg's life, her fight for opportunities for women, and her jurisprudence symbolized the struggle and victory of liberal feminism. That movement was embodied in her three initials and a white lace collar she typically wore with her judicial robes. Now, it would be replaced by a new vision, one articulated by a very different female judge, whose own three initials represented a different feminism and a different view of the Constitution. A mother of seven from the heart of American Catholicism. The woman Trump had said he was saving for Ginsburg.

Trump introduced Amy Coney Barrett as his nominee in the Rose Garden, in the same place where Bill Clinton had introduced Ginsburg in 1993, after the Year of the Woman. Back then, Dannenfelser was twenty-seven, barely beginning with her shoestring sisterhood and hoping to carve a more powerful place for conservative antiabortion women in Washington. That was half a lifetime ago. Now, at fifty-four, she and those women sat in the Rose Garden watching Barrett become the new symbol of the culture they wanted to usher in for America.

"While I am a judge, I'm better known back home as a room parent, carpool driver, and birthday party planner," Barrett said, looking at her seven children and husband taking up the entire front row next to the First Lady, Melania Trump. Seeming to preempt the criticisms of Democrats, Barrett directly addressed the American people. "If confirmed, I would not assume that role for the sake of those in my own circle and certainly not for my own sake," she promised. "I would assume this role to serve you."

Barrett knew her Catholic faith would be a public lightning rod. When Trump considered her in 2018, after the Dianne Feinstein "dogma lives loudly within you" incident, she went to great lengths to avoid giving the media a chance to take a photo of her religious observance and potentially paint her as a zealot. One Sunday morning after Mass, when she realized the press was outside the front of the church, she hopped a fence and landed in a vegetable garden. The yard was her associate pastor's, who, she said, "helped me make my escape."

Barrett's garden diving didn't hide her beliefs. She was a member of an antiabortion faculty group, and in 2006, she signed a newspaper ad from the local Right to Life group opposing "abortion on demand" and defending "the right to life from fertilization to natural death." Roe was "very unlikely" to be overturned, she told a group of students in 2013 when the ruling turned forty. The best way to reduce abortion in the United States, she said, was to support poor single mothers, who are likely to choose the procedure. It was an argument that antiabortion pregnancy centers had made time and again. "Motherhood is a privilege, but it comes at a price," she said. "A woman who wants to become pregnant accepts this price, but in an unplanned pregnancy, the woman faces the difficulties of pregnancy unwillingly."

The antiabortion movement had accomplished a giant feat—the first mother of school-aged children to serve on the Supreme Court also opposed abortion and was a devout Christian believer.

"Goals," Lila Rose, the post–Roe generation antiabortion activist, wrote on social media with a heart-eyed emoji, above a clip of Barrett walking with four of her seven children, all dressed up for her nomination ceremony in the Rose Garden. At age forty-eight, Barrett was poised to become the youngest justice on the bench, positioned to shape a generation of American law—or, if she lived as long as Ginsburg, two.

Barrett was both Christian supermom and high-powered legal scholar, elite and outsider in her own way, a combination of the more secular conservative Federalist Society credentials and the beliefs of the emerging Christian legal movement. None of this was the conservative femininity of Phyllis Schlafly, who rose to power as a homemaker arguing against the advancement of women outside the domestic domain. This new iteration of conservative feminism didn't argue that women's gains should be rolled back or that women should not be professionally ambitious. But it wanted those advancements not to come at the expense of ideals of motherhood, Christian morality, and the centrality of married, heterosexual parents raising children. This conservative feminism believed that the legalization of abortion had hurt women, not liberated them.

What America was watching at the court, though few realized it at the time, was the secular feminist world represented by RGB being supplanted by a new symbol for American womanhood: ACB.

But for all their planning, once again, antiabortion leaders had also gotten extraordinarily lucky. Not only would they get three Supreme Court justices, they could flip the court. It was yet another moment they could have never orchestrated and that they interpreted as a sign of divine intervention.

THE CONFIRMATION WAS madness from the beginning. Trump formally selected Barrett a day after Ginsburg lay in state at the Capitol, the first woman and first Jew to receive the honor. Barrett's nomination ceremony in the Rose Garden turned into a COVID superspreader event, landing the president himself at Walter Reed National Military Medical Center. Leo's groups, especially the Judicial Crisis Network, quickly devoted $10 million to the campaign to confirm the nominee—just as they had for Gorsuch and Kavanaugh. At Trump's reelection rallies, supporters debuted a new chant—"Fill the seat."

The confirmation process, once again, chipped away at the court's ability to position itself as above politics. Republicans wouldn't give Garland a hearing, but here was McConnell pushing Barrett through as the presidential race reached the final stages. The process was partisan and polarizing, and split the nation once again. Vast majorities of Republicans—83 percent, according to one CNN poll—wanted Barrett confirmed, while only 8 percent of Democrats did. Independents were split.

As they sprinted to her confirmation hearings, Republicans took pains to play down Barrett's potential impact on Roe. In the first presidential debate, three days after Barrett's Rose Garden nomination, Trump was uncharacteristically reticent on the issue.

When Biden said Roe was on the ballot, Trump shot back. "There's nothing happening there," he said. "You don't know her view on *Roe v. Wade*. You don't know her view." Once again, Mike Pence played down the issue, refusing to say during the vice presidential debate whether he would want Indiana to ban abortions if the court overturned Roe. Kamala Harris, for her part, also skirted a parallel question about whether California should have no restrictions.

But a small number of Republicans said what the antiabortion movement believed to be true about Barrett. It was the reason they had wanted her all those years earlier, when Trump picked Kavanaugh. "This is the most openly pro-life judicial nominee to the Supreme Court in my lifetime," Missouri's Josh Hawley, one of the senators who had won his seat in the 2018 social conservative backlash to the Kavanaugh episode, said in a speech on the Senate floor supporting her nomination. "This is an individual who has been open in her criticism of that illegitimate decision *Roe v. Wade*."

Like so many nominees before her, Barrett offered few hints about her legal position in her hearing. During the hours of questioning from Democratic senators, she refused to say whether Roe was correctly decided. When pressed on whether Roe was a "super-precedent," she evaded a direct answer by citing the fact of the question. "Roe is not a super-precedent because calls for its overruling have never ceased, but that doesn't mean that Roe should be overruled," she said.

Eight days before the election, on October 26, Leo tuned in from his home in Maine to watch his old friend Clarence Thomas swear Barrett into the court. Watching her raise her right hand, it felt like the culmination of his entire project. It was "exhilarating," he said. The John Roberts vote was suddenly less essential. There could now be more consistent rulings that upheld the original meaning of the Constitution, he thought, decisions against abortion rights, race-based affirmative action, gun control, and other priorities. Richards, of course, saw the moment differently. The confirmation was "a suspension of everything we believed to be true," she said. The Supreme Court was not above politics, she thought, nor did it even try to be anymore. "I was naive," she said of her decades of faith in those judicial and political norms. "This is a Republican Supreme Court."

Trump would go on to lose the White House to Biden. Dannenfelser's political prediction that a third justice might boost moderate support for Trump was wrong. Suburban women voted for Biden in droves, boosting him into the Oval Office. But she was right where it mattered. Leo, Dannenfelser, and Pence got their biggest prize with eight days to go.

Trump, whom Dannenfelser stuck with through "Grab 'em by the pussy," ended up as the most successful antiabortion president America had ever known. His administration transformed the judiciary, shifting power toward opponents of abortion for a generation. Trump appointed nearly 230 judges to the federal bench, just one fewer powerful federal appeals court judges in four years than Obama appointed in eight, and three judges to the Supreme Court. Of the judges he appointed to the highest courts—the Supreme Court and circuit courts—86 percent either had been or were Federalist Society members. And with his speech to the March for Life and graphic comments in his State of the Union about how abortion providers "execute a baby," he changed political expectations for Republican presidents. What Trump and his Republican allies had done was to lay the groundwork for long-term cultural change, not by winning hearts and minds but by leveraging political force to conquer the courts.

Dannenfelser saw her decision to stand by Trump in 2016 as now justified. "We'd never get this court," she said. "Maybe never again."

Some in her movement wouldn't accept that Trump lost. By now, many antiabortion believers had embraced the Trump era's new right-wing conservatism and election denialism, a cause that struck at the foundation of American democracy Abby Johnson, a former clinic director for Planned Parenthood who quit to become an antiabortion activist, spoke at a rally that opposed the certification of Biden's victory, wearing a pin that said "1972"—signaling America before Roe—along with a founder of the Oath Keepers, the far-right group, and Alex Jones, the conspiracist.

What had started as an effort to gain a foothold in the Republican Party after the post-2012 autopsy had ended in a takeover. Trump had promised conservative Christians that "Christianity will have power." And now that vision of Christian power was at the center of a Republican Party they had remade.

27

The Coup

Ilyse Hogue watched the siege on the Capitol in horror, unable to tear her eyes away from the footage of attackers storming into buildings and destroying the hallowed grounds of American democracy. She had spent years trying to warn about the marriage of right-wing extremism with the antiabortion cause. Now, she was watching their violent merger in real time, as new radicals tried to overturn the results of the 2020 election.

Her phone started exploding with messages. Abortion providers and clinic operators traded texts about faces they recognized in the grainy close-up photographs and jerky video footage from that horrible day. They saw Tayler Hansen, the antiabortion activist who painted "Baby Lives Matter" outside clinics from Salt Lake City to Richmond, filming a woman named Ashli Babbitt as she lay dying on the floor of the Capitol.

There was John Brockhoeft, who firebombed a Planned Parenthood clinic in Cincinnati, posting a video of himself describing Trump as "our beloved president" as he stood outside the Capitol. And there was Derrick Evans, a fixture at a West Virginia clinic with a reputation for such intense harassment of patients that a volunteer escort obtained a restraining order against him. Now a member of the West Virginia House of Delegates, Evans live streamed a video of himself, helmet-clad, joining the mob pushing its way into the

Capitol. He was arrested two days later, pleaded guilty to civil disorder, and was sentenced to three months in jail and a fine.

At NARAL, Hogue had her staff collect the accounts in a research report, eventually turning their work into a digital ad. A few, mostly liberal, publications picked up on the ties between antiabortion activists and the violence. The ties evoked the long history of violent action from parts of the antiabortion movement, from the clinic bombings of the 1980s and 1990s to the killing of Doctor George Tiller, an abortion provider in Wichita, Kansas, shortly after Obama took office. "This was a movement that embraced political violence long before Trump," she said. "It's not like some of them had to be acculturated to it."

Before members of the far-right Proud Boys marched toward the Capitol, they stopped to kneel in the street and prayed in the name of Jesus. A group called the Jericho March, which had led a series of demonstrations for "election integrity," marched around the Capitol seven times, modeling their protest on a biblical battle in which the Israelites marched around the city of Jericho until its walls crumbled, letting their armies take the city. Jericho marches were used by the antiabortion movement dating back to the 1970s, where protesters marched around abortion providers' homes and offices.

The morning of January 6, at the Save America rally on the Mall, Abby Johnson, the post–Roe generation antiabortion activist, addressed the crowd—"all of you fine Patriots," she called them—to defend Trump and unborn babies, just as she had at the Republican National Convention. "Christians in this country are too quiet. They are not crying out and demanding justice for our modern-day Holocaust that is taking place," she declared to cheers. When Trump arrived at the rally, she took a selfie in the front row, the president behind her riling up the crowd before he urged everyone to march to the Capitol.

As the attack escalated that day and Trump refused to stop it, Marjorie Dannenfelser texted Mark Meadows, Trump's chief of staff. "Violence in pursuit of upholding justice and the dignity of the human being is nonsense at best. What is happening in the Capitol now is not reflective of prolife Americans and Trump supporters who align with his call to support police today," she wrote, sharing a link to the statement she had released publicly.

Leaders of other major antiabortion groups also disavowed the attack. But the crowd standing inside and outside the Capitol that day included plenty of their own, showing how the more radical elements of their movement could eclipse them with their own tactics. Over four years, much of the antiabortion Christian coalition that pushed Trump and Mike Pence into office had become entangled with the conspiratorial beliefs that the president helped foster on issues like election denialism and opposition to public health mandates. Their spiritual and political mission to end abortion had become intertwined with the causes that animated Trumpism, now the defining ideology of the Republican Party. As the new party radicalized, so did their movement. Positions once relegated to the fringes of American political life—overturning an election or overturning Roe—suddenly seemed possible.

Republican senators who objected to the election results had long been among the most outspoken abortion opponents, including Senators Josh Hawley, Ted Cruz, and Cindy Hyde-Smith of Mississippi, a longtime SBA ally who was from Becky Currie's hometown. But their ecosystem reached far deeper into American life. One city council member from Hillsdale, Michigan, who traveled to Washington to protest election fraud on January 6, returned home and helped propose an ordinance to outlaw abortion in his city.

"It is no different from the Right to Life march in January," the councilman, Greg Stuchell, said of his fellow January 6 marchers. "For every one that was there, there's probably another one hundred that wished they could be."

But unlike the March for Life, a peaceful annual protest where families carried red roses, the Capitol siege was violent and extreme.

Pence, long a champion of the antiabortion movement, was threatened by the crowd, as some called for his execution after he promised to uphold the election results. The attack pushed the bounds of political life in a way that was easy to recognize as radical, with potential to transform the country. A group of mostly men storming a government building with guns and assaulting about 140 police officers. It was a scene familiar from foreign countries or television shows. Macho extremism, ripped from an action film.

What was harder to see was how the slow, steady drumbeat—of litigation, appeals and stays, laws and confusing medical jargon, discussion of precedent and super-precedent and congressional rules—could actually add up to even more lasting change. The legal, political, and scientific maneuvering of the antiabortion movement, often with a feminine face, used democratic tools to transform American life from the inside. The tempo of that drumbeat was speeding up and couldn't be easily stopped by simply electing a new president. It was a quieter change, one not expressed with smashed windows and shouts, but one that could also restructure a nation by controlling its most basic unit: parent and child. It was a transformational coup, and an entirely legal one.

Two days after the January 6 attack, the Capitol grounds now ensconced in barricades, the Supreme Court justices had a private meeting. Three of them—Samuel Alito, Clarence Thomas, and Neil Gorsuch—wanted to take up the Mississippi case that term, as soon as possible. That would likely mean delivering a decision in June 2021, less than a year after Ginsburg's death.

But Brett Kavanaugh suggested an unusual and misleading alternative: vote to hear the case, but withhold the public announcement they had done so. The court could keep the case on its public docket week after week, he explained, giving the impression that no decision had been made. In the spring, the court would formally announce that it would hear the case, pushing oral arguments into the next term. The later schedule would allow more time for other abortion cases to move through the lower courts and would provide cover against allegations that the court's new conservative majority was taking advantage of Ginsburg's death. It would also give them some distance from the Capitol siege.

Amy Coney Barrett, just weeks into her new job, sided with Kavanaugh. If the case were going to be heard that term, she would vote against hearing it at all. Lacking the votes to move forward, Alito agreed to Kavanaugh's conditions. Their plan was set. They would hear the case—but not tell anyone just yet.

Less than two weeks later, the Trump administration ended. Dannenfelser announced an "election transparency" campaign with her friend Frank Cannon's American Principles Project to pass new restrictions on voting, after states loosened some voting rules during the pandemic. Prioritizing issues around Trump's falsehood that the election was stolen was a way to keep donors, voters, and Trump's biggest supporters engaged in their antiabortion mission.

ADF's CEO, Michael Farris, who had initially opposed Trump in 2016, now secretly worked to block the election results. He sent draft language for a potential lawsuit to Republican attorneys general, fishing to get one of them to file suit against states like Pennsylvania, Georgia, and Wisconsin to try to keep Trump in office. Texas ultimately did. It was similar to ADF's model legislation effort to overturn Roe—handing allies a ready model to enact ADF's ideological goals—though Farris said he acted in his personal capacity.

Leonard Leo quietly took control of one of the largest pools of political money in American history, with help from a secret \$1.6 billion donation from a little-known conservative donor, Barre Seid. The intensely private Chicago-based electronics manufacturing mogul had spent decades quietly funding conservative causes. Now, at ninety, he had entrusted his legacy to Leo through a series of opaque transactions over a two-year period that allowed him to avoid as much as \$400 million in taxes. There were few legal limitations—and little sunlight—on how Leo could use the money to influence American politics. The donation transformed Leo into a power broker who could steer the conservative movement and, perhaps, the future of the country. He started looking beyond the courts into pressing his conservative agenda on issues like education, election fraud, and diversity initiatives in corporations.

Abortion-rights activists began to feel some relief. Now Democrats held the trifecta of power in Washington—controlling the House, Senate, and White House—for the first time since 2010. Alexis McGill Johnson told the Associated Press she was "able to breathe in hope and possibility." Biden moved quickly to reverse Trump policies in the early months of his administration. He rescinded the Mexico City policy, the rule blocking foreign nongovernmental organizations from providing information about abortion. On International Women's Day, he signed an executive order establishing the Gender Policy Council, putting a longtime ally of the abortion-rights movement at the helm of a new office that aimed to protect sexual and reproductive health at home and abroad. That spring, he took steps to roll back the restrictions on Title X funding that had prompted Planned Parenthood to drop out of the program and lose tens of millions in federal money. And after some lobbying, his first budget proposal dropped the Hyde Amendment, which banned the use of federal dollars for abortions, fulfilling his campaign promise.

It wasn't quite the Clinton dream that thrilled abortion-rights activists back in 2016. Biden still didn't talk about abortion much. The new conservative supermajority on the Supreme Court and the Republican state legislatures remained a serious threat. Yet for the first time in many years, abortion-rights advocates felt some relief.

But their four years in the wilderness had already cost them so much. Even with their new power, they were limited in what they could do to stop the march on Roe. In the Senate, the Democratic majority lacked the votes to eliminate the filibuster and codify abortion rights into federal law.

State legislatures in more liberal states across the Northeast and West had begun enacting policies to protect abortion rights, but those could not compare to the national protection of Roe or compete with the large swaths of the Midwest and South where legal abortion could become largely unavailable. Democrats had never fully recovered from their brutal losses across the country during the Obama years. After the 2020 elections, Republicans still held unified control of state governments in more states, dominating twenty-three states compared to fifteen states controlled by Democrats.

Outside Washington, many people felt free to tune out what had felt like a never-ending noise of political news. Exhausted and overwhelmed after years of pandemic schooling, health precautions, and economic uncertainty, they took a break from politics. Biden had pledged to protect abortion rights. Now, he was elected and many voters assumed those rights were secure, particularly Roe, which most never really believed was at risk in the first place.

Besides, the court didn't seem to be moving quickly when it came to Roe—at least in terms the public could see. The justices kept rescheduling consideration of Lynn Fitch's petition to hear the Mississippi fifteen-week case. Week after week, Nancy Northup, the head of the Center for Reproductive Rights, which was suing Mississippi over the ban, checked the list of cases to see if the court would take up theirs. There was never an answer. The court just kept the case on their agenda for the next conference session when they considered what cases to accept for review. The extended delay was noteworthy, Northup thought. Both lower courts had unanimously rejected the law. It was blatantly unconstitutional under Supreme Court precedent of Roe and Casey. "They should have swatted away with no thought whatsoever," she said.

She wondered about her opponents' plan. They rarely took big swings. Typically, they inched forward, chipping away at abortion rights, and there were ways they could do that now too. They could prioritize one of the bans on abortion in cases of Down syndrome or race or sex selection, laws that might seem more reasonable to many Americans than a total ban at fifteen weeks. Why would they change course, she asked herself, when they were so close to the ultimate victory? "They've been very successful about being under the radar," she said.

Even now, the biggest actions on abortion rights were happening under the radar. The powerful antiabortion network of the Trump years left executive power, but it had not been dismantled. It simply found new roles in new seats of influence.

As Biden took over, one promising conservative lawyer packed up his office in Washington, rented a car, and started driving south along the Blue Ridge Mountains. He was the exact kind of lawyer Leo had devoted his life to raising up. He was an originalist. A Stanford Law School graduate. A former Thomas clerk.

He was Scott Stewart, the Trump administration lawyer who had tried to stop Jane Doe from getting her abortion. Fitch had offered him a job, crafting strategy for her biggest cases. He headed toward Jackson.

PART IV

THE FATE OF THE NATION

JUNE 2022

Jackson, Mississippi

The Pink House Defenders were surprised by how calm the day was turning out to be. There was no shouting over their walls. Not even a sidewalk sermon. Just one lone protester, an older man in a camping chair outside the entry gate.

"This is not normal," said Derenda Hancock, who led the group of activists who guarded this abortion clinic. "It's strange as crud."

In court filings and newspaper stories, the low-slung, bubblegum-pink building with the lime-green roof was known as Jackson Women's Health Organization, the only abortion clinic in Mississippi. Hancock called it the Pink House. They all did.

Every day the clinic was open, the Defenders put on their rainbow-striped traffic vests, blasted their '90s alt-rock, and maneuvered patients' cars around the protesters, through the metal gates covered in black tarps, and into the twelve parking spots. Hancock waited tables a couple of days a week, but her main job—her mission—was guarding this small stretch of pavement. "Somebody needs to be out here," she said. "Patients shouldn't have to deal with all this with no one out here to help them."

It wasn't easy for Hancock and her team, standing for seven hours in the sweltering sun, fighting the street preachers, the religious homeschoolers with their packs of children, and the abortion abolitionists. This morning, suffocating heat blanketed

Jackson, shimmering off the asphalt in radiating waves, as they helped the women enter for their appointments. After that, there was nothing much for the escorts to do but sit in the shade of their portable tarp, light a cigarette, and talk. The topic today—and every day—was the case aimed at shutting them down.

"Oh, honey, this isn't about abortion," said Kim Gibson, a former paralegal. "This is low-hanging fruit they've been working on. This is the wedge that's going to open the door for the rest of it."

Gibson had come to the Pink House every week for the past five years. But she saw herself as fighting an organized movement far greater than just their handful of regular protesters.

"Christian nationalism. That's their goal," she told the group, leaning back in her camping chair. "These are religious laws that are passed, but 'it's for the welfare of the mother.' The fuck it is."

She paused. The song "Better Man"—Pearl Jam's requiem to abused women—boomed from the speaker, floating across the asphalt. "I'm on a rant today, y'all," said Gibson. Hancock chuckled. "But it's the truth."

The truth was that Gibson was furious. She was enraged by the churchwomen holding their signs outside and the guys on the ladders who screamed damnation over the gates. But she was also angry at the people who were supposed to be fighting for her: the Democrats, national reproductive rights organizations like Planned Parenthood and NARAL, even some of their local activists. They had all failed to save them, she believed.

"It's all been 'We'll do it in the courts,'" she said. "That was a total failure for years, and they just kept buying and kept doing it, kept on. There's this avalanche of loss since 2010."

The "antis," as they called the antiabortion activists, had a plan. "And we can't get our shit together for anything," she said. "They did the work we didn't do."

Hancock and Gibson knew the end was near. They saw the flood of women from Texas and Louisiana, states where abortion had become functionally illegal with bans after six weeks of pregnancy, coming to the Pink House. They maneuvered around the crush of media in their parking lot, getting in the way with their cameras and microphones. And on top of everything else, they heard the gloating of the protesters, already crowing about the Supreme Court decision that would effectively ban abortion in Mississippi and beyond. "They offer us, every day, post-Roe grief counseling," Hancock said bitterly. "They're just swimming in their victory."

Sitting in the shade of the tarp, Hancock suddenly glanced up from her phone. The court just added tomorrow as a decision day, she announced to the group. "You know what's gonna happen, right? Everyone's throat is going to be cut. The axe is going to drop," she said.

"The shoe is going to fall," added Gibson.

"In the meantime . . ." Hancock trailed off. Gibson picked up. "We keep going."

Inside the doors of the Pink House, Dr. Cheryl Hamlin met with groups of women to give them mifepristone—or, as she called it, "mify"—the packet of pills that would end their pregnancies. She had delivered these instructions so many times in this small room with salmon and lavender walls that she had lost count.

"The pill you are taking today has no side effects," she began. But once you swallow it, a nurse warned the women, there's no reversing: if you don't complete the process with the second set of pills, you will either lose the fetus anyhow or keep the pregnancy and could have an abnormal baby.

It's with that second set of pills, Dr. Hamlin explained, that they would start to feel their abortion begin. After about three to four hours, there would be bleeding and cramping. "You'll pass clots the size of a lemon," she said. "At some point, you're just going to be sitting on a towel or on the toilet. It's going to be more than bothering with a pad." The blood will decrease dramatically after two hours. After two weeks, it should stop completely. You can start your birth control as soon as you stop passing tissue, she said.

If it doesn't happen that way—maybe there's only a little spotting or no bleeding at all—don't wait the suggested two weeks for the follow-up visit, she urged. "Pretty good sign it didn't work," Dr. Hamlin said. Give the clinic a call right away. "It probably means you're still pregnant," she told the group.

"Okay, I'm going to pass out your pills," Dr. Hamlin said. "You're free to go, but I'll stay here and sign your charts for a few minutes, if you have questions."

The clinic made the women deposit their phones in a basket outside, a security precaution to protect their privacy. As they waited for the pills, the women discussed their miscarriages, pregnancies, and childbirths. They described the bleeds they'd had, whether their water broke or had to be broken. They talked about how much work they had missed and how much they expected to miss after they took the second dose. One woman mentioned her three sons. She had her first child at fifteen, and now he was about to graduate from high school. "They done wear me out," she said. And for the past few weeks, she reminded everyone, there had been a baby formula shortage. "I ain't going through that shit," she declared, taking the packet.

Everyone swallowed their first pill. Dr. Hamlin and the nurses offered stern warnings: if they failed to take their second pill and had to come back to start again, they would be charged again. A woman who felt nauseous was urged to wait in the clinic after her dose. If she threw up the pill after she left, it would be another hundred dollars to restart the process, Dr. Hamlin explained. The woman had traveled three hours from Louisiana and it was the trip on the potholed roads that did her in, she said. "Yeah, you gonna rock and roll here in Mississippi," a nurse said.

After they took their pills, some of the women asked Dr. Hamlin questions. "Can I still breastfeed while taking this?" wondered a woman with a four-month-old at home. "What about marijuana edibles"—her treatment for anxiety and depression—"is it safe to keep up the standard dosage?"

"Neither should be a problem," she told them.

Dr. Hamlin had never been to Mississippi until deciding she wanted to help the Pink House after Trump won the 2016 election. Since then, once a month, Dr. Hamlin had made the 1,255-mile trip from her home in Boston to Jackson for her three-day shift. Over that period, she typically saw nearly one hundred women for counseling, medication abortions, and surgical abortions. At the clinics around Boston, she saw about fifteen patients on a busy day. There was no mandatory counseling. No speech that she was required to say by state law, informing women that having an abortion would increase their risk of breast cancer—an inaccuracy she immediately corrected every time she said it. No need to mark the official start of the required twenty-four-hour waiting period.

Recently, she had started telling the women in Mississippi about the coming Supreme Court decision, warning them that this clinic and almost every other one in the Midwest and South would likely close soon. Most didn't know anything about the case. Dr. Hamlin urged them to vote and wished she could recommend some other steps to take. She knew there were none.

In an office down the hall, behind a desk piled with paperwork, Shannon Brewer, the clinic director, sorted through her papers. Her eyes darted, every few seconds, to check the monitor on her right—a video feed of eleven security cameras in and around the building. It was a habit developed over a lifetime in the Pink House, always watching and waiting for the next crisis to come.

Brewer had started part-time in 2000. Her aunt, Betty Thompson, was the director then and needed help. Brewer had six children and was barely making it. She had no furniture in her apartment, just a mattress from the Salvation Army that she shared with the kids. She had almost given up her fifth, a son, for adoption. But when the time came to hand over her new baby, she couldn't do it. "If you have an abortion, you don't even know who this would have been. So that's totally two different things. That's what people don't get," she said in a 2016 documentary about the clinic. "It's harder to see your child and then just hand your child away to somebody else. I believe in abortion because no woman should have to feel the way that I felt."

Brewer believed that working at the Pink House was what she was meant to do. She was there in 2004, when it became the last clinic in the state, and in 2010, when Susan Hill, the first owner, was dying of breast cancer and sold her business to a friend. When the new owner, Diane Derzis, decided to repaint the beige building that bubble-gum pink, Brewer was skeptical. She worried the color would make it even more of a target. After it happened, she realized that it didn't matter; the clinic already stood out in the conservative Christian stronghold of Jackson.

The Pink House almost closed its doors after a 2012 state law required its doctors to have admitting privileges at a local hospital, a standard the clinic couldn't meet because none of the hospitals would agree. A court eventually blocked the law, and they stayed open. Brewer kept working.

And in 2018, when state representative Becky Currie pushed the fifteen-week ban through the state legislature, Brewer wasn't worried. The bill was a clear violation of Roe. Just like in 2012, she thought, their lawyer at the Center for Reproductive Rights would sue, and there would be a court ruling blocking the law. She never expected the Supreme Court would actually take up the case. But it did. And here she was, racing the clock to decision day. "It's the waiting," she said. "I feel like they are playing a game with me."

Unlike Hancock and her escorts, Brewer thought the justices would wait until the final day of their term to release their ruling. But in the meantime, she was drowning. The clinic expanded its hours to accommodate the influx of patients from out of state. She thought the media requests would stop if she just did a round of interviews. It didn't work. There were just more patients, more paperwork, more press, and an onslaught of need that felt never-ending.

"It's not as shocking as people think it is," she said with a sigh, her eyes flitting to the video screen as her hand signed another set of papers.

Everyone kept asking her how she was feeling. How Brewer was feeling was tired.

2021–2023

28

The Brief

Scott Stewart barreled down the highway, Washington fading in his rearview mirror. He had never set foot in Mississippi. But Donald Trump's defeat had thrust him into the job market, and Lynn Fitch, the state's attorney general, had reached out. She needed a new solicitor general to lead the state's biggest cases. The spot had been open for months, ever since Trump had nominated Kristi Johnson, who helped write the Dobbs cert petition, to become the first female judge for the Southern District of Mississippi. Fitch's team found his name tucked into a pile of résumés from the Republican Attorneys General Association (RAGA), a group that had received more than $13 million from Leo's network of organizations and whose executive director used to work for the Federalist Society. Fitch hadn't heard of Stewart. When he interviewed via Zoom over Christmas, he didn't realize his camera was off. It didn't matter—Fitch liked what she heard.

Stewart was thirty-eight, mobile, not yet married, and most of all ambitious. Over the past decade and a half, the job of state solicitor general had become a higher-profile slot for ambitious young lawyers, even a path to more prominent posts like judgeships. For Stewart, the opportunity was ideal—a Republican state with a Democratic president in the White House offered lots of potential for conflict, interesting arguments, and high impact. And there was the lure of the Dobbs case, potentially his first chance to argue a case at the Supreme Court.

When he got the job, a friend he had worked with at Gibson Dunn, a law firm known as a conservative powerhouse, reached out to congratulate him and shared advice on being a new solicitor general. It was Misha Tseytlin, who had brainstormed the fifteen-week concept. The network, as always, was tight.

Behind the wheel, Scott had a thousand miles and two long days of driving to think about how to apply all he had learned in Washington to a state that Washington often forgot about. If the Trump administration had taught him anything, it was to hold the line. Trying to stop Jane Doe from getting an abortion was just one example. He had defended some of Trump's most controversial immigration policies, including the legal fallout from the policy to separate children from their parents at the border.

Jackson, Mississippi, he knew, would be like no other place he had lived. Tall and fit, with sandy-brown hair, Stewart was a California kid. His father coached tennis to Hollywood stars, and Stewart learned the game on their backyard court sandwiched between the beach and steep canyons of Malibu. But Stewart was not part of the California that conservatives often criticized for liberalizing America's sexual values and imposing them on the country. His family was among the conservative minority.

Stewart was used to standing for conservative values in liberal elite culture, places like Princeton, which recruited him to play tennis, and Stanford, where he kept his views largely to himself amid what he saw as the stark ideological uniformity of the place. In Portland, Oregon, he clerked for Judge Diarmuid O'Scannlain, a pugnacious voice for right-wing judicial thought on the liberal Ninth Circuit. Stewart parlayed his conservative credentials after his Clarence Thomas clerkship, the year Antonin Scalia died, into a post on Trump's transition team, assessing the legality of various potential policies.

He crossed the state line into Mississippi, entering the poorest and hungriest state in America, with an old-money class steeped in the traditions of the Deep South, like Fitch. But there was one major way he fit in: for the first time in his life, Stewart now lived in a place where he was in the political majority.

Until it looked like the Supreme Court would actually take up the Dobbs case—if it ever did—it seemed prudent to focus his attention on other pressing issues at work, Stewart reasoned. At home, he looked for a church, and settled on a Presbyterian congregation, an evangelical offshoot that did not ordain women as pastors.

Just like Nancy Northup, Fitch and Scott watched the court seem to ignore their case for months, never offering a decision on whether to take it up. And like their opponents, they found the seeming indecision strange. Everyone had a theory about why the justices were dragging their feet. Maybe John Roberts wanted to give time for Amy Coney Barrett to settle into her new job, fearing the case was too political too soon after she was seated. Or perhaps the court wanted a different Roe test case, one that wasn't as clear-cut a shot at the viability standard. Or maybe the justices wanted the political drama from the election to settle down before embarking on a controversial ruling.

Maybe they would not hear the case at all.

THE SILENCE BROKE one morning in May 2021.

Fitch was on her way to the airport after attending an event hosted by RAGA. That weekend, the organization had an exclusive gathering at a private island on the secluded coast of southeast Georgia nestled between the marsh and the sea. The three-day retreat at the Cloister, with its grand verandas and luxe accommodations, was a perk for the most elite donors to the organization—the kind of weekend typified by golf, cigar-and-whiskey receptions, and the spa. There, corporate bigwigs schmoozed with top state law enforcement leaders, people like Fitch, who would often determine the fate of their interests in America's highest courts.

But during this weekend, the organization was in disarray. Major donors were fleeing after learning that its policy arm authorized robocalls urging supporters to march on the Capitol on January 6. Staff and leaders were stepping down in protest, and its chairman had resigned. But the group had an angel investor: its biggest funder was the Judicial Crisis Network, one of Leo's signature dark-money nonprofit groups—which had been rebranded as the Concord Fund. The fund was part of Leo's ballooning web, a constellation of organizations that through name changes and difficult-to-trace spending—and with help from the secret $1.6 billion donation from Barre Seid—circulated money to accomplish the conservative agenda. The fund had stepped in with a $2.5 million check.

Fitch stared at the text from her chief of staff, Michelle Williams, trying to process the magnitude: *We just got cert.*

The Supreme Court had agreed to hear the case that could strike at Roe. Williams knew the significance of the words she had sent. She was part of Marjorie Dannenfelser's original sisterhood back in the 1990s and even babysat her children in the early SBA years, before becoming Representative Michele Bachmann's chief of staff with the Tea Party rise. In the Trump administration, she was chief of staff at the Office of Management and Budget to Russell Vought, a longtime abortion opponent who had enacted the Trump policy to defund Planned Parenthood.

By the time Fitch got to the airport terminal, she saw her own face and blonde bob—an annoyingly old headshot, she noted to a staffer—on what felt like every television screen. It was happening. The hopes of the conservative movement, and fears of the abortion-rights world, rested with Mississippi.

That evening, Scott Stewart, now the Mississippi solicitor general, pulled up *Roe v. Wade* for the first time in a long while. He had a lot of reading to do. He had never really studied abortion cases before, except for Roe and Casey. It was a strange area of law—there had been so many cases, over so many years, and almost none of them had a unanimous decision. One, *Stenberg v. Carhart*, had eight opinions for nine justices.

He was clerking for Clarence Thomas when the Supreme Court struck down the Texas abortion restrictions in Whole Woman's Health, the ones that Wendy Davis had filibustered—except for the twenty-week limit. Thomas dissented, arguing that the full law should stand because courts should defer to legislatures regarding abortion. And there was the case of the pregnant detained Jane Doe. But other than that, abortion had not come up often in his career. The legal arguments he made in the Jane Doe case were not primarily about Roe but about whether the girl had constitutional rights given her undocumented status.

Now, Stewart had to move quickly. Mississippi would have barely two months to submit a written brief to the court to present its case. And he would have just a few months after that to prepare for oral arguments scheduled for the court's fall term. It was the biggest case of his life.

He had to decide on a strategy. Plenty of people in the antiabortion and conservative legal movements had ideas about what he should do, including ADF's flotilla of lawyers. By 2021, they had spent years seeding the fifteen-week law, first by adopting Tseytlin's idea to find a strategic number of weeks, then crafting the model legislation and working with state representative Becky Currie and Jameson Taylor to push it through the legislature, and then creating additional paths in Utah and Arkansas. They felt a strong sense of ownership over the case. But so did Fitch and Stewart, and unlike those state legislators who just adopted ADF's bills, they had already begun crafting their own plans.

Fitch's original cert petition had focused on upholding the Mississippi law, and mentioned the possibility of overturning Roe just as a footnote, buried after eighteen pages: "If the Court determines that it cannot reconcile Roe and Casey with other precedents or scientific advancements showing a compelling state interest in fetal life far earlier in pregnancy than those cases contemplate, the Court should not retain erroneous precedent."

He knew a lot of lawyers would encourage him to continue down that easier path: to simply argue that Mississippi's law should be upheld. To not push for the whole overturn of Roe but to chip away—as the movement had for so many decades—and get the court to undo the viability standard.

But for Stewart, that was thinking too small, too safe. This moment was different from all those decades past. Trump had pushed their cause from the biggest bully pulpit in the land. Conservatives now had a majority on the court that seemed to be on their side.

It was not a moment for compromise, Stewart reasoned. It was a lesson he had learned from Thomas, his old boss, who was known to hold the line without deviation. Stick with a position, take the heat, and never budge. It was a trait Stewart found rare and admirable.

When you believe something, he had learned, you go all the way. His argument had to be bigger, bolder. He would be steadfast: Roe and Casey were wrong and must be reversed.

It did not take long for top Alliance Defending Freedom lawyers to book flights to Jackson. They saw Dobbs as their project, going all the way back to that idea at the Federalist Society meeting after Trump's election to find a strategic number of weeks. If they played this case right, they might not need the circuit split they were trying to provoke with Utah and Arkansas. This case alone could accomplish their objective of undercutting Roe's viability line.

It was a crucial moment for the entire antiabortion coalition—the most significant abortion case of the new Trump court. But even after years pushing for a singular goal, the coalition was not a monolith, especially on strategy. Stewart wanted to openly ask the Supreme Court to overturn Roe. ADF, of course, wanted Roe overturned—its ultimate target was to ban abortion nationwide at conception—but it favored a more limited, less risky approach. Now the group just had to make sure that Stewart and Fitch didn't jeopardize the plan they started laying almost six years earlier, at cocktails with Tseytlin in the Mayflower Hotel.

The ADF lawyers rode the old mirrored elevators of the Walter Sillers State Office Building to the twelfth floor, ready for a private summit with Fitch and Stewart. Mississippi was their client, and ADF had been checking in, making loose plans in case its petition was taken up. This could be the case of a generation, and ADF wasn't about to cede control.

ADF's soon-to-be new president, Kristen Waggoner, brought a core team of top-notch attorneys and media experts, including a new lawyer ADF had hired—Erin Hawley, a graduate of Yale Law School who had clerked for Chief Justice Roberts. She was married to Senator Josh Hawley of Missouri, who had openly advertised Barrett's antiabortion views and punched his fist to the sky on January 6, in apparent support of then-peaceful demonstrators, before he had to flee the Capitol for safety. Overturning Roe was a joint mission for the Hawleys, who had met as clerks for Roberts. "He likes to take credit for our marriage," Josh Hawley later joked of the justice, as the couple sat onstage at a meeting of socially conservative activists. "And we like to say to him that we're the most conservative thing he's ever done." The Dobbs case, Erin Hawley said, was about "the heart of a nation." The Constitution said nothing about abortion, she would say, but the Bible was clear that it was morally wrong. Like so many evangelical believers, she would cite Psalm 139:13: "For you created my inmost being; you knit me together in my mother's womb."

Squeezed around a long table, with swivel chairs that felt slightly too big for Fitch's small conference room, ADF lawyers lined up on one side and the Mississippi team on the other. The room was sparse, save a large painting of Fitch behind the head of the table, with narrow windows that looked down onto the Mississippi

Supreme Court. This private meeting, one kept secret from the press, top politicians, and even other allies in the antiabortion coalition, would mark a pivotal turning point in the strategy of their movement.

The ADF lawyers outlined their thinking. Their original plan was to find the magic number of weeks that would trigger this exact court case, to get the court to remove the viability line as the limit for when states could ban abortion. When the Supreme Court agreed to hear the case, it said it wanted to hear just one of the three questions in their brief: "Whether all pre-viability prohibitions on elective abortions are unconstitutional." To ADF, that signaled that the justices wanted to address the viability line specifically.

Priority number one, ADF lawyers argued, was to get rid of the line. Removing that limit—about twenty-three weeks—would open the door to all kinds of restrictions being upheld by lower courts. It would be a huge victory for their cause. It was a backdoor way of gutting Roe, invalidating the central principle of the original decision, without fully requiring the justices to take the thornier step of overturning fifty years of precedent. They all had to stick to the plan, a new version of the strategy their movement had adopted for decades: move incrementally and chip away.

Stewart listened as they urged caution. He already had his own plan to strike directly at Roe. He disagreed with the team around the table from ADF. The lawmakers of Mississippi had enacted a law, and that law was fundamentally incompatible with Roe, he argued. "The people of Mississippi are pro-life. They enacted this law. It is my duty to defend it to the best of my ability, and the right thing to do is to ask the court to overturn Roe," he told the room filled with strategists who had worked on this issue for decades, according to Erin Hawley. The only effective strategy, Stewart said according to participants, was to target the very heart of it all—the right to abortion that the court had found in the Constitution in 1973. The best argument was not that this law was fine under Roe, he decided. It was that Roe was wrong.

Some of the ADF lawyers bristled. Stewart's plan felt risky, and aggressive. If the court wanted to use this case to overturn Roe, it could, argued the ADF team. But to ask for that explicitly could be going too far, too fast even for this new court. It would raise the risk that they could be told no. A defeat would be devastating, potentially even going so far as to reaffirm abortion rights in some way and create another precedent to fight.

There was a lot to consider. It wasn't totally clear that they had five votes to fully overturn Roe right now. Certainly, it was the best court they'd faced in a long time. But the 6–3 conservative majority was still new, and the country was still reeling from the contentious Supreme Court battles of the Trump era. ADF lawyers suspected that Roberts feared such a dramatic reversal. Roberts had a reputation as an institutionalist, sensitive to decisions that could threaten the court's already-shaky public standing.

Brett Kavanaugh remained another unknown. He had sided with Stewart in the Jane Doe case, but, as social conservatives had pointed out during his confirmation fight, he didn't have a long record of rulings on abortion cases. He dissented in *June Medical Services v. Russo*, the Louisiana case, taking a view that encouraged abortion opponents, but his short opinion just said that the doctors should try harder to get admitting privileges to local hospitals and didn't make a major statement about Roe. Barrett's personal opposition to abortion was well known, but to ask for a full reversal of Roe seemed to put a lot of faith in her originalist credentials.

And looming over the conversation was the reality that Stewart had never argued a case at the Supreme Court. By this point, ADF lawyers had argued and won twelve Supreme Court cases, dealing with questions of contraceptive access under Obama's health care law mandate and anti-LGBT discrimination in public accommodations, among other topics. Their victories consistently carved out additional space for Christianity in American public life and pushed for greater religious freedom.

The ADF lawyers' message was clear: the safest path to victory was their plan. They should simply ask the court to uphold their fifteen-week law. Ending the viability standard was as far as they could get right now.

Fitch's team was grateful for ADF's help. But this had the feel of a power grab—a bunch of Washington lawyers coming down to Jackson to take over once the job became a chance to make history. This was Fitch's case. She had chosen Stewart, and Stewart was determined. There was magic in boldness, he believed, and too often, even clever litigators held back and missed having a massive impact. Mississippi would forge its own path.

"Like everything else, you get four attorneys in a room, you're going to get ten opinions," Kevin Theriot, an ADF lawyer who dialed into the summit by phone, said later. "It's not that our original strategy went out the window. It was just that instead of making 'You should overturn Roe' the second argument, they made it the first argument."

He added, "God had created a team that was capable of doing some really good stuff."

It was decided. Mississippi would go for Roe. Leaving the meeting, the dynamics were clear: ADF would take a back seat to Stewart and Fitch's bolder approach. Later, ADF played down the divide. "They were the final decision-makers on whether they were going to go for it or not," Waggoner said. "We were happy to play a supportive role."

Stewart's thinking reflected the shifts that had overtaken the antiabortion movement and the conservative legal project during the Trump administration. For four years, they had gone bigger and bolder than what had previously felt possible. Their work didn't always succeed: Jane Doe got her abortion. The new Biden administration rolled back their administrative actions. Courts blocked many of their state abortion bans.

But the efforts themselves had changed the window of possibilities. To overturn Roe, conservatives had to directly ask the court to do so. ADF may have been skittish about making the request, but Fitch and Stewart were not. Their decision to disregard ADF's incremental advice set the terms for everything that followed.

STILL, ADF WOULD keep its promises to be involved. Waggoner offered any and all assistance to Mississippi. ADF loaned Hawley to Stewart and Fitch as an adviser. She could pull back the veil on Roberts's thinking and the political landscape, particularly the Senate. The case was something her husband "really cares deeply about" too, she said, adding that "we didn't discuss anything confidential."

They needed two plans: one to manage the court, and another to manage the public. The plans had to work together, a wholesale legal and marketing strategy to present one clear, united, and unassailable front. Everything had to be controlled. They could not risk igniting a political firestorm—the court had already become so politicized. Everyone would stay quiet, functionally downplaying the case.

Even after all the power they had gained during the Trump years, there was a persistent belief in the antiabortion community that they were David fighting Goliath—that they were outsiders, small and disparate, versus their mighty opposition. Many in the movement still saw Planned Parenthood, the ACLU, and the Center for Reproductive Rights—what they called the "abortion lobby"—as the collective powerhouse, with centralized messaging, backed by white-shoe law firms ready to do pro bono work, in coordination with allies in the media. It motivated them to work harder, to be craftier, to persist at all costs.

But the reality was different now. While their antiabortion views still represented a distinct minority of the country, they had built their cause into an elite legal and ideological system, with a sprawling ecosystem of activists, organizations, lawmakers, and pro bono lawyers. They were all driving, working together on the single goal of undoing Roe and remaking the country. Their policy arms churned out legal arguments and medical studies. Their lawyers argued their cases, and their judges ruled on them, all fostered by the bench Leo built. And their allied lawmakers pushed their agenda in statehouses and Congress. Yet despite their overwhelming success, the left largely continued to underestimate them. It was their greatest strength.

Behind closed doors, Fitch's team drew up a nine-slide blueprint, marked "Confidential": a twelve-month political and public relations strategy in the run-up to the expected court decision on Dobbs in June 2022. "Strategy to maximize impact at SCOTUS," it began. The whole operation was surprisingly low-budget, estimated at about $231,000, to be paid out of the attorney general's office and Fitch's political fund.

The case wasn't just good policy for Fitch. It seemed like good politics, too, a chance to build a conservative brand that could boost her political career. Already, there was chatter in the state that she could run for governor. But first, this had to be managed perfectly. They shared the plan over email, with a link to contribute to her campaign.

Point one: "Ensure strongest possible legal strategy."

That would be Stewart's job, whose smiling headshot appeared on slide four. They needed to determine what objections each justice might be considering and then strategize to address those vulnerabilities in their legal argument.

Point two: "Communicate a positive message that echoes our briefs and creates the right overall environment for targeted Justices."

The goal was to limit discussion of the case in the press to avoid spooking the justices about the risky politics of the case, and avoid drawing public attention to their plans. Williams, Fitch's chief of staff, would take the lead. Fitch would not go on Fox News frequently to talk about the case. Instead, they would orchestrate a very specific media plan. She and her team would not use the word *abortion*. Their message would be upbeat. Fitch would cast the case as a defense of "a law to safeguard women's health and protect life after 15 weeks gestation." Their slogan would be "Empower Women, Promote Life." Winning meant not letting abortion-rights advocates monopolize the narrative on women's rights. Venue mattered too: Fitch prioritized op-eds instead of interviews, so her full words would be less likely to be edited. They would focus on outlets their fervent supporters watched, like EWTN, the Catholic television network, and conservative outlets where she would predict "a lot of celebration" once Roe was overturned.

Point three: build "a coalition of voices with diverse messages all feeding into that same echo chamber."

The echo chamber was essential. This was their ecosystem, an effort to amplify the voices of their allies and create the impression that their community of supporters was more vast than polling indicated. Like so many activist movements, the antiabortion coalition had been strengthened in this social media decade, using the online platforms to project their rallying cries. Posts on Twitter and Facebook could take on lives of their own, and moments could go viral online. As often proved the case with social media, the effect suggested greater power disproportionate to their real-life support, at times furthered by bots and trolls. They would target three key media moments: filing the brief, oral arguments, and the expected decision.

On the day of arguments, they organized an Empower Women Promote Life Rally in front of the Supreme Court, featuring largely female lineup of speakers, including Dannenfelser and Hawkins. Williams and her team planned for every possible contingency, down to their opposition cutting their power lines. Speakers would be racially and religiously diverse, avoiding the depiction of their mission as a solely white or Christian project, and include a doctor, an atheist, a Black Democratic state lawmaker, and a mother of a child with cystic fibrosis—the wife of a top Trump official.

The whole network of people and institutions, tightened over a decade, was coming together. The Dobbs campaign would be a full-scale assault by their movement's legal experts, conservative academics, and especially female voices who would argue the case in the court of public opinion. Fitch would craft her personal story of conservative womanhood as the ultimate vision of what they saw as possible for mothers, even single ones like her. On a trip to Washington, they filmed her slowly walking in front of the steps of the Supreme Court in a light blue suit and chunky block heels—gathering footage that seemed designed more for a campaign video than a legal case.

Fitch was the main political face, but Stewart drove the legal argument. In the weeks that followed, Stewart quietly mapped out Mississippi's case. Meanwhile, Tate Reeves, the governor of Mississippi, was on cable news, arguing that the case wasn't about Roe but the science of when a fetus could live outside the womb—essentially the viability line.

"Let me just tell you that for people such as myself that are pro-life, I believe that the Supreme Court made a mistake in the 1970s," Reeves said on CNN in June 2021. "But that's not the issue at stake that is before the court, hopefully, when the arguments are heard sometime in the fall."

But up on the twelfth floor of the Walter Sillers Building, where Stewart and Fitch refined their plans, Roe was the central issue. For Stewart, the Dobbs case needed to be more Iceman than Maverick, a reference to characters from the movie *Top Gun*. Disciplined and academic, not reckless and heated. Calculated, planned in its entirety.

He tapped the movement's network for advice, consulting allies from government to academia to think tanks. Stewart talked with fellow Republican solicitors general, religious liberty lawyers, and academic attorneys, like Barrett's friend and neighbor Carter Snead at Notre Dame.

For Fitch, it was important that the legal argument be a continuation of her political ethos, encompassing the conservative vision of womanhood that had defined much of her career. If they could show how the country had changed for women since 1973, they could argue that Roe was no longer needed for gender equality—a foundational part of the argument made by abortion-rights organizations. The precedent could be undone because America had changed. And Fitch, with her professional success story as a single mother, could be the face of that shift.

To make that argument, Fitch and Stewart drew from the work of Erika Bachiochi, a Catholic scholar and conservative expert in feminist legal theory whose work was inspired by her conversion after a largely secular childhood. She was part of a small but rising group of conservative female scholars who had been laying an intellectual framework to invert the feminist argument of equal advancement into a case against abortion. Bachiochi saw the sexual revolution of the 1970s not as liberating women but, instead, empowering men. She believed the invention of the birth control pill decoupled sex from marriage and marriage from child-rearing, and as a result, women, she said, were brought down to "men's standards of freewheeling quick sex." In her thinking, it became easier for men to refuse commitment to marriage or family life, and that led to more single motherhood, which created more poverty and struggle for women.

Abortion, she thought, incentivized damaging "sexual risk-taking." Women needed to "take their place again as gatekeepers of sex." If abortion were banned, the potential costs of sex would increase. Criminalization of the procedure would "empower women" to expect more from men—commitment, support—and basic things like "a job, to expect them to get off their computers and get off porn and all sorts of things." And that, she said, would force a "real maturation of men," restoring the primacy of the family, and decreasing poverty rates. Bachiochi encouraged the antiabortion movement to advocate for pro-family policies, such as paid leave, which would make it easier for working women to have babies.

Still, she was making a philosophical case that to many in the mainstream seemed disconnected from the lived realities of modern sex, relationships, and family economics. Even when abortion was illegal, the "costs" of a possible pregnancy didn't stop sex outside of marriage. And politically, there was little reason to believe that eliminating federal abortion rights would prompt action to improve policies for American families and pregnant women. Federal efforts to require businesses to offer paid parental leave died in the Senate during the Trump administration. And of the states with trigger laws on the books in 2021 that would quickly ban abortion if Roe were overturned, none had mandated paid leave.

Bachiochi wrote one of a flood of amicus briefs sent to the court. In an apparent milestone, there were more briefs filed by abortion opponents than abortion-rights advocates—86 to 52. The overall explosion of commentary from historians, elected officials, and medical experts was a trend that reached beyond just Dobbs, marking a larger shift in how advocacy groups tried to influence the Supreme Court. There were 23 "friend of court" briefs filed in Roe and more than 140 filed nearly five decades later in Dobbs.

The antiabortion movement flooded the court with its version of historical narratives, scientific data, and legal scholarship. It marked the fruition of a decade of new organizing and groups' coming to organizational and political maturity. The scope of their lobbying effort revealed how the network was remaking legal thinking. Brief after brief was authored by organizations and individuals who placed their Christian vision at the center of their work. It was a reflection of the work they had done since Obama's 2012 victory, expanding the reach of their own institutions and building greater political power. Leo himself was at the root of much of the lobbying of the court, with dozens of amicus briefs connecting back to him as a board member, financial supporter, or official of the organizations writing the briefs.

Legal scholars who had worked with Justice Barrett at Notre Dame argued that the court's abortion precedent was unconstitutional. Dannenfelser, along with seventy-nine female state legislators, wrote that since 1973, women had increased their political representation in politics and could now advance the policy preferences of their gender legislatively and did not need to rely on the court. Medical associations that were founded to oppose abortion made the case that abortions after fifteen weeks posed significant physical and mental health risks. More than 550 elected officials, including governors, US senators, House members, and state legislators, signed onto briefs, as did twenty-four states with similar laws restricting abortion.

David Daleiden, who was then facing criminal charges in San Francisco Superior Court related to his Planned Parenthood sting, wrote a brief and cited his surreptitiously obtained quote from Dr. Deborah Nucatola twirling her salad at lunch, saying, "A lot of people want intact hearts these days." Courts had found him and the Center for Medical Progress liable for more than $16 million in legal fees and costs and damages to Planned Parenthood, but he repeated his argument for the justices. (As of this writing, a trial on the criminal charges was scheduled for March 2024, and an appeal was still pending as to the award of attorneys' fees and costs.)

At the Supreme Court, the relationships between the authors of some of the briefs and the justices they were trying to convince ran deep. Lawyer after lawyer had clerked for the justices or worked with them before they joined the bench. It wasn't just conservatives; attorneys on both sides of the aisle often argued before the justices for whom they had clerked. That was simply how the court worked. In any other American courtroom, jurors and the judge typically recuse themselves if they have any personal relationship to one of the parties involved. But at the Supreme Court, such connections were not only considered standard—but an asset.

STEWART FILED THE new brief for the state of Mississippi in July, and Roe was no longer just a minor footnote. Now, he mentioned it 144 times. His argument was a full-scale assault on a precedent that had defined American life for nearly half a century, in plain language.

"Roe and Casey are egregiously wrong," he began. "The conclusion that abortion is a constitutional right has no basis in text, structure, history, or tradition."

His language was unrelenting: Roe was "hopelessly unworkable." It had "inflicted significant damage" with "a jurisprudence that is at war with the demand that this Court act based on neutral principles." He argued that the ruling had warped the democratic process by removing the issue from the legislature and weakened the court.

"Roe and Casey are unprincipled decisions that have damaged the democratic process, poisoned our national discourse, plagued the law—and, in doing so, harmed this Court," Stewart wrote.

He had planned to be Iceman, and in many ways, he was. The strategy was targeted, he was clinical and academic. But this was a Maverick brief, a moon shot that bucked the longtime incremental strategy of many leaders of the antiabortion movement, even as it stated what they truly believed.

His approach was the culmination of a decade of conservative escalation, dating back to 2010 when the Tea Party lawmakers rushed into Congress and demanded immediate, sweeping change. Their hard-line ethos gave rise to Trump, the conservative transformation of the court, and the no-holds-barred rhetoric of infanticide and baby executions. And now, to this radical brief.

Stewart argued that the Mississippi law was not discriminatory toward women but instead promoted women's health and "protects unborn girls and boys equally." He cited science doubted by much of the medical establishment, referencing advancements that raised questions about whether the court should address a state's interest in preventing "fetal pain." The statement implied fetuses could feel pain before fifteen weeks—a position now inched up five weeks from the twenty weeks in the Texas law—and still one that no major medical organization had accepted for years. But most striking was Stewart's framing that overturning Roe, one of the legal decisions most associated with the feminist movement, would be the true liberation of women. Roe said that an unwanted pregnancy could lead women to "a distressful life and future." Casey expanded on that thinking, saying that Roe was needed for "women to participate equally in the economic and social life of the nation." For decades, the antiabortion movement had countered those decisions with arguments about the immorality of abortion and the rights of the fetus.

Stewart took a radically different approach, imbuing his brief with the conservative vision of womanhood that Fitch elevated. The world had changed and women no longer needed abortion to provide equality, he said.

Women had advanced to the "highest echelons" of economic and social life, Stewart noted. Progress toward gender equality with laws prohibiting pregnancy discrimination and expanding paid leave meant a pregnancy would not hamper women's economic and educational advancement, he wrote. Adoption and contraceptives were accessible, so an unwanted pregnancy was less likely, he argued. "States should be able to act on those developments. But Roe and Casey shackle States to a view of the facts that is decades out of date," the brief concluded.

The reality was much more complicated. While women were likely to be more educated than their male partners, and female representation in public life had reached historic highs, American women had not reached parity with men. There was a robust body of data showing that becoming a mother had a significant—and negative—economic impact on women's lives, particularly for low-income women, who faced the biggest barriers to abortion access. Some studies showed that both the employment rate and earnings of women dropped as much as thirty-five points when their children were born, compared with those of men. Childcare was unaffordable for nearly half of American families, and the country's paid leave policies remained some of the weakest in the world. Despite laws banning pregnancy discrimination, it was rampant in the country's biggest corporations. His argument also glossed over the fact of pregnancy itself, the physical and emotional costs of the nine-month period when a woman grew another being in their body—a state men never experience.

Stewart's arguments about Roe and women's advancement were bold. But they also echoed words from 1973. In their dissent to Roe, Justices Byron White and William Rehnquist cast the decision as "an exercise of raw judicial power" with no basis in "the language or history of the Constitution." Stewart argued much the same.

"The national fever on abortion can break only when this court returns abortion policy to the states—where agreement is more common, compromise is often possible and disagreement can be resolved at the ballot box," he wrote.

If there was a "national fever" over abortion rights, it wasn't one that had infected a majority of Americans, who thought the issue of Roe had been settled long ago. But it had infected key justices on the court. And for now, at least, they were the only votes that mattered.

A SENSE OF resoluteness swept over Nancy Northup of the Center for Reproductive Rights as she read Stewart's argument. Finally, there was clarity. For the Pink House in Mississippi, and for clinics across the country, her lawyers had fought restriction after restriction over the past decade. The drumbeat of incremental litigation was so ever present that it faded into background noise, making it hard to convince people that the antiabortion forces were gaining tremendous ground. But now, there could be no more confusion over what was at stake. Stewart made the true target clear. Roe. The most foundational abortion right. It would come down to Stewart's argument versus the ones Northup's lawyers at the Center would make.

Mississippi's new brief left her team with a decision to make, the exact inverse of the choice made by Stewart and ADF. In their response to Stewart, Northup and her lawyers could offer the court an off-ramp, a way to avoid the thorny question of Roe. If they gave the court an option to uphold the law and avoid fully striking down Roe, they could potentially save the right to an abortion before fifteen weeks—when more than 90 percent of abortions occurred—at least for a while, until the next case reached the Supreme Court.

But Northup did not see a path for compromise. She knew that the fifteen-week cutoff was arbitrary, with no basis in medicine or the law. Though Northup and her lawyers didn't know the particulars of ADF's plans, they realized the line was a litigation strategy.

Even though the original decision skirted the issue, to Northup and her team, Roe wasn't an abstract legal question of whether a right was explicitly mentioned in the Constitution. The precedent was about whether women, just as men, had control over their bodies. To them, Roe was about whether women had a constitutional protection of liberty and equality.

As a result, the center's response to directly defend Roe was a no-brainer, at least to Northup. They could not argue for a fifteen-week standard that had no basis in medical reality or in how women experienced pregnancy, childbirth, and their economic lives. Besides, Northup believed that the only justice remotely inclined toward a compromise that would uphold the fifteen-week ban but keep Roe was John Roberts, an institutionalist who was perceived to be uneasy about upending nearly a half-century-old legal precedent. If another justice—maybe Alito or Thomas—wanted to rally the conservative wing around the idea of overturning Roe, he could try to do so without the center suggesting it. Why set up a loss before you actually lost? Northup thought.

"There are no half-measures here," the center wrote in its brief. "Each of the State's purported alternatives would upend the balance struck in Casey and ultimately extinguish 'the woman's liberty to determine whether to carry her pregnancy to full term.'"

Citing a barrage of studies, the center's brief argued that women who are denied the ability to end a pregnancy face greater health risks and lost education and career opportunities. Those women are more likely to experience domestic violence and economic insecurity, and to raise their children in poverty. "The State's suggestion that gains in women's status somehow support taking away their right to make basic decisions about their lives and their bodies is nonsensical," it said.

Roe couldn't be outdated, they argued, because women plan their professional and personal lives knowing the right to an abortion exists, even if they never exercise it. Maybe that means trying for another child, even if the pregnancy could be risky, or being sexually active knowing that if a condom breaks, there is a backstop to having to stay pregnant. After two generations, women had come to depend on the right to a legal abortion. The passing decades had only made Roe "further cemented as critical to gender equality," the center's lawyers wrote.

"Accepting Mississippi's request to abandon the viability line would turn back the clock for generations who have never known what it means to be without the fundamental right to make the decision whether to continue a pregnancy," they wrote. "Any answer to the question presented other than a categorical 'yes' would shatter the understanding women have held close for decades about their bodies, their futures, and their equal right to liberty."

And just like Mississippi, though in slightly smaller numbers, the center had dozens of amicus briefs filed to the court that supported its arguments. The American College of Obstetricians and Gynecologists and other prominent medical organizations wrote that the fifteen-week ban had no grounding in medicine or science. Childbirth "they wrote" was far riskier than an abortion. "Risk of death associated with childbirth is accordingly approximately 14 times higher than any risk of death from an abortion," they wrote. Seventy-three women's rights organizations, led by the National Women's Law Center, argued that abortion was crucial to personal freedom and economic advancement—particularly in Mississippi, where women made up more than 71 percent of low-wage workers. Reproductive justice law scholars, racial justice groups, and economists pointed to the discriminatory nature of the ban, which would disproportionately affect low-income women and women of color.

More than 235 members of Congress and twenty-two states signed on to the center's effort, as did organizations of female lawyers and more than five hundred female athletes, who provided firsthand testimony arguing that without a constitutional right to abortion, "women's participation in athletics would suffer." The Biden administration wrote its own brief and asked the court if its solicitor general, Elizabeth Prelogar, could argue alongside the clinic. The effort amounted to the full force of liberal America dismissing Mississippi's conservative vision of gender progress.

This case, Northup was certain, was the final fight. If Stewart won, Roe would fall. A victory by Mississippi could make abortion illegal in about half the country. At least thirteen states already had trigger bans on the books, making them certain to move quickly to ban abortion, with very limited exceptions. And another thirteen states were likely to follow quickly with their own restrictions.

The court set oral arguments for December 1. One side represented a minority of Americans, the other mainstream public opinion. They would face off as equals before the justices. The clock started to tick.

29

Texan Revenge

Yet, Stewart and the center wouldn't be the only ones making their case about abortion rights to the Supreme Court in the summer of 2021. Two days after the Supreme Court agreed to hear Dobbs in May, the governor of Texas signed the newest, most restrictive abortion ban in America. Suddenly, Mississippi's law looked almost moderate. Texas now outlawed abortion after about six weeks of pregnancy, with no exceptions for rape or incest. With its new law, the state that gave America Roe in 1973 had found its own novel way to take it away.

The law—SB 8—included an unconventional mechanism to circumvent Roe by giving the power of enforcement not to state officials but to ordinary citizens. It created a new class of citizen-policers who could sue people they believed might have helped a woman get an abortion—anyone from doctors and clinic leaders to Uber drivers who transported a woman to her appointment. Anyone inside or outside of Texas could become a potential bounty hunter and get a $10,000 reward if they won their lawsuit. The only people involved with the procedure whom the law protected were the abortion patients themselves, who could not be sued. Rapists could not sue providers or others who helped with the abortion, to prevent an assailant from cashing in on an assault, but "an angry ex-boyfriend" could be considered an "appropriate plaintiff"—

a provision that underscored the twisted enforcement mechanism of the law.

Typically, abortion-rights supporters sued state officials—like Dobbs in Mississippi—to block restrictions in federal court. Judges in those courts could strike down the laws on constitutional grounds, arguing they were clear violations of Roe. The state would appeal, and the cases often took years and cost millions to resolve.

Even some antiabortion Republicans in the Texas legislature weren't eager to pay millions defending another restriction. SB 8 was designed to assuage some of those concerns. The elimination of state officials as legal enforcers could make it harder for the abortion-rights lawyers to sue in federal court, pushing the cases into Texas state-level courts, where conservative judges were typically friendlier to the antiabortion cause—potentially limiting the length of the litigation and the cost of appeals. Even better, the law could be enacted more quickly because any legal challenge would have to wait until a citizen brought a lawsuit.

Abortion providers, once again including Whole Woman's Health, sued in federal court anyhow, naming officials who were not directly tasked with enforcing SB 8 but still had authority over related laws. The new law, they wrote, "flagrantly violates the constitutional rights of Texans seeking abortion and upends the rule of law in service of an anti-abortion agenda." To much of the public, SB 8 seemed shocking. It had seemingly emerged from nowhere and went into effect so quickly. The law was widely unpopular, including among Republicans and white evangelicals. A majority of Texans had supported the twenty-week ban that Wendy Davis filibustered in 2013. But now, 69 percent of adults in the state said that this near-total was too restrictive. Those results foreshadowed the changing political reality as the laws grew far more aggressive: even in deeply conservative states, opposition to abortion had limits.

Still, the Texas law quickly became a new template for antiabortion activists. The National Association of Christian Lawmakers, a group started by Arkansas state senator Jason Rapert, who had championed ADF's eighteen-week bill, made the Texas law its first piece of model legislation in July. Soon, more than half a dozen states put forth similar bills. The law's enforcement mechanism, boasted Rapert to the *Deseret News*, was like "putting a SCUD missile on that heartbeat bill—they can't stop it."

For years, people like Leonard Leo, Marjorie Dannenfelser, and the ADF lawyers had carefully plotted their way toward overturning Roe. But this law marked a transition to a new, more radical approach. What was happening in Texas was a different version of what Scott Stewart was trying in Mississippi, an effort by the post-Roe generation of lawyers, lawmakers, and activists to accelerate the strategy of their movement's elders.

Donald Trump's embrace of the fringes of conservative politics and his transformation of the Supreme Court had emboldened this new generation. Stewart pushed the bounds of the conservative legal project fostered and grown by ADF, Leo, and the Federalist Society. Whether intentionally or not, his brief made common cause with antiabortion activists who had long been frustrated by the movement's incremental approach. The most conservative of this new cohort often called themselves "abortion abolitionists" and crusaded through Southern churches, legislatures, and college campuses preaching that the movement needed to end all abortion from conception. The remade antiabortion movement pushed states to introduce more than 660 abortion restrictions that year, and 108 laws were enacted in nineteen states—the highest total since 1973. Some instituted tight restrictions that would go into effect if Roe were overturned. Others tried to advance their own strategies to overturn Roe or gut it. Six states banned mail-order abortion medication. Arizona enacted a ban on abortion for reasons of genetic abnormalities. Just as Republican officials could no longer control their Trump wing, Dannenfelser, Leo, and their Washington world—what the abolitionists derisively called the "pro-life establishment"—were watching their carefully laid plans be taken over by an unruly fringe. Victory seemed closer than ever, and it energized the abolitionists to charge ahead to the broader movement's underlying ultimate goal: to criminalize all abortion. The fringe was becoming the mainstream.

THE RADICAL TEXAS law meant that just weeks after Stewart filed his brief, an entirely different abortion law was fast-tracked for Supreme Court review. Northup and the center filed a last-minute emergency motion to block the Texas law from going into effect on September 1. But this was a new Supreme Court, one where a conservative majority held sway. The deadline passed, and the court said nothing. Just before midnight, the justices formally denied the motion in an unsigned, bitterly divided ruling. John Roberts dissented, calling the law an unprecedented "statutory scheme." But the law was allowed to go into effect—even as it denied Texas women the constitutional rights that Roe had established.

"What a pity that we cannot do the right thing," wrote Sonia Sotomayor in a one-line email to Samuel Alito sent minutes before the law would go into effect, begging the court to issue a decision.

America now had its first post-Roe state. The nearly seven million women of childbearing age who lived in Texas would no longer be allowed an abortion, unless they knew they were pregnant almost immediately.

Despite the massive scope of the ruling, there was no questioning of lawyers at oral arguments and no monthslong grappling with the decision. Instead, the law went through the "shadow docket," a quicker decision-making process that was traditionally used by the court to deal with urgent matters, like issues related to elections, voting, or capital punishment. During the Trump administration, the court started using the process to deal with less pressing but more politically charged issues like regulatory actions that would be challenged by advocacy groups or liberal states—sometimes even before the appeals court had a chance to issue a decision.

The shadow docket shielded justices from individual criticism. The only reason the public knew the precise vote on the Texas law, 5–4, was that each of the minority justices wrote a signed dissent, suggesting the depth of their disagreement. The majority's 401-word, single-paragraph ruling amounted to a constitutional dodge, a way to ban abortion and violate the standard set in Roe while circumventing the thorny legal issues such a ruling raised.

"The Court's order is stunning," fumed Sotomayor. "Presented with an application to enjoin a flagrantly unconstitutional law engineered to prohibit women from exercising their constitutional rights and evade judicial scrutiny, a majority of Justices have opted to bury their heads in the sand."

Some conservatives saw a different, quieter sign in the ruling. The Mississippi case was just three months away from oral arguments. Why would the court uphold a six-week ban if it planned to strike it down in their Mississippi ruling? The conservative majority must be leaning toward overturning Roe. Conservatives now stood, as one evangelical adviser to Trump put it, at the "one-yard line."

TEXAS OFFERED A preview of what a new America would look like if Roe fell. And it showed just how little abortion-rights activists could do to stop the forward momentum, despite a sudden flurry of efforts.

The day after the ruling, President Joe Biden pledged "a whole-of-government effort," directing the Department of Health and Human Services and the Justice Department to identify federal measures that could ensure abortion access for Texas women. The Justice Department sued the state of Texas asking to immediately block the law. It was the first lawsuit by the federal government challenging the constitutionality of a state abortion restriction. Biden's attorney general, Merrick Garland—the judge Republicans had blocked from a Supreme Court hearing when Antonin Scalia died—said the law was "clearly unconstitutional under longstanding Supreme Court precedent."

Representative Diana DeGette, the co chair of the Pro-Choice Caucus, called House Speaker Nancy Pelosi and told her she had a bill ready to enshrine abortion rights into federal law. It was a version of the Women's Health Protection Act that Northup had unsuccessfully pushed on Capitol Hill during the Obama administration. But now, with an abortion-rights majority in the House, it had 203 cosponsors. When Pelosi brought the bill to the floor three weeks later, it passed with the support of nearly every Democrat.

Vice President Kamala Harris invited abortion providers and patients into her offices—the first time they were welcomed into Biden's White House for a public meeting. The fact that it happened eight months after he took office cut a striking contrast from the overwhelming welcome antiabortion advocates received during the Trump administration, when Mike Pence immediately addressed the March for Life.

But the problem Democrats faced was simple: they were too late. Their efforts might have seemed like action, but they were futile compared to the systematic, all-encompassing campaign antiabortion activists had waged over the past decade. Republicans had the state legislatures. They had a top-to-bottom network. They had the court. They had the power they needed to change American life.

The Supreme Court refused to halt the Texas law three different times in the following months, dismissing the Justice Department's appeal in a one-line, unsigned ruling. The Democratic legislation to codify Roe into federal law failed in the Senate that winter, after Senator Joe Manchin, a Democrat, and Republican senators Susan Collins and Lisa Murkowski opposed it. Collins and Murkowski later introduced their own bill, a narrower approach that they said would protect health care providers who do not want to perform abortions, like Catholic hospitals. That legislation failed to gain enough traction with Democrats.

Once again, abortion-rights advocates tried to mobilize the majority of Americans who backed the cause against this new round of abortion restrictions. Thousands marched in Washington that fall, wearing shirts emblazoned with "1973," under a banner reading, "Rally for Abortion Justice." But those kinds of public protests hadn't worked in the past. Wendy Davis filibustered; the twenty-week ban still stood. The Women's March was the largest single-day protest in American history; the Trump administration became the most successful antiabortion administration in history.

As the Mississippi case moved toward the highest court, the groups most devoted to Roe's defense were spending significant time mediating wrenching internal disputes. While their opposition had worked with singular focus to take down Roe, abortion-rights advocates were fighting for intersectionality, an attempt to strengthen their movement by expanding alliances with other progressive allies.

At Planned Parenthood, as Texas lawmakers were preparing their law, Alexis McGill Johnson was restructuring her organization along those very lines. She wrote an op-ed for *The New York Times* disavowing Margaret Sanger's association with eugenicists, saying Planned Parenthood's founder courted white supremacists. "What we have is a history of focusing on white womanhood relentlessly," McGill Johnson wrote. "By privileging whiteness, we've contributed to America harming Black women and other women of color. And when we focus too narrowly on 'women's health,' we have excluded trans and nonbinary people."

McGill Johnson promised new support for the Black Lives Matter movement and transgender rights and pledged to fight "the many types of dehumanization we are seeing right now." If Sanger was "Karen's godmother," as she had told her staff, Planned Parenthood had to stop being an "organizational Karen"—showing up, asserting itself, and telling everyone else where to march—leveraging its privilege, she wrote. "What we don't want to be, as an organization, is a Karen. You know Karen: She escalates small confrontations because of her own racial anxiety."

The piece prompted a furious backlash from historians and biographers, who argued that Planned Parenthood was imposing a twenty-first-century understanding on Sanger's twentieth-century beliefs. McGill Johnson's focus on reconciling Planned Parenthood's complicated legacy around race spoke in the language of the moment about a cause that was roiling liberals across America. But as McGill Johnson announced Planned Parenthood's new trajectory, also notable was what she left out. The flood of new restrictions—and the incoming threats of laws like in Texas and Mississippi—appeared only as a clause, a sixteen-word aside about "relentless attacks." What Planned Parenthood faced in that moment was so much more than just "relentless attacks." It was an entire network pushing to undercut the very purpose of their organization, women's health and sexual freedom. At a moment of ultimate vulnerability for so much that they had championed, McGill Johnson did not mention Roe at all.

She was not the only one in her movement focused on the intersection of race and abortion rights. When a group of abortion-rights activists, progressive allies, and White House aides got on a call to figure out a response to the Texas law, shortly after the Supreme Court's terse ruling, at least one activist said their central goal should be to eradicate "white supremacy." To reproductive justice advocates on the call, Roe had never fulfilled the promise of accessible abortion in communities of color. Tackling structural racism was the new foundation they needed before they could make progress on anything else. Yet, for other movement stalwarts, the call to focus on race sounded like a shift in mission, away from fighting for Roe and all it stood for, at the very moment they were on the verge of losing everything.

Debates over race weren't the only divisions exposed by the movement's new push toward intersectionality. Driven by transgender activists, abortion-rights groups had increasingly adopted gender-neutral words to talk about their issue. The shift in language consumed an outsize amount of media attention, at times overwhelming public discussion of Roe's fragile status. After Representative Cori Bush of Missouri, a progressive Democrat, used the term *birthing people* in a congressional hearing about Black maternal mortality, it erupted into a mini-uproar on social media—one that subsumed coverage of the actual topic of the hearing.

For some, like Diane Derzis, the owner of the Pink House and Northup's client in the coming Mississippi case, all the drama over language seemed like a distraction from their most pressing issue: the end of a foundational constitutional right for women. "I'm all for trans and gay rights, but them and abortion don't go together. They're not similar, they're totally different," she said. "That's hurt us." The issues, she believed, had become linked in a way that she feared would alienate more moderate supporters of abortion rights. She worried that political correctness was endangering their cause. "We're too PC to say it," she said. "I support your right, but don't put it with mine."

Still, after decades of largely white, straight leadership, the abortion-rights movement had changed. The three most powerful liberal women's political groups—Planned Parenthood, EMILYs List, and NARAL—were now all headed by women of color. Planned Parenthood had McGill Johnson. EMILYs List selected Laphonza Butler, a former union leader who grew up in Mississippi, as the first Black woman—and first mother—to lead the organization. And at NARAL, Mini Timmaraju took over for Ilyse Hogue, who'd left a few months after the election. The daughter of Indian American immigrants, with a background in working to preserve reproductive rights in Texas, Timmaraju joined the organization from roles overseeing diversity hiring for the new Biden administration and Comcast.

In the fight over abortion rights, the intersection of women's rights and civil rights was brought to a head. To some, it felt like there was something slightly unfair about the transition. Non-white women had spent decades fighting for their place in the movement. Now, these leaders were finally getting the mantle when all seemed nearly lost.

And in Texas, abortion rights were crumbling before their eyes, remaking decades of reproductive health care in an instant. A law didn't stop women from getting pregnant. Or from wanting abortions. In one high-profile incident, sheriffs in the Rio Grande Valley arrested a twenty-six-year-old woman and charged her with murder for a self-induced illegal abortion. Few details were made public, including how the abortion was performed, but the situation prompted protests outside the jail and confusion among local prosecutors. The district attorney later dropped the charges and issued an apology. But the arrest illustrated the power rogue prosecutors could suddenly have over women's reproductive lives when abortion laws changed.

Some doctors, fearing running afoul of the vague Texas law, began talking in coded language to their patients about their health care options, saying things like, "The weather's really nice in New Mexico right now. You should go check it out," or "I've heard traveling to Colorado is really nice this time of year." Clinics in surrounding states were inundated with patients, creating a domino effect that decreased the availability of appointments in those places, drove up costs of procedures, and pushed some residents to also travel out of states where abortion was still legal for their procedures.

Some Texas women drove all the way to the Pink House—the Jackson, Mississippi, clinic that the Dobbs case was trying to shutter. "That just shows you how desperate it's going to be," Cecile Richards said, the irony not lost to her.

But despite those harrowing and chaotic scenes, the idea that a constitutional right could be removed seemed unbelievable to many on the left. Roe had been part of women's reproductive planning for two generations. It was hard to reimagine a world without it.

Even after the Texas law, only one in three Democrats thought the Supreme Court was likely to overturn Roe, according to a Planned Parenthood poll of voters in states expected to have some of the most competitive races in the 2022 midterm elections. The survey was conducted in November 2021, just twenty days before Stewart and Northup's lawyers would face off in oral arguments at the court. The vast majority of people that Planned Parenthood expected to be on their side were not only unprepared for what was coming, but felt no real political urgency around it.

"Strategic Imperative," the Planned Parenthood pollsters wrote in an internal memo. "In the coming months, it will be important to remind voters what is at stake in the impending Supreme Court decision on Roe vs. Wade, including the potential for restrictive laws in their own states."

30

The Argument

The night before oral arguments at the Supreme Court, scheduled for December 1, Marjorie Dannenfelser introduced Mike Pence at an event at the National Press Club in Washington. Standing at a podium with a sign that said, LIFE IS A HUMAN RIGHT and that depicted a glowing spaceman-like fetus like the one on the *Life* magazine cover all those years ago, he ticked through all the movement's talking points and his administration's accomplishments.

All the speeches he'd given about abortion for decades culminated in this moment. It could be the beginning of the new nation Pence and his movement wanted to create. He asked the court to overturn Roe.

"The question before the court, and before the American people, is no less than this: What kind of nation do we want to be?" he said. "This is about saving the lives of millions of children yet unborn. But make no mistake about it: This is also about justice and the future of this nation."

Early the next morning, Scott Stewart knotted his lucky tie—blue with white dots, the one he wore to argue cases. He headed up the steep steps of the Supreme Court alongside Lynn Fitch, in her blue suit, past the protesters jostling with their shouts and bullhorns. Normally, people would have waited in line for hours, even overnight, for a chance to get a seat inside for such an important case. But the COVID-19 pandemic meant that only the lawyers, clerks, court personnel, and the media would be allowed in.

A woman in a mask and a green winter hat—the color of the abortion-rights cause—held a giant piece of cardboard with big black letters, "WHERE DOES THIS END?" Antiabortion activists came with Bibles and crosses to proclaim a "post-Roe generation." They carried signs too: "Abortion Is Murder," with bloody red handprints. "Civil Rights Begin in the Womb." Police kept watch at the barriers and guarded the steps.

Nancy Northup stood on the steps of the court with Shannon Brewer, the director of the Pink House, before dark teal banners proclaiming, "Abortion Is Essential." The Center for Reproductive Rights' lawyers had come to the court three times over the past six years to argue for abortion rights. But this fourth trip was different, thought Northup as she prepared to speak.

To the abortion-rights activists, the antiabortion crowd seemed chaotic, rougher than normal. "They've got the court at their back, and it's a different scene than it was even just a couple years ago," reflected Amy Hagstrom Miller, the founder of Whole Woman's Health. "This is about controlling women. It's about power."

This could be the battle that could mark the end of the era that defined her life, Northup knew. "We are here to win," she told the crowd, who were gathered for a rally organized by Liberate Abortion, a new coalition of more than one hundred abortion-rights groups. Yet, despite her conviction, Northup hinted that a different future could be coming. "I pledge to you, that no matter the outcome of this court case, the Center for Reproductive Rights will use every legal lever to make sure that abortion access is protected for all," she said.

People across America put in earbuds. Before the pandemic, the court did not allow cases to be recorded or streamed. But the crisis forced a technological change. Audio of the arguments would be live streamed, and the entire nation could listen. Waiting inside the lawyers' lounge before walking into the courtroom, Stewart told

Fitch he needed to pace. He'd gone over his argument again and again, in eight practice sessions with legal allies of the movement. He knew many in the circle of conservative lawyers who followed the Supreme Court still worried he was going too far. In the final weeks, allies had pushed him to give the justices an off-ramp, even just for ten seconds of his two-minute opening statement. Days ago, he had walked the streets of Northwest Washington, wondering if the experts were right.

Then it was 10:00 a.m. The gavel sounded. Stewart took off his mask.

A half century earlier, the Texas assistant attorney general opened his argument in Roe with a line that would go down as one of the worst wisecracks in legal history. "It's an old joke, but when a man argues against two beautiful ladies like this, they are going to have the last word," said Jay Floyd, referring to Sarah Weddington and Linda Coffee, the lawyers who won the case for Norma McCorvey—the woman who became widely known as Jane Roe.

But Weddington and Coffee didn't get the last word. Stewart was standing in the same courtroom, arguing against that old decision. As in Roe, two women were the state's opposing counsel: the US solicitor general, Elizabeth Prelogar, and Julie Rikelman, the center's senior litigator, who argued and won the case striking down Louisiana's abortion restriction the previous year. But this time a woman also sat on the anti-Roe side: Fitch. The room was somber and tense. No one was joking.

"*Roe v. Wade* and *Planned Parenthood v. Casey* haunt our country," Stewart declared, standing behind the wooden lectern. "They have no basis in the Constitution. They have no home in our history or traditions. They've damaged the democratic process. They've poisoned the law."

Stewart gave no off-ramp. It was all or nothing. He spoke directly to the nine justices before him. There were two whom both sides were watching most of all: Roberts, the institutionalist, and Kavanaugh, the wild card. The others seemed like sure bets. Justices Alito, Thomas, Gorsuch, and Barrett likely wanted to overturn Roe. Sonia Sotomayor, Stephen Breyer, and Elena Kagan would defend it. If Kavanaugh and Roberts seemed to embrace a narrower reading of the case centered on the fifteen-week law, Roe might stand. If not, Stewart and Mississippi would likely be heading toward victory.

Thomas jumped in to pose the first question to Stewart, one of his "kids," as he called his former clerks. He wondered what Stewart would suggest if the court wanted to uphold Roe and Casey. Stewart didn't stumble: The best course of action would be to overturn the rulings. But short of that would be to functionally gut Roe without completely overruling the decision by eliminating any viability standard—a decision that would allow restrictions at any point in pregnancy.

Sotomayor pushed back. "Will this institution survive the stench that this creates in the public perception that the Constitution and its reading are just political acts?" she said, wondering when the "life of a woman and putting her at risk enter the calculus." Fifteen justices over thirty years had upheld Roe and Casey, she argued. This matter was only before the court because the balance shifted with the new justices. What message would that send?

Listening in a conference room to the live stream of the arguments with her team of lawyers, Northup was ready when Rikelman came up after Stewart to make her argument. The center's goal was to bring women's voices into the room and ensure that the real-life impact of taking away a right would be felt amid the abstract discussions of legal theory. Rikelman did not mince words. The ban was "flatly unconstitutional" under the precedents of Roe and Casey, she said. "For a state to take control of a woman's body and demand that she go through pregnancy and childbirth with all the physical risks and life-altering consequences that brings is a fundamental deprivation of her liberty," she said. "Eliminating or reducing the right to abortion will propel women backwards."

Some listening that day noted a shift in the court's usual restraint. The oral arguments offered plenty of hints of how the court might rule. Alito's words rang through the air when he cited the language in the center's brief that there were "no half measures," telling Rikelman that "the only real options we have" are to reaffirm Roe or overrule it.

Listeners got subtle—and not-so-subtle—glimpses into the thinking of Trump's picks. Kavanaugh wanted Rikelman to respond to the idea that "because the Constitution is neutral"—in other words, that the document doesn't specifically mention abortion—"that this Court should be scrupulously neutral on the question of abortion, neither pro-choice nor pro-life." His words echoed the originalist position championed by Leo. Rikelman quickly disputed his contention, arguing that abortion was part of the Constitution's "guarantee of liberty." But the question itself hinted that he might not be such a wild card.

Rikelman doubled down, arguing that outlawing abortion would force women to take on the burden of parenthood. It was an argument that other new members of the court were quick to dispute. "Why don't the safe haven laws take care of that problem?" Barrett wondered, referencing laws that allow women to legally and anonymously relinquish their babies at fire stations and other public places. The inquiry shocked and outraged abortion-rights supporters. It was a fantasy to believe that adoption eliminated the price of pregnancy itself—the economic costs, physical toll, and emotional burden, they argued. But it was a line of reasoning that was common in antiabortion circles, including the world Barrett came from at Notre Dame.

Rikelman shot back with statistics. It was seventy-five times more dangerous for women to give birth in Mississippi than have an abortion before viability, she said, risks that disproportionately impacted women of color. "Pregnancy itself is unique. It imposes unique physical demands and risks on women and, in fact, has impact on all of their lives, on their ability to care for other children, other family members, on their ability to work," she said.

As the argument wound to a close, the chief justice offered his views. "The thing that is at issue before us today is fifteen weeks," said Roberts. His words seemed to embrace a compromise.

But a ruling that upheld fifteen weeks would be no compromise at all. Such a decision would gut Roe without saying the words by eliminating the viability line that was the heart of the legal precedent.

But it could, Northup realized, offer a more politically palatable argument for conservatives to make. The public barely believed Roe was at risk. Explaining that the decision was functionally gone without the words of the court putting it plainly for America to see would be difficult for abortion-rights advocates, Northup knew. The delusion of the security of Roe was so entrenched in the thinking of many Americans that it could very well continue. Still, it wasn't clear that Roberts would be able to muster a majority behind a compromise approach that would leave any piece of Roe standing.

Then it was finished, 114 minutes after it began. The justices filed off the bench. Stewart, Rikelman, Fitch, and the other lawyers exchanged polite handshakes. The audio stream went silent.

THE WHOLE THING felt "chilling," thought Cecile Richards. Barrett's remarks, in particular, were like hearing the shots of an invading army. "We just live in a completely different world than the world that she sees," she said. "And she's a young justice and she's going to be on there for a long, long time." Richards hadn't been surprised when she saw the antiabortion movement's arguments on display in the Texas statehouse with SB 8 or the Mississippi legislature with the fifteen-week ban. But to see them at the Supreme Court felt like a gut punch, an erasure of the vision of gender equity her mother fought for all those decades ago.

"I always sort of held out hope that there was going to be an adult in the room, not necessarily the Supreme Court, but at least within the Republican Party, that would say, 'Look, I understand that's been our rhetoric for all these years, but in fact, that's going too far,'" she said. Now, after oral arguments, she was no longer hopeful.

Standing in her kitchen in Texas, listening as she unpacked boxes in her new condo, Wendy Davis began to sob. In that moment, she realized that what had seemed impossible when she stood for all those hours in her pink sneakers was about to be the new reality. "I always thought the Supreme Court was going to save us," she said.

That evening, leaders of the pro-life movement gathered at the JW Marriott in Washington for an invite-only banquet sponsored by ADF. Everyone seemed to be there, and ADF gave out party favors of small wooden plaques, depicting a pregnant woman leaning against a Supreme Court column. The mood was celebratory even though the decision wouldn't come for another six months, as the justices' words seemed to confirm that Stewart's approach was not the misstep ADF initially worried it might be. There was Marjorie Dannenfelser of SBA, David Daleiden, who ran the Planned Parenthood video operation and Mary Taylor from Pro-Life Utah, who had wanted a fifteen-week ban instead of eighteen. There were authors of the amicus briefs, and Becky Currie, who believed she had developed the idea of the fifteen-week law in Mississippi. And for all the network's strength, it was strikingly diffuse. Many participants knew only the small part they played, and did not know how the whole fit together. Currie met Stewart briefly that night for the first time. "He couldn't pick me out of a crowd," she said.

On the stage, Lynn Fitch, Scott Stewart, and Erin Hawley sat proudly as they described how they had gotten to this moment. "First of all, to God be the glory," Fitch began.

"We all prayed, worked so hard for this day. It all came together because everyone here, everyone that's been involved across our country, we're believers, and we knew this day would come," she said. "God selected this case. He was ready. The justices were ready to hear what we were all going to be talking about."

For those listening, the people around them in that ballroom and all they accomplished represented a vision of the kingdom of God coming on Earth, as Jesus's prayer taught in the Gospels. They were also a living example of religion's powerful function as a conservative force: It conserves. Across time, religion maintains a way of life, tradition, culture, and power, for better or worse.

Their work offered a vision of what a modern Christian empire looked like. It did not involve violent crusaders or declaring an official state religion. It was not clerics instituting a theocracy. The antiabortion movement had used the existing system to define the Constitution the way it saw fit. A right was not being taken away from women, the movement argued, because it never should have existed in the first place.

If they won, abortion rights would no longer be constitutionally protected at the federal level. Conservatives would have clarified the kind of Constitution they believed America had, different as it might seem from the one the court saw back in 1973. As a foundation of American democracy, the Constitution is the guiding document of the country's shared values, and of who is included and excluded in those rights. In a fundamental way, the Supreme Court's interpretation of what that means would declare who America was in 2022, even if a majority of the nation disagreed.

ADF's strategy on Dobbs reflected how it believed it could reshape America. There's a saying that law is downstream from culture, said Greg Scott, a longtime communications strategist for ADF, explaining the idea that a cause gains popular support first, and then the law formalizes those beliefs. "I actually reject that," he said. "We are in this feedback loop and this ecosystem where frequently that is true. But then at other times, the law does drive culture."

And now, amid the applause, ADF leaders looked ahead. By their internal calculations, if the court overturned Roe and the issue was sent back to the states, thirty-one states would or could soon ban abortion. That meant they needed just seven more states to reach eighty-eight: the number required to pass an amendment to the Constitution and ban abortion entirely.

But even that was just the beginning. ADF's ultimate goal was sweeping cultural change across America to preserve the values of conservative Christians. They were, after all, a "religious ministry," not just a law firm, as Kristen Waggoner said. Ending abortion was the first target, but ADF had already begun planning for four more.

According to a strategy document, ADF leaders set out to achieve what they called "generational wins," victories that would change the law and culture of America for an entire generation. After each win, ADF would work to fortify that change so it would last for generations to come.

ADF lawyers would work to reverse the Supreme Court's decision in *Employment Division v. Smith*, to "fully protect the free exercise of religion," the strategy document explained. That decision, authored by Antonin Scalia, ruled that religious beliefs did not excuse disobeying valid laws. The issues around the case had particularly inspired Stewart in law school. They would file lawsuits to build a legal case against it.

They would pursue litigation to enforce free speech rights on college campuses. They would push legislation to protect the freedom of association there as well, to eventually overturn a decision that Ginsburg had authored called *Christian Legal Society v. Martinez*. The ruling had allowed a public university not to recognize a Christian student group that excluded gay students. Alito called the decision a "serious setback for freedom of expression."

They would target LGBTQ rights and protections, and "stop efforts to elevate sexual orientation and gender identity to protected-class status in the law akin to race." They would "work to restore an understanding of marriage, the family, and sexuality that reflects God's creative order."

And they wanted the court to strengthen parental rights over state authority by having the court revisit a case called *Troxel v. Granville*. ADF would work to pass state legislation, similar to its approach on abortion, effectively rolling back the expansion of transgender rights to prevent parents from "being coerced into consenting to life changing, ill-advised surgeries and procedures in the wake of gender dysphoria."

It was an enormous agenda, one that not even everyone in the ballroom knew. And even that was just in the United States. ADF was also building an international arm to oppose abortion in European countries.

Onstage, Fitch beamed. The hundreds of faces looking back at her represented a core of their movement. Many believed there would have been no Dobbs without "a cultural swell in favor of protecting innocent unborn life, beginning in 1973," as one ADF lawyer put it.

But that "cultural swell" was still a minority, and even more so than a decade ago. Just 8 percent of Americans wanted to ban abortion at conception with no exceptions, half of the 16 percent who said the same in 2012. Another 29 percent believed it should be illegal in "most" cases. The reality was that there would have been no Dobbs without a coordinated, sniper-like strategy to take down Roe. A mission that went against the wishes of a majority of Americans.

"This has been certainly a God thing," Fitch told the audience. "We've all been called. We've all been waiting."

Now, she said, they could not stop. "We've got tough times ahead, but we're ready," she said. "Everyone in this room, you're ready."

31

Disbelief

Nancy Northup wanted to leap through her Zoom screen. It was March 2022, three months after the Dobbs oral arguments. The White House had called this meeting, during Women's History Month, to celebrate new legislation making it easier for sexual assault victims to sue their employers.

The administration had invited the country's leading abortion-rights advocates—Northup, Alexis McGill Johnson, and Mini Timmaraju—along with women's organizations and groups that worked on issues like domestic violence, to meet with Ron Klain, Joe Biden's chief of staff, and other aides. McGill Johnson was in the Zoom box next to her. Timmaraju was inside the room in the Eisenhower Executive Office Building, across from the White House.

Biden, unsurprisingly, was not there. He rarely talked about abortion. In fact, as president, he'd never uttered the word or met with the leaders of their organizations—a striking contrast with Dannenfelser, who met with the president frequently during the Trump administration. His joint address to Congress—his version of a State of the Union that first year in office—did not mention the threat to abortion rights, referring only in passing to "protecting women's health." Vice President Kamala Harris, fairly outspoken on the issue during her primary campaign, had made no notable remarks about the topic since taking office.

And even now, abortion rights didn't top the agenda for this meeting.

It was infuriating, thought Northup. Texas had already criminalized nearly all abortion. Other states, like Arizona and Florida, were moving forward with new bans. A decision on Dobbs was imminent, and from the moment she left the steps of the court that cold day in December, Northup knew Roe was over. She didn't know precisely how: Would John Roberts get support for a fifteen-week compromise? Or would Roe be completely overturned? But it didn't matter. Federal abortion rights would soon be lost, perhaps at least for a generation.

After all this, it seemed impossible that the White House—and its Democratic allies—still did not understand the force of what was about to come. She remembered explaining the case and the likely outcome to a Democratic senator after oral arguments. The senator had responded, "Wow, I thought you were going to have better news for me."

Northup couldn't take the Democratic disbelief anymore. She did not know how to be clearer. There was no path to victory. Roe would fall. There were no more briefs to save it. No appeals left to file. She jumped in. "I am going to say something I have never said in twenty years running the center," she said.

"We are going to lose this case," she blurted out.

A heavy silence settled over the room. It felt different hearing it out loud, thought Timmaraju, even if she knew what was coming.

Klain and the other administration aides in the room offered promises. They were working on plans. The president had directed the Gender Policy Council, which he had established when he entered office, to start looking at ways to blunt the impact of a decision. The administration had created a task force to draft plans to advance access to reproductive health. They wanted to keep in close contact, the aides said. We'll stay in touch, they promised.

Northup closed her Zoom window. Democrats controlled the executive branch, the House, and the Senate, and abortion-rights advocates couldn't get their own meeting at the White House. Planned Parenthood, NARAL, and the entire abortion-rights movement had rallied their supporters, raising money and lending their extensive field operations, to elect Biden and other Democrats. Where were those Democrats now, when their movement needed them? Still, in front of them all, Northup had done her duty from her computer screen. She delivered her message. Hopefully, she thought, Biden and his team would listen.

In the Manhattan offices of the Center for Reproductive Rights, her lawyers had begun preparing for this new era. Northup knew that ending Roe wouldn't end abortion. It would just relocate it. Since the Texas abortion ban became law, studies indicated that around 1,400 women were leaving the state monthly for abortions. If Roe fell, abortion would move from clinics in Jackson and Sioux Falls to bedrooms, across state lines, and into emergency rooms when women's health reached the stage of critical care.

Already, the center was working with Planned Parenthood and the ACLU to sketch out litigation plans. They were exploring ways to keep clinics open, challenge trigger bans, and exploit any possible ambiguity in the decision. Their maps were the reverse of the whiteboard hanging in Dannenfelser's office, charting out safe-haven states, middle ground, and at-risk areas.

Where Dannenfelser's map was imbued with her vision of political possibility, theirs showed a nation closing its doors to abortion rights and women's health. Even with unified control of Washington, there was little Democrats could do to save Roe. Since 2019, over a dozen liberal states had escalated their efforts to protect abortion rights and expand access. One striking example was in Michigan, where Democratic governor Gretchen Whitmer had filed a preemptive lawsuit to overturn the state's trigger law, a process she began after Ginsburg died. But, at best, that was less than half the country.

The Biden administration had called on Congress to codify Roe into federal law, but it hadn't proposed specific legislation or unveiled any strategy to advance such a bill. Truthfully, the effort was futile. Given the continued support for the filibuster, the only way abortion-rights supporters could move forward with a bill enshrining Roe in federal law was with sixty votes in the Senate. They had fifty-two votes for abortion rights, counting Susan Collins and Lisa Murkowski. Winning eight more seats in such a divided country would be nearly impossible.

Democrats and their allies on the left weren't blasé about abortion rights. But like much of America, it was hard for them to see clearly—and even harder to believe—what was coming. The antiabortion forces had done their job well. They didn't conceal their ultimate aim; they had talked about undoing Roe for decades. The Federalist Society had made clear its intention to reorient the court around a new set of conservative principles that would make the justices more willing to undo precedents of the past.

But the storm of laws and litigation, proposals and policies over the past decade had made it easy to dismiss the antiabortion movement's efforts as just another round of incremental steps. The laws seemed like small actions by fringe Republican state legislators, who were powerless to change national policy. All that noise drowned out the bigger picture of how a decade of work was leading to a new kind of court.

The antiabortion movement took advantage of the country's complicated views about abortion to strike at what Americans didn't find complicated at all: Roe. In the weeks after oral arguments, a CNN poll found that nearly 70 percent of Americans wanted Roe to be upheld, a number that had stayed broadly consistent since Alito was put on the bench in 2006. In April, nearly the same majority—62 percent—said they were unaware of any laws passed by their state making it harder to get an abortion. The conclusions were clear. Most Americans supported abortion rights. And most Americans didn't realize they were at risk.

That disconnect had created a believability gap that had endured through the past decade. The antiabortion forces crept forward, but the broad sense of Roe's inviolability never changed. Not after Donald Trump won. Not after Brett Kavanaugh and then Amy Coney Barrett joined the court. Not after oral arguments. And not now, even as they waited for the decision. It was like that old maxim about a frog in a pot of cold water, the temperature rising slowly, as the frog sat unaware, slowly boiling alive.

It all left Cecile Richards contemplating where the America that her mother had promised had gone. She remembered when the religious right defeated Ann and all those other Democratic lawmakers in 1994. She had underestimated them. "The folks that took over the Republican Party in Texas that year are really running the show all over the country," she said. The power of a majority wasn't enough to overcome the "raw, bare-knuckled politics, of a minority exercising its power over a majority," she wrote in *The New York Times.*

"I had faith that if we provided excellent health care and showed how access to reproductive rights had helped women, as well as our economy, and if we kept most of the country on our side, this, too, would pass," she wrote. "I was wrong."

32

The Leak

Every Monday night, for weeks that spring, Marjorie Dannenfelser invited a famous ally to pray with her supporters for the outcome of the Dobbs case—Mike Pence, Lynn Fitch, David Daleiden of the Planned Parenthood videos, and others.

On the evening of May 2, she was sitting in her car, leading the weekly prayer call. The guest was Frank Pavone, leader of Priests for Life, an incendiary Catholic priest and religious adviser to Donald Trump who, in the 2016 campaign, live streamed an event in which he placed an aborted fetus on what appeared to be an altar. (Pope Francis would later remove him from the priesthood, citing "blasphemous communication.")

The prayer calls were a reminder that for so many in the anti-abortion movement, the battle was about more than just politics. Spiritual forces were at work, Dannenfelser told participants. She said they were standing for good and against evil. "Each Supreme Court justice is under incredible pressure," Dannenfelser said. "There is a hidden and visible assault on the part of the dark side. Let's name him: the Devil."

The ping of a notification on her phone interrupted her. She was slightly irritated. Her staff knew she was praying. She ignored it. It was late and most of Washington was powering down for the day. But another came. And another. Within minutes, she had dozens of missed texts.

She broke away to see what was happening. A news story had been published by Politico, an online publication best known for covering the minutiae of politics. It included an attachment, scanned and slightly crooked, titled "scotus-initial-draft.pdf." It was a leaked draft of the Dobbs decision.

This sort of thing didn't happen with the Supreme Court. It happened in Congress, the White House, even the Pentagon. But not at the highest court. A leak like this was extraordinary, shocking.

Dannenfelser had planned for all sorts of outcomes, but not this. She scanned the text. The Supreme Court had decided to overturn *Roe v. Wade* in its entirety, ending nearly half a century of American law. The words were there, printed in traditional Supreme Court font, for all to see. It was stamped in the top-right-hand corner with all the justices' names and the date it was allegedly circulated, February 10, 2022, three months earlier. It was ninety-eight pages long.

Politico's story didn't just include the draft. It contained details about the court's internal discussions. According to "a person familiar with the court's deliberations," five of the justices—Samuel Alito, Clarence Thomas, Neil Gorsuch, Brett Kavanaugh, and Amy Coney Barrett—had voted to overturn Roe in the conference held after oral arguments. The three liberal justices—Stephen Breyer, Sonia Sotomayor, and Elena Kagan—were working on their dissents. It remained uncertain whether John Roberts would join the majority who were ready to end Roe and if he would write his own opinion, according to the article.

Dannenfelser dialed Leonard Leo. Whether this was real or fake, they needed a messaging strategy. Frantic calls, group text chains, and hastily scheduled Zoom strategy sessions spread like wildfire across the entire antiabortion network. It looked credible, everyone agreed. But there were so many questions. Was it timed to influence Roberts? But toward which outcome? Did the disclosure come from the left to outrage people? Did it come from the right, to try to lock in a justice? Justices could change their minds on a case up until the last minute.

Dannenfelser started texting and calling everyone she could think of—leaders, coalition partners, politicians—with the same message: Don't say anything until the official ruling. "To say nothing is the most important thing you can do," she said. "This is something that is going to last generations." ADF issued the same set of marching orders: "Until the court rules, the court has not ruled," Kristen Waggoner, the group's president, said. Until they saw the final decision, they would not dare celebrate. The memory of what happened in 1992 with the Casey decision was still seared in the memories of so many in the movement: news reports revealed that Justice Anthony Kennedy had flipped his vote, leading to a result that affirmed Roe instead of overturning it. That formative year, the one also dubbed the year of the Democratic women, was what prompted Dannenfelser and so many others to devote their lives to this cause in the first place. Anything could happen behind the court's closed doors. All she could do was be ready.

Dannenfelser had spent months organizing supporters and allies for the decision to come in late June, when the court's biggest rulings typically were released. Like Nancy Northup, she was convinced after oral arguments that the justices would rule in favor of the antiabortion movement. That spring, Dannenfelser had taped videos in front of the Supreme Court to distribute on social media after the decision came—one for if the court upheld the Mississippi law and another for a complete reversal of Roe. There was no pretaped video for the court completely ruling against her. It just didn't seem likely.

For months, she had organized meetings with nearly every Republican governor, senators and their staff, and dozens of representatives. She had contacted everyone she suspected might run for president, more than a dozen state attorneys general, Senate Republican leader Mitch McConnell, and the head of the Republican National Committee. Dannenfelser urged a comprehensive Republican communications strategy and made a mock-debate video training for members on how to talk about Dobbs: they should focus on the humanity of the child and note that the decision was democratic, restoring the right of the people to make laws.

Eliminating Roe had been a central goal of her movement, but the ultimate goal was to end abortion. Dannenfelser also needed to teach state Republican attorneys general about the process for moving trigger bans and other restrictions quickly forward in conservative states.

Her team worried about the other half of the country, places like New York, California, Illinois, and other liberal states that were taking steps to expand abortion access in anticipation of the ruling. So they partnered with Chris Christie of New Jersey, a longtime ally, who joined Dannenfelser on calls with governors from more moderate states to share how he navigated the issue as a "pro-life governor" in a liberal state. But to stop abortion in those places, their movement would need to go further than just the right words. They would need a national ban.

In April, Dannenfelser and her allies made the rounds of the Capitol repeatedly, pushing for federal legislation that would ban abortion across the entire country. In a meeting with the Republican Study Committee, the largest conservative bloc in the caucus, she discussed the options of both a fifteen-week federal ban and a six-week one. Others in the coalition, like Kristan Hawkins of Students for Life, pushed for the six-week ban. But Dannenfelser saw the goal as long-term, to build support for such bans over time, so that if Republicans ever won a filibuster-proof Senate majority, they could pass it. For now, she argued that a fifteen-week federal ban would allow Republican states like Texas and Oklahoma to keep more aggressive limits, while also setting a baseline in blue states like California, New York, and Illinois. Unlike bans earlier in pregnancy, polling showed a majority of voters supported restrictions around the start of the second trimester. Plus, it was five weeks earlier than the twenty-week bans passed by the House since 2013, which did not become law.

In a private call with donors after one such meeting on Capitol Hill in late April, Dannenfelser and her top political strategist,

Frank Cannon, urged their staunchest supporters to get ready for the fights to come. In the coming days, "the prolife movement of the last fifty years ceases to exist," and a state by state battle will replace it, Cannon said. "Those fights will begin immediately, a lot of them will take years to play out, they will be intense from the very beginning."

Dannenfelser pointed donors to an editorial recently published in *The Wall Street Journal*. The piece, just 825 words, was easy to miss and went largely unnoticed, even among official Washington. But buried midway into the article was an eyebrow-raising piece of analysis.

The editorial said that five justices—Kavanaugh, Barrett, Thomas, Gorsuch, and Alito—seemed likely to vote to overturn Roe and Casey. But, it implied, Roberts could be trying to persuade another justice to adopt his compromise position of upholding the fifteen-week law and leaving Roe untouched. If he failed, the editorial speculated that Alito would draft the opinion eliminating Roe. "He may be trying to turn another Justice now," the editorial said of Roberts. "We hope he doesn't succeed—for the good of the Court and the country."

While couched in speculative language—"our guess," wrote the author—it was an odd comment. Deliberations inside the justices' chambers were notoriously secret. They were not, generally speaking, printed in the pages of major newspapers. The information seemed like it was from an authoritative source, Dannenfelser told her donors. "They communicated what we think we've been hearing as well," she said of the piece.

Now, four days after that small bit of analysis buried in the editorial pages, here was what appeared to be a credible court document. An opinion overturning Roe, authored by Alito—just as the editorial suggested.

Opinions were closely held until they were ready to be released to the public, as were details of the judges' private conferences and negotiations over cases. That sense of omertà was the reason almost no one, even Scott Stewart and Northup, knew for certain why the court took so many months to agree to hear the Mississippi case. The court depended on that secrecy to maintain a sense of judicial fairness, an image of a temple of discretion unswayed by the political fervors of the moment or the personal beliefs of the justices. A leak like the one in Politico—the disclosure of an entire opinion—was an unthinkable breach of trust.

Yet that image of the court's impenetrability wasn't completely accurate. There had been leaks before. And the most detailed, at least in the modern era, had happened during deliberations in another contentious abortion case: Roe.

On July 4, 1972, six months before the decision was released, *The Washington Post* published a story about the court's internal deliberations. It included details of a memo from Justice William O. Douglas to his colleagues describing what he saw as Chief Justice Warren Burger's improper power plays to try to delay a decision until President Richard Nixon could fill two vacancies on the court. The story was unusual—no byline, no named sources, and published on a national holiday—and it revealed a striking amount of detail about the court's private negotiations, including the date of the conference where the case was discussed. It was certainly a leak from inside the court, perhaps even, historians later speculated, from Douglas himself.

After nearly one hundred interviews and months of forensics, an investigation commissioned by Roberts came up short, unable to identify the person who caused what the justices declared to be "a grave assault on the judicial process." The question of who leaked the document was an irresistible one, but the more significant meaning could be found in the fact that it was leaked at all. The focus on the leaker served—once again—to obscure the power of abortion as a symbol, one so fundamental that it could shatter the court. Abortion was so much more than a medical procedure or even an electoral rallying cry. For so many in the debate, abortion stood for the bedrock values of America—what it meant to have the unalienable rights of life, liberty, and the pursuit of happiness. Both sides believed that a grave miscarriage of justice, and thus of the future life of the nation itself, was on the line, for different reasons.

The stakes were so great that they broke the democratic traditions of the last remaining branch of government where such norms still held significant sway. It was the power of abortion, and all it stood for, that changed how Americans saw the very legal foundation of their democracy. It was the case about abortion—not decisions on guns or immigration or the January 6 investigations—that prompted one of the "worst breaches of trust" in the court's history, as the report from the Roberts investigation described the leak.

Americans' faith in the court collapsed with shocking swiftness. Before Barrett was confirmed, in the fall of 2020, broad swaths of Americans—70 percent in one survey—said they had confidence in the court. In the days after the leak, registered voters swung to being evenly split on the question, and the decline grew over the coming weeks. Poll after poll showed that a clear majority no longer trusted the court. Opinions split by party. Immediately after the decision, 14 percent of Democrats and 37 percent of independents said they had confidence in the court; among Republicans, that figure was 71 percent.

The leaked decision over Roe transformed public perception of the court into that of an institution as partisan as nearly any other in American politics. Before the leak, the court largely stood apart, above the rough-and-tumble dysfunction of Congress and the White House. Afterward, the court was plunged into the political morass. In the months and years that followed, there would be investigations into the justices' ethics and political associations, calls for a new ethics code and greater disclosure of their personal spending.

Thomas, whose acceptance of large gifts from rich conservative donors was suddenly under fresh examination, described the incident as a "kind of an infidelity" that destroyed the trust among the justices. In remarks to conservative thinkers and activists, he questioned how long such a Supreme Court could survive. "I wonder how long we're going to have these institutions at the rate we're undermining them," he said. "And then I wonder when they're gone or destabilized, what we're going to have as a country."

The court was the last sacred institution in American political life. And now, because of the power of Roe, it had become as broken as everything else.

WITH THE LEAK, the spell of denial shattered in an instant. Americans everywhere read the draft, texting it to friends with exclamation points and, depending on their ideological persuasion, expletives or prayers. The believability gap was blown wide open. For a decade, large swaths of Americans didn't fully register the slow erosion of abortion rights, and they certainly did not know the extent of the antiabortion network that fought to create this moment. Now public opinion jolted with startling speed: within days, the number of Americans who identified as "pro-choice" jumped dramatically, rising six points to 55 percent—the highest Gallup had measured in nearly three decades.

Protests exploded on the steps of the Supreme Court and across the country. "I am angry!" shouted Senator Elizabeth Warren, standing on the steps of the court in a hot-pink blazer. "An extremist United States Supreme Court thinks they can impose their extremist views on all of the women of this country, and they are wrong."

Outraged women cornered their elected representatives, flooding their offices with calls and messages. On a flight from Detroit to Washington, two strangers—both women who said they were Republican and "pro-life"—approached Representative Elissa Slotkin, Democrat of Michigan, with their fears about a trigger law banning abortion in their state. Slotkin, as shell-shocked as her constituents, started calling everyone she knew with a connection to the abortion-rights movement asking how she should proceed. A former CIA officer, she was used to conducting constant security assessments of future possibilities. Where was the plan for this "black swan event"? she wondered. Would there be a press conference in front of the Capitol? Several days of marches?

"In fifty years of Roe being on the books as legal precedent, we had never codified it in law," she fumed. "The other side for fifty years has had a legal strategy—where is our fifty-year strategy?"

The answer would infuriate Slotkin. The three major abortion-rights organizations had mobilized, but broader political efforts remained fairly discreet. There was no party-wide strategy to capitalize on the moment. No organization in place for several days of marches, a messaging push, or new legislation responding to the crisis expected to come.

The legal arm of the abortion-rights movement—Nancy Northup, Brigitte Amiri, the ACLU lawyer who defended Jane Doe, and their allies—had spent months preparing a legal strategy to challenge trigger bans in court. Planned Parenthood and other abortion providers had begun shifting resources to accommodate patients, opening new facilities like a regional logistics center in southern Illinois, a centralized call center to help organize travel and lodging help for women traveling to the state for abortions. In March, billionaire philanthropist MacKenzie Scott made the largest ever single donation to Planned Parenthood, giving $275 million to be divided between the national office and twenty-one regional affiliate organizations. McGill Johnson earmarked the national funds to tackle racial equity issues. The regional affiliates devoted their money to improving the medical services in their clinics.

Some Democrats in Washington, like Diana DeGette and others at the party's campaign committees, had met to strategize about the possible electoral impact on their midterm candidates. But for the most part, they were unprepared.

After months of disregarding Northup's warnings, Democrats scrambled to respond. The day after the leak, staffers for Harris tore up the top of her planned remarks for a speech to EMILYs List that evening, remaking her words to fit the reality that the country suddenly saw. "Now we enter a new phase," she told a ballroom of supporters in Washington. "There is nothing hypothetical about this moment."

At the Capitol, Senate Democrats rushed to put together a meeting. Prominent Democratic senators could not remember any time in the past decade when their full caucus gathered to exclusively discuss the issue of abortion rights. Democrats, Chuck Schumer told abortion-rights advocates in a separate meeting, needed to do three things—"vote, vote, vote." On social media, some liberals scoffed at the party's plan to just "vote harder." Democrats controlled the House, Senate, and the White House; why couldn't they do something, they asked? Why was the answer, yet again, to elect Democrats? That hadn't worked to preserve Roe.

The Department of Homeland Security warned of rising threats from both sides. In Wyoming, a masked woman set fire to an abortion clinic the month before it was scheduled to open. Vandals spray-painted antiabortion pregnancy centers from Florida to Michigan. Protesters disrupted services at the evangelical Lakewood Church in Houston, stripping down to their underwear and screaming, "My body, my choice!" with expletives. Even the justices were not immune: Protesters gathered weekly in front of Alito's and Thomas's homes, chanting and shouting in their quiet suburban neighborhoods. A few weeks after a security fence was erected around the court, an armed man was arrested near Kavanaugh's house after saying he wanted to kill him over Roe.

Dannenfelser urged Republicans to shy away from openly discussing the full impact of what was to come. Establishment Republicans largely followed her advice. "You need—it seems to me, excuse the lecture—to concentrate on what the news is today," McConnell told reporters. "Not a leaked draft but the fact that the draft was leaked." Donald Trump, whose administration appointed the crucial votes, stayed largely silent, making only passing reference to abortion at his first rally after the leak.

But it was hard to maintain any message discipline across the party. Where longtime antiabortion movement leaders saw political danger, the post-Roe generation saw new possibilities. Mississippi's fifteen-week law and other similar limits "served their purpose in leading us to where we are today," wrote Hawkins, the head of Students for Life, in a letter to Republican members of Congress. But now it was time to go further, she argued.

The post-Roe activists wanted bills that would outlaw abortion starting at six weeks, criminalize some forms of contraception, and ban the distribution of abortion pills. "We press on toward the goal to win the prize, leaving old legal tools behind," wrote Hawkins, alluding to words from the apostle Paul in the Bible. "We ask you to join us in ensuring that the strongest measures possible are employed to achieve life, liberty, and the pursuit of happiness for every American, from conception to natural death."

Abortion abolitionist campaigns spread across the country. Days after the leak, the state legislature in Louisiana advanced a proposal to classify abortion as murder, with commensurate punishments for women who have the procedure. Similar abolitionist efforts were pushed in Arizona, Texas, and Oklahoma. They reflected Trump's 2016 argument that women who had abortions should receive "some form of punishment," which he quickly walked back after a sharp response from women leaders in the antiabortion movement. Now, unlike the careful effort to put women at the front of the movement, these campaigns were led largely by men.

The rightward shift meant that for Republican politicians, simply declaring oneself "pro-life" and opposing Roe was no longer enough. To win primary races and prove their conservative credentials with the rising fringe of their party, Republicans embraced six-week bans with no exceptions for rape, incest, or the life of the mother. These hard-right stances would have been considered disqualifying just ten years earlier. And as Texas had recently demonstrated, they still remained deeply unpopular with a majority of voters.

But this new moment also showed that Todd Akin, the congressman who torpedoed his 2012 Senate campaign, had perhaps come just a decade too early. Instead of being a relic of the past, he had actually been a harbinger of the future, one that the mainstream America of his day did not see coming. The Republican candidates of 2022 were going far beyond Akin's comments about "legitimate rape" by embracing total abortion bans with no exceptions and paying no price with their party. Akin did not live to see the new world that he foretold. He died of cancer two months before the oral arguments in Dobbs. Until the end, he maintained that the mistake was not his comment but his apology.

33

The Obituary

Roe v. Wade fell on June 24, 2022. It had lasted forty-nine years.

The seminal ruling, which remade American politics and society, was gone. The 1973 decision that most American women believed had granted them a sense of autonomy and equality—and that had pushed Christian conservatives to war—was over. After decades of legislation and lawsuits, failures and victories, politicking and prayer, the country finally split in two. A fault line became a chasm. With the words on the Dobbs opinion's first page, a new America was born:

> Held: The Constitution does not confer a right to abortion; Roe and Casey are overruled; and the authority to regulate abortion is returned to the people and their elected representatives.

The Dobbs ruling was the final cause of death for a right that had been growing weaker for decades. For half a century, America's highest legal authority understood that a right to an abortion was rooted in the Constitution's promise of liberty and implied right to privacy. This new court declared that reasoning was wrong and reversed Roe entirely. The vote tally was 6–3, and Samuel Alito wrote the opinion. The final copy was nearly unchanged from the leaked draft, save for the addition of the opposing arguments.

"Roe was egregiously wrong from the start," Alito wrote. "The Constitution makes no reference to abortion, and no such right is implicitly protected by any constitutional provision." Casey, the decision that affirmed that women had a right to end their pregnancies until a fetus could survive separately from a woman's uterus, fell completely too.

For decades, Roe had been a symbol of American ideals. Its fall was a symbol, too, of a new set of values that had taken power in America. Roe, understood for years by liberal America as an embodiment of freedom and equality for women, was replaced by Dobbs, a decision that conservative Christians saw as a manifestation of the primacy of life and that conservative lawyers believed corrected the legal overreach of the 1960s and 1970s.

All six justices who undercut Roe were Leonard Leo mainstays: he had been involved in confirming Clarence Thomas, John Roberts, Samuel Alito, Neil Gorsuch, Brett Kavanaugh, and Amy Coney Barrett. All were in the Federalist Society mold. And all were conservative Catholics, though Gorsuch attended an Episcopal church later in life. It was a vast shift from 1973, when all the justices were Protestant save one—and the sole Catholic justice sided with the majority in favor of Roe.

With one ruling, this new court created a new country. How women thought about birth and motherhood, their health, families, child-rearing, and finances was transformed based on geographic location. America was not divided by North and South but in a state-by-state patchwork where women and their fetuses had different rights depending on where they lived. A woman in Wisconsin would have dramatically different choices than one across the border in Minnesota. The ability to receive a specific medical procedure would shift based on where a woman entered a clinic or hospital, or called a doctor. In one state, abortion providers could be put in prison for ninety-nine years; in another, they would be heroes. Disparities had existed for years, given the successful effort to chip away at abortion access in Republican states and for low-income women. Now the court's opinion made those differences a stark national reality.

"Abortion presents the Court a profound moral question," Alito wrote for the majority. "The Constitution does not prohibit the citizens of each State from regulating or prohibiting abortion. Roe and Casey arrogated that authority."

Alito's decision was steeped in the originalist philosophy, or as he described the legal theory in a 2021 town hall at Thomas Aquinas College, a conservative Catholic private school, the idea that the Constitution "means what people would have understood it to mean at the time it was written."

The new court majority washed away the "super precedent" of Roe, which had guided so many decades of confirmation hearings. "Precedents should be respected, but sometimes the Court errs, and occasionally the Court issues an important decision that is egregiously wrong," wrote Alito. "When that happens, stare decisis is not a straitjacket."

Yet it wasn't simply one ruling that birthed this new country. The fall of Roe was the culmination of a targeted—and in key moments, startlingly lucky—campaign over a tumultuous decade by an under-the-radar network of elite conservative lawyers, Christian activists, and Republican politicians in key positions of power, built over years. A small but powerful coalition, determined to end abortion rights, conducted a coordinated and sweeping operation across courts and legislatures, Congress and campaigns, to topple Roe and remake American culture. They had found the levers of power and pulled them.

The impact of their work on the nation went far beyond questions of medicine and childbirth. Abortion was the screen onto which the country projected some of its greatest anxieties about religion and family, medicine, and the role of women in American life. For conservatives, abortion rights amounted to the nation abandoning not just state power but also families, unborn children, and morality. For liberals, those rights were the foundation of ensuring women's status as free and equal citizens, of their right to control their own bodies, and therefore, their destinies.

ALEXIS MCGILL JOHNSON was wrapping up a meeting with the board of Planned Parenthood's political arm when she heard the news. They'd been planning for the midterm elections and the escalation of threats they expected to come if Republicans retook control of Congress. The group took a break at 10:00 a.m. to engage in what had become a ritual in recent weeks, refreshing the Supreme Court website.

When she saw the decision, fog enveloped her brain. This was not the first time this country had taken rights away from people, she thought. Now it was happening to women. "There is nothing more fascist than taking away people's right to control their own bodies," she said. The right, she thought, created a world where "the tyranny of the minority" could dominate.

It felt devastating, watching the court ignore the views of the majority of Americans, she thought. Roe might never have been grounded in real freedom, real equality, she thought. The decision might have been little more than an empty promise for low-income women and women of color since nearly the day it happened. But she saw this outcome—the overturning—as a slide into autocracy. "We are watching the destruction of our democracy in slow motion," she said.

Nancy Northup was sitting in the Center for Reproductive Rights' quiet, mostly empty offices in New York. The networks kept calling to get her on TV. But her first thought was her four children. She texted them a simple message: "They did it."

If the words were expected, the timing was a surprise. Northup, and her whole team, thought the decision would be released the following week and planned for Julie Rikelman to travel from Boston then. She did not understand why the decision came on June 24, not the last week of the term as was typical for major rulings.

Northup had many losses before, but this one felt all-encompassing. Things she had believed had been crumbling in America, like the separation of church and state, and the idea that America was a pluralist country and not a Christian nation, were actually far more unsettled, she thought. Northup had lived her entire reproductive life with Roe as the law, from before she got her first period until after menopause. Her kids were in their twenties. This was about their generation, their reproductive choices, she thought. "They are facing just a dreadful world ahead," she said.

Cecile Richards was home in her apartment on the Upper West Side when the decision came. The night before she had been on a call with activists in Texas discussing how they would react to the ruling. Despite their preparation, the ruling felt "devastating," nearly "unimaginable," she said. She thought of her mother, as she always did in these big moments. The decision of this court indicated opposition to voting rights, LGBTQ rights, and so many other causes that her family held dear, Richards thought. "Abortion is just the canary in the coal mine," she said. "We're just the beginning."

Mini Timmaraju from NARAL called her husband, then texted their nanny and begged her to come over. She had just arrived home in Philadelphia from Washington the night before and had planned to return the next week for the expected decision. Now she rushed to get back to march to the Supreme Court with protesters. She thought about 2016 and all her colleagues who had worked for Hillary Clinton. If the outcome of the election had been different . . . The memory made her want to punch things. All she could do, she thought, was keep trying to fight.

Her mother sent her a text, moments after the ruling. Chaya Timmaraju was her daughter's first feminist role model. Timmaraju remembered watching how impressed her mother was with their new country when they moved to Texas from India back in 1979. That was not long before Ann Richards became state treasurer.

"This is no longer a country for women," her mother wrote. All Timmaraju could muster in response was a heart emoji reaction to the message. It was only then that her tears finally came.

The day unleashed the pent-up momentum of the antiabortion movement. Abortion rights in Republican states fell like dominoes. In Alabama, a federal judge lifted an injunction on the state's near-total abortion ban, considered the most restrictive abortion law in the country when it passed three years earlier. In South Dakota, a trigger ban from 2005 instantly made performing an abortion or supplying abortion pills a felony, punishable by two years in prison and a fine. In Virginia, Governor Glenn Youngkin tapped four Republican lawmakers to write a bill banning abortion after fifteen weeks. Old laws banning abortion—even from the Civil War era—could potentially be enforced, carrying mandatory prison sentences. In Oklahoma, where the Republican governor had signed five conflicting abortion bans into law over the past thirteen months, even some legislators were unable to explain what was now illegal.

Lawyers for abortion clinics rushed to file emergency injunctions. Swearing out loud to herself in her home office, Brigitte Amiri, who fought for Jane Doe, called one of her clients in Kentucky, EMW Women's Surgical Center, and told the clinic workers to turn away the women sitting in the waiting room. "You've got to cancel all patients now," she instructed. Then she rushed to file a lawsuit in Kentucky state court to block the state's trigger ban.

No one had to read the full 213-page decision or sift through the complex legal arguments to understand what had happened. Americans flooded into city parks and streets and outside federal courthouses. In Phoenix, police deployed tear gas after protesters started banging on the glass of the state capitol. In Silicon Valley, Meta executives issued orders prohibiting employees from openly discussing the ruling, to avoid creating a "hostile work environment." Other companies—Macy's, Vox Media, and Goldman Sachs—announced plans to cover travel expenses for employees to get abortions.

For weeks, the White House counsel had told administration aides that the decision could come any day, but that big decisions like this one most often came in the final week of the term before the justices left town for the summer. Her message had filtered through Democratic circles, and it became a kind of gospel that the ruling would be released on the final day. No one knew why it actually came that day, June 24, and not at the end of the term. But almost immediately, there were far more pressing concerns, like getting the president and other top officials before cameras to meet the moment.

Almost no one was ready or in the right position. Joe Biden's health secretary was touring a Planned Parenthood clinic in Saint Louis when Missouri's trigger ban was enacted, forcing the center to immediately halt appointments. As a group of House Democrats gathered on the Capitol steps and sang "God Bless America" to celebrate the passage of gun control legislation, shouts from abortion-rights protesters echoed in the background.

At her weekly press conference in the Capitol, a visibly shaken Nancy Pelosi read a poem by the Israeli poet Ehud Manor. "I have no other country even though my land is burning," she read. "Here is my home. I will not be silent for my country has changed her face." She repeated the line in a quiet voice. It was the same poem she read after the January 6 siege, during Donald Trump's second impeachment, when she asked her Republican colleagues to "finally open their eyes and hold this president accountable" before they acquitted him.

When Biden spoke from the White House more than two hours after the ruling was released, a cluster of top female officials double-clutched their cell phones, frantically toggling between their personal and official devices. Their summer Friday outfits—red flowered dresses, bright yellow capris, and striped T-shirts—were a sign of just how unexpected the timing was. For them, it was a moment of mourning, a black suit kind of day, and they were not prepared.

No executive action could restore Roe. Democrats didn't have the sixty votes in Congress to codify Roe, nor did they have the votes to eliminate the filibuster and pass such a law with their slim majority. The president was impotent to stop the fallout. With few options, Biden reran the same appeal Democrats had been making for decades: protect abortion rights by electing more Democrats. "With your vote, you can act," he said. "You can have the final word. This is not over."

The protests outside the Supreme Court sprawled from the steps, guarded by security barriers and armed police, across the Capitol plaza. Representative Alexandria Ocasio-Cortez tried to rally the crowd through a bullhorn. "What can you do in Congress?" a woman finally shouted. "Right now, elections are not enough," Ocasio-Cortez replied. "We have to fill the streets."

But filling the streets could accomplish very little. By the end of the day, abortion would be illegal in at least eight states. Within three months, the procedure would be banned or limited in seventeen states. On June 24, 2022, there were about 65 million women of childbearing age in America. Within two months of the decision, about one-third—20.9 million—would live in states where abortion was a criminal act.

None of this came as a shock to one Democrat, whose vision for the nation had promised another direction. Hillary Clinton read Alito's words in frozen fury. The decision was, in her legal opinion, "terrible," "poorly reasoned," and "historically inaccurate," she said. Its meaning to her was clear: women were not equal.

"It says that we are not equal citizens," she said. "It says that we don't have autonomy, agency, and privacy to make the most personal of decisions. It says that we should be rethinking our lives and our roles in the world."

As secretary of state, Clinton had tried, in the best way she knew how, to protect Roe, not only in America but across the globe. She warned of what was coming when she ran against Trump, even when she was dismissed as alarmist or hysterical. But now it was undeniable. Democrats had failed.

"One thing I give the right credit for is they never give up. They are relentless. You know, they take a loss, they get back up, they regroup, they raise more money." She added: "We have nothing like it on our side."

Clinton thought about how the three Trump justices answered questions about Roe in their confirmation hearings, testifying about precedent and suggesting the ruling was not at risk. "They just flat out lied. And Democrats did nothing in the Senate," she said. Those justices, she said, "were all teed up to do the bidding of political, ideological, religious organizations and leaders that they are beholden to. It's just truly remarkable."

Yet she understood why it was so hard for many Democrats to see what was happening along the way, how they could so easily suspend disbelief even as the evidence grew all around them. It seemed contrary to the last half century of law, the rulings that legalized contraception and same-sex marriage. It defied what she believed were the rights of women and rights of privacy.

"We didn't take it seriously and we didn't understand the threat," she said. "Most Democrats, most Americans, did not realize we are in an existential struggle for the future of this country."

TWENTY-SIX MINUTES AFTER the ruling, Marjorie Dannenfelser got a text from Mike Pompeo, the former secretary of state under Trump—"The Lord is good." Soon a flurry of missed calls back and forth from Mike Pence, Leonard Leo, Lynn Fitch, and Mississippi governor Tate Reeves. The RNC blasted out an email that could have been her own views: "Americans overwhelmingly support pro-life policies." But the most meaningful message was just two words. It was from her father: "You won!" It made her emotional. Her father, the doctor, now eighty-nine, still disagreed with her and still loved her. For her, it was a family story after all, leaving her Southern Episcopal family for this cause they had opposed, for a God they had not understood.

The ruling felt like an answer to prayer for many in the movement, going back to John C. Willke's vision so long ago. The national right to abortion disappeared at 10:10 a.m., as the pages of the decision were uploaded to the Supreme Court's website. Even the exact time felt like a sign for true antiabortion believers. They texted one another the words of Jesus, found in Bible verse John 10:10: "The thief comes only to steal and kill and destroy; I have come that they may have life, and have it to the full."

Across the country in Orange County, California, David Daleiden remembered his Planned Parenthood video sting as he drove down the freeway. He turned on an ancient Gregorian chant, rolled down his windows, and raised the volume for all to hear: "*Te Deum laudamus*," or "God, we praise you."

Kristan Hawkins of Students for Life declared that the total abolition of abortion would be next. "Today, life won," Pence proclaimed, calling for a national abortion ban. Mitch McConnell said the court "corrected a terrible legal and moral error, like when *Brown v. Board* overruled *Plessy v. Ferguson*."

Even Trump, who had been mute after the leak, took a victory lap, applauding himself for appointing the three conservative justices. "I think, in the end, this is something that will work out for everybody," he said in an interview on Fox News.

When Roe was established in 1973, front-page columns of *The New York Times* and other major newspapers headlined the reaction of Catholic cardinals. Half a century later, it was not official church leaders but the laypeople—the conservative politicians, and activists—who stood at the forefront. The church's social and political power had transferred from bishops to the enormously powerful, if small, group of conservative Catholic operators like Leo, Dannenfelser, and Hawkins who worked outside official religious structures. The shift revealed how the societal clout of the official Catholic Church hierarchy had diminished over the past fifty years, even as the power and ideological hold of its conservative wing grew stronger. Now Catholics and conservative evangelicals were merging not on religious grounds but around political ideology, fueling the Trump movement and setting out to transform America.

ADF's and Mississippi's teams pumped out op-eds and interviews framing the decision as a win for democratic values. Dobbs remade more than law; it remade the national view of motherhood, Erin Hawley said on *Fox News*. "This decision doesn't take rights away from women," she said. "It allows states to protect the unborn—and also to empower women."

Fitch declared the victory was not just for women but for the court itself. "The task now falls to us to advocate for the laws that empower women—laws that promote fairness in child support and enhance enforcement of it, laws for childcare and workplace policies that support families, and laws that improve foster care and adoption," she said. It was a tacit acknowledgment that a number of low-income women, who could not afford to travel out of state for an abortion, would be forced into motherhood without the resources to care for their children.

Inside Dannenfelser's headquarters in Arlington, Virginia—newly renamed Susan B. Anthony Pro-Life America to reflect their new fight—staff busted out a bottle of Dom Pérignon that a donor had sent a few years back. They had saved it for this moment. A team alerted Dannenfelser each time another state's trigger law went into effect.

She watched the scenes of women protesting at the court. Dannenfelser saw the ruling as a legal victory built on years of changing the culture. It was a mission that could be traced from Willke and his wife's speaking tour through church basements to the online exposé of Planned Parenthood videos, to the broadcasting of their message from Trump's bully pulpit. In that telling, Dobbs was the result of a passionate grassroots transformation of the hearts and minds of America. "The experience of abortion was not the great liberator that women were told it was going to be," she said. "They've never acknowledged that there were two people to contend with in any unexpected pregnancy."

But American support for Roe had never changed. This was a story of planning, to be sure, of a broad network pulling together across courts and country to change the nation. But Dannenfelser's win—their win—was also due to a series of extraordinary lucky breaks from shocking deaths on the highest court, a surprise presidential victory, and opponents who did not realize the true stakes until it was too late.

Before heading over to the Fox News studios to appear on *Tucker Carlson Tonight*, Dannenfelser plopped into a red leather booth at a nearby restaurant and chatted with Frank Cannon, her strategist who had vowed with her to fight their way back into the Republican Party after Obama won reelection. So much had changed over ten years. She thought of her daughter with special needs. Just this week, she had graduated and gone to the prom. If it had not been for her, Dannenfelser said, she might have given up years ago.

She reflected back to 1992, when her movement lost Casey and when SBA began. "Each time that there was a problem, we got stronger," she said. "And that is not humanly possible. I don't think we could have done that without the aid of the Holy Spirit."

Dannenfelser recited words from Henry Hyde, the creator of the Hyde Amendment that the reproductive justice movement fought for so many decades. It was a fragment of one of his old speeches that she had printed on the wall of her conference room, about meeting God after death. "'When the time comes as it surely will when we face that awesome moment, the Final Judgment, I've often thought, as Fulton Sheen wrote, that it's a terrible moment of loneliness," she said. "You have no advocates. You're there alone, standing before God and a terror will rip through your soul like nothing you can imagine. But I really think that those in the pro-life movement will not be alone." She choked up.

"I think there'll be a chorus of voices that have never been heard in this world, but are heard beautifully and clearly in the next world. And they will—" She struggled to continue, her voice breaking. "They'll plead for everyone who has been in this movement. They will say to God, 'Spare him, because he loved us.'"

She grabbed her things to leave as ABBA's "Dancing Queen" played over the restaurant's speakers. In this post-Roe country, Dannenfelser believed not just the laws but the politics of abortion would eventually shift in her favor. Democrats who opposed abortion would reappear over the next decade, she thought, emboldened to share their true views by the court's ruling. With Roe gone, she believed that America would finally build their culture of life, as more voters would realize they were supporting morality and human decency. That was the nation Dannenfelser saw coming.

If the Supreme Court leak had shocked Americans, the decision's final text was a revolution of its own. Dobbs was more than a cut-and-dried legal opinion. It was a declaration, written in the language of the movement that created this new future. Where Roe discussed the fetus as the "potentiality of human life," Dobbs now referenced the "unborn human being"—the language of the Mississippi law. A footnote cited research from the Charlotte Lozier Institute, the think tank founded by SBA to provide studies and research to bolster their cause.

The outcome on June 24 was not simply a fait accompli when Ruth Bader Ginsburg died and Amy Coney Barrett joined the court. Behind closed doors, the justices debated fiercely. Roberts was a holdout, as suggested in *The Wall Street Journal* and Politico. If he convinced another conservative justice to join him, there would be no majority, and his opinion would control the deeply fractured decision. He tried to win over Kavanaugh to his fifteen-week compromise position and worked with Breyer, the liberal justice nominated by Bill Clinton, who considered joining Roberts to preserve some form of Roe.

The antiabortion forces had argued against Kavanaugh's selection to the court, hoping for Barrett instead. Yet in the final count, he was their pivotal ally. When Kavanaugh convinced the court to adopt his plan to keep the case a secret for four months, Barrett initially agreed.

But then, sometime before the public announcement, she changed her mind, voting against taking up the case at all.

Ultimately, it didn't matter: the court needed only four justices to agree to hear the case. It was Kavanaugh who provided the fourth vote. Those four men—Thomas, Alito, Gorsuch, and Kavanaugh—overruled the concerns of the court's three women, including the one woman in their own ranks, the pride of the conservative antiabortion movement and the only mother among all the justices. And despite what Senator Susan Collins said Kavanaugh had promised in their private meeting—his assurances that he would respect the precedent of Roe—when offered the option of a compromise, he refused Roberts and sided with the bare majority voting to overturn Roe altogether.

Roberts wrote a concurring opinion that he would have taken "a more measured course"—upholding Mississippi's fifteen-week ban but leaving Roe alone. "Surely we should adhere closely to principles of judicial restraint here, where the broader path the Court chooses entails repudiating a constitutional right we have not only previously recognized, but also expressly reaffirmed applying the doctrine of stare decisis," Roberts wrote in his own concurring opinion. "The Court's opinion is thoughtful and thorough, but those virtues cannot compensate for the fact that its dramatic and consequential ruling is unnecessary to decide the case before us."

In the final count, it was the Trump justices—Gorsuch, Kavanaugh, and Barrett—who gave Alito and Thomas the majority to overturn Roe. If Ginsburg had lived another four months and two days, the ruling would have almost certainly been 5–4 in the other direction—if the court had even taken up the case. This reality was not lost on much of the country, which had lived through three polarizing confirmation hearings over four years. When asked in surveys, nearly six in ten Americans said they believed the decision was "mostly based on politics"—not in the law. For many Americans, the speed of the upending of Roe, less than two years after

Republicans procured their conservative majority on the court, undercut their belief that the court was impartial.

Alito saw it differently from much of America. To him, the court was creating a better, more equal America by correcting a moral wrong. He compared the ruling to *Brown v. Board of Education*, equating overturning abortion rights with ending racial segregation. There were significant differences: Brown expanded rights for existing classes of citizens; Dobbs curtailed them. Brown aligned with public opinion; Dobbs flouted it. But perhaps most significantly, the court agreed on Brown, ruling unanimously to overturn that precedent. The consensus sent the message that the decision was based on strong legal reasoning that stretched across ideological lines—not just the politics of the parties that voted the justices onto the court.

But in this decision, this court was fiercely divided. For the liberal members, an America without abortion rights was not a country they recognized, as they made clear in a scathing and sorrowful dissent. By eviscerating Roe, the court essentially ruled that a state could force a woman to give birth, transforming "what, when freely undertaken, is a wonder into what, when forced, may be a nightmare," Breyer, Sotomayor, and Kagan wrote. Some rights, they argued, were too valuable to be entrusted to voters and majority rule. "Even in the face of public opposition, we uphold the right of individuals—yes, including women—to make their own choices and chart their own futures," they wrote. "Or at least, we did once."

While the dissenters anticipated a darker future, the majority opinion looked to the past. Roe had been rooted in an evolving concept of liberty, an interpretation of the Fourteenth Amendment, which granted all citizens "equal protection of the laws." To reexamine the legal basis for Roe, Alito delved into British common law starting in the 1200s and moving through the centuries, citing treatises written in outdated English—"abortion of a quick child was 'murder' if the 'childe be born alive' and a 'great misprision' if the 'childe dieth in her body,'" he wrote, referencing a seventeenth-century legal writing. He devoted particular attention to the mid-1800s, when the Fourteenth Amendment was ratified. During that period in American history, states passed a series of restrictions on abortion rooted in the values of female purity, submissiveness, and Christian piety of the Victorian Age.

Alito devoted pages to the laws passed before 1868 and little more than a paragraph to the laws that came after. For the decades of the early republic, abortion had been largely permitted until "the quickening"—the time when fetal movement is detected by a woman, typically around fourteen to twenty weeks into a pregnancy. Still, Alito's findings were clear: "The inescapable conclusion is that a right to abortion is not deeply rooted in the Nation's history and traditions."

In some ways, it was not a surprising conclusion. The men who shaped English common law and wrote the Fourteenth Amendment did not view women as full and equal citizens. At the time, women had no legal existence separate from their husbands. They could not vote or, in most states, own land. A husband could rape or beat his wife with no legal consequences because she was considered part of her husband's property. Women's economic and legal freedom, their very bodily autonomy, would not come until the 1960s and 1970s, with rulings granting a constitutional right to use birth control and have an abortion.

And it wasn't just abortion rights that weren't "deeply rooted in the Nation's history and traditions." There were a number of what legal scholars called "unenumerated rights" that were not explicitly articulated in the Constitution but that previous courts had judged to be an extension of the right to liberty in the Fourteenth Amendment. Assessed through the thinking of the 1800s, contraception, interracial marriage, and same-sex unions were not "deeply rooted" in the founding documents. All—like equality for women—were rights that came centuries after the crafting of the Constitution.

Alito tried to reassure Americans that those other legal precedents were not at risk by his opinion. "Nothing in this opinion should be understood to cast doubt on precedents that do not concern abortion," he wrote. But that position didn't track with the legal reasoning of his writings, as Thomas made clear in a frank concurring opinion. "In future cases, we should reconsider all of this Court's substantive due process precedents," he wrote, listing decisions that guaranteed rights to same-sex intercourse and marriage, and contraception.

But the law is based on logic—not assurances, as the liberal justices pointed out. Future courts would be governed by Alito's reasoning, not one sentence in his 108-page decision. Already, they noted, some conservative lawmakers were pushing to move a right to contraception from being grounded in the Fourteenth Amendment to being regulated by states. "Rights can contract," the dissenters warned. "We cannot understand how anyone can be confident that today's opinion will be the last of its kind."

THE NIGHT OF June 24, Dannenfelser left the Fox television studio, after filming an interview with Tucker Carlson, and got into her security detail's truck. She worried about people finding her home address. They pulled away, the Capitol large and white against the black sky.

At a crosswalk out beyond the windshield, three young women stepped into the headlights. They carried signs, homemade with markers, to protest the decision Dannenfelser had devoted her life to winning. The first grabbed the hand of the second, who reached out for the hand of the third. They crossed together, and disappeared into the night.

Dannenfelser got a text. It was Father Paul Scalia, Justice Antonin Scalia's son. She read it out loud: "At long last, Thanks be to God."

It was a day she could only have imagined all those decades ago at Duke, when she wrote a letter to the school newspaper and publicly declared her life's new mission.

Forgotten to history was the other letter, the one that pushed Dannenfelser to write in the first place, from a woman she did not remember.

That letter was written by another student, Stacy Pollina. Back then, Pollina marched with friends in a Take Back the Night campaign, to protect women after a string of sexual assaults on campus. After graduation, she became a midwife, hoping to do everything she could to help women get pregnancy care where it seemed most urgent. She worked with immigrants and low-income families. By the time of the Dobbs ruling, she led a reproductive and sexual health program at a community health center, in a tiny town on the rural coast of Northern California.

Abortion would remain legal in California in this new America. But even that didn't mean accessing it was easy—nor, for that matter was getting any obstetrics care at all in Pollina's community. The local hospital—the California-based Adventist Health—was a faith-based system affiliated with the Seventh-day Adventist Church, which opposed abortion in almost all circumstances. There was a Planned Parenthood down the street. But it only performed abortions until about twelve weeks of pregnancy. If a woman needed a surgical abortion, she had to go to another clinic two and a half hours away. At the local high school graduation ceremony every year, Pollina watched girls cross the stage and counted the ones she had helped to get an abortion so each could finish her education.

Pollina had voted for Hillary Clinton. She had worried when McConnell held open Scalia's seat, refusing to hold hearings for Merrick Garland. But as the court changed in Washington and Mississippi passed its ban, she kept doing the work she could thousands of miles away, helping women directly, hoping to make a difference. Roe fell anyway.

She reread her letter to the Duke paper from thirty-five years ago. "To make abortion illegal is only to rape women of what freedom they already have—the freedom to choose to have an abortion or not, in accordance with their own moral values," Pollina read.

"To make it illegal is to impose certain moral values upon every women in the form of control over her body through legislation."

Pollina didn't remember writing the letter, and she did not remember that a senior then named Marjorie Jones wrote a letter in response. In fact, she didn't remember Dannenfelser at all.

She pulled up Dannenfelser's bio on Wikipedia and grew quiet. "This is what I've done," she said. "And she's done a little bit more."

34

The Heart of It All

Despite her hope that the country would eventually turn her way, Marjorie Dannenfelser's America was not the America most of the country wanted. It was a triumph of a largely conservative Christian minority over a more secular and pluralistic majority. And it was a tragedy to much of that majority. Roe was gone and the country was shaken by its loss.

The new legal reality transformed America with shocking speed. Within two months of the decision, about one-third of American women had lost all access to elective abortions in their states.

The country's politics reeled in response. The first post-Roe vote happened in Kansas, where voters overwhelmingly rejected a referendum removing abortion-rights protections from their state Constitution by eighteen points, running up margins not only in swing suburban areas but in redder rural counties. Even Planned Parenthood was shocked by the scale of its victory in a conservative state. "Kansas is a model for a path to restoring reproductive rights across the country through direct democracy," said Alexis McGill Johnson. "We know that Kansas will not be our last fight or our last victory."

Suddenly, it was Republicans who found themselves scrambling to address new levels of opposition, and not just in Kansas. Activists in Michigan, who had been working on a separate pro–abortion rights referendum, saw a similar increase in interest. Seemingly overnight, millions of dollars in donations poured into Democratic campaign coffers and abortion-rights groups.

Though it carried a political cost, Dannenfelser had achieved her goal of becoming like the NRA. And Leonard Leo had created a court that was reversing the legal rulings of the 1960s and 1970s with striking speed. The day before the decision in Dobbs, the court had struck down a New York law limiting gun licenses, offering a selective read of history that found gun control—like abortion rights—not deeply rooted in the text of the Constitution or American history. The two rulings showed how the Federalist Society judges, led by Samuel Alito and Clarence Thomas, were taking originalism from legal theory to national reality. All signs pointed it to being one of the most transformative eras of the court in American history. The new direction was a result not solely of the court itself but a giant web of outside actors that had locked in power to transform America, a network that was significantly motivated by Roe.

A few weeks after Roe fell, Alito flew to Rome and delivered an address to an audience at a private palace, the Palazzo Colonna, as part of an event sponsored by Notre Dame's law school. The speech was not heavily publicized and kept private until a week after it happened, when Notre Dame posted the video on its website. In his remarks, Alito gave the impression of a justice unbowed by the public outcry. He took shots at foreign leaders who condemned his opinion in Dobbs, even slamming Britain's Prince Harry, who had compared the "rolling back of constitutional rights" in America with the Russian invasion of Ukraine. "I had the honor this term of writing, I think, the only Supreme Court decision in the history of that institution that has been lambasted by a whole string of foreign leaders," Alito said defiantly.

But his overarching concern that day was the decline of Christianity in public life. Alito told the audience he saw a "growing hostility to religion, or at least the traditional religious beliefs that are contrary to the new moral code that is ascendant."

He called the room to action. Defending religious liberty was of utmost importance, he said, because Christians were vulnerable, with their free expression of belief subject to attack. The Declaration of Independence said men were endowed by their Creator with unalienable rights, but now not everyone believed there was a Creator, he noted. Protecting nearly unchecked religious freedom would encourage people of faith to speak out more forcefully on social issues. "People with deep religious convictions may be less likely to succumb to dominating ideologies or trends, and more prone to act in accordance with what they see as true and right," he said. "Civil society can count on them as engines of reform."

Alito's version of reform resonated with Leo, whose vision for America was always bigger.

Four months after the ruling, Leo donned a tuxedo and returned to the Mayflower Hotel as he had for so many years for the Federalist Society meetings. This time he came for a private dinner with behind-the-scenes Catholic power brokers, lawyers, donors, and activists, many of whom had prayed and worked for the end of Roe.

The Catholic Information Center, the Opus Dei–run group where Leo had long served on the board, was giving him an award. Opus Dei placed special importance on the work of laypeople, who it believed had a particular role to transform the world. If anyone had accomplished the Opus Dei mission—to use one's ordinary, daily work to sanctify the world for Christ from the inside out—it was Leo, and through him the entire conservative network he created.

For Leo, like many others in the antiabortion movement, the mission to end Roe came from a desire to shift how America interprets the Constitution. But those legal goals were difficult to untangle from deeply religious, and Catholic, convictions about what it means to be human, to be male or female, and how that understanding should ground society. The fight against abortion rights was a part of a broader battle against the secularization of an America that had turned its back on Christian concepts of morality, including the "holiness" of human suffering. "Human suffering completes Christ's salvific act," Leo explained.

That night, a testimonial video flashed photographs of Leo laughing with Clarence Thomas, shaking hands with Neil Gorsuch, posing with Brett Kavanaugh, and dining with Samuel Alito. Antonin Scalia's wife, Maureen, praised his "wonderful, deep, and comfortable faith." Carrie Severino, of the Judicial Crisis Network, Leo's vehicle for funding court nomination campaigns, praised him for a unique ability to identify the problems of society and to solve them with Christ's message.

William Barr, Donald Trump's former attorney general and a former Catholic Information Center board member, said he could think of no one else who had lived his faith more powerfully. "It is particularly fitting that the very year in which Dobbs was decided, we are honoring Leo," he said. "Because no one has done more to advance traditional values, and especially the right to life, than Leonard."

Another image appeared. It was of Leo and his daughter, Margaret Mary, about fifteen years earlier, before she died. She and her father were together in the Diplomatic Reception Room at the White House, with President George W. Bush kneeling beside her wheelchair. Leo had a realization in caring for his daughter, Father Paul Scalia said in the clip, "that the faith is the means by which we best help those who are in need."

This award was about both of them—father and daughter. Earlier that day, Leo and his family gathered at the CIC to unveil the portrait of "Margaret Mary of McLean" on the wall.

Like the saint she was named for—Margaret Mary, a paralyzed girl hundreds of years ago who had visions of the Sacred Heart of Jesus—Margaret Mary of McLean and the miracles her parents and their friends believed followed her death became a sign to Leo of the intervening love of Jesus.

Standing at the podium, his hair gone gray, Leo pushed his distinctive round glasses up on his nose. He rarely spoke publicly of his daughter and would not that night.

The award was to recognize Leo's part in the New Evangelization, an effort popularized by John Paul II in the early 1980s for Catholics to re-evangelize a secularized and de-Christianized world. That movement in America, along with the modern Christian right wing well beyond the Opus Dei faithful, had just won the victory of a lifetime. They had ended a ruling as deeply entrenched in American life as it was opposed in Catholic doctrine.

But Leo's speech that night was no victory lap. The battle for American culture, politics, and government continued. The Church was entering its third millennium, he said, and lay Catholics needed to step up their efforts even more. Even though a majority of the Supreme Court and many public officials were "faithful Mass-attending Catholics," Leo warned, Catholicism and its faithful were under attack, especially after the Dobbs decision. Catholics were being "censored," "canceled," and fired from jobs for speaking out about their faith.

"Our culture is more hateful and intolerant of Catholicism than at any other point in our lives," he said. "It despises who we are, what we profess, and how we act." Leo rattled off a list of persecutions of Catholics throughout the centuries, and urged his listeners not to despair. The Church had always survived, he said.

The losses in the months after Dobbs couldn't compare to the bloodshed of earlier eras, when priests and nuns were killed in the French Revolution or American Catholics faced persecution by the Ku Klux Klan. But even that fall, it was already clear that the antiabortion forces were losing politically, facing a massive backlash from liberal and independent voters who strongly disapproved of the ruling. Their Republican allies, including Trump, were running away from the issue, some disavowing earlier promises to restrict abortion. And Democrats were pounding their opponents with accounts of the most catastrophic outcomes, cases of raped children and women facing life-threatening complications.

Their current-day opponents were "just as myopic and ignorant as their counterparts from earlier ages," who burned and banned and killed, Leo said. They were immoral "barbarians, secularists, and bigots," who vandalized churches and harassed Catholic public officials at restaurants and their homes—referencing protesters who went to Kavanaugh's and Thomas's homes after Alito's opinion leaked. They were "a progressive Ku Klux Klan" that repeated "the KKK canard that Catholics want this country dominated and controlled by a theocracy, which no well-informed Catholic should ever support."

He added, "They are conducting a coordinated and large-scale campaign to drive us from the communities they want to dominate. . . . They control and use many levers of power."

It was a description that his opponents could easily say applied to Leo, and to the entire antiabortion movement, to the conservative lawyers and lawmakers, activists, and donors.

For years, the antiabortion movement had built a powerful identity on the belief that Christians did not have power. They argued Christians were besieged, crushed by a rising liberal America. The story of the fall of Roe revealed the opposite to be true. Their brand of conservative Christianity built enormous power where it mattered most. They did not have to be the majority to be the ones now crushing liberal America—all they had to be was a powerful, well-positioned minority.

At its core, Roe was a "question of power," Leo later reflected: Was it state legislatures or the Supreme Court who decided what women did with their bodies and when "life can be terminated"?

"It's all questions of power, right? Almost anything involving the dignity and worth of the human person is a question of power. I mean, that's not anything earth shattering," he said.

Over the past decade, Leo had certainly learned a few things about power. As the country moved into the new, post-Roe era, Leo, like ADF, was only expanding his reach. The fall of Roe was a beginning, not an end. The entire Roe era had created rights that were unmoored from the country's traditions and Constitution, he had told the Hillsdale College students back in 2018, from legalized contraception to same-sex marriage to affirmative action. The fall of Roe was the start of those liberties being unwound, and the America that the conservative Christian movement believed the founders intended could begin again. It was about legal interpretation. But it was also bound up in a religious quest, aimed at pushing back the growing forces of secularism.

Already Leo was building new institutions for his bigger battle, reaching far beyond abortion rights to grow conservative power and transform broad swaths of American life. He aimed to adapt his successful revolution of American law and apply it to the entire country—to build more networks of conservatives to enact wholesale cultural revolution.

A new organization was in place to do just that. The Teneo Network, with Leo as a new board member, aimed to replicate the success of the Federalist Society to a broader swath of American culture—from corporations to media to higher education. They could "crush liberal dominance" across American life, Leo would say, by connecting the forces of conservative elected officials, political aides, activists, federal judges, state attorneys general, media figures—even pro athletes and business leaders. They had members already—people like Senator Josh Hawley, former Trump administration aides, Republican Attorneys General Association leaders, staff for 2024 presidential contenders—all expanding their reach.

The story of the fall of Roe pressed forward. But for Leo and the movement he represented, the fall of Roe was part of another story far greater than the future of America. It was a story that reached back beyond the past decade or the fifty years of the sexual revolution or the founding of the nation. It was a story that rippled back beyond even the five-hundred-year story of the Protestant Reformation, and beyond the millennia-long story of Christian empire. It was a story that began with a young girl named Mary, who faced an unplanned pregnancy and gave birth to a baby who saved the world. It was a story of the fate of Christendom.

At the Mayflower that night, the forces of secularism that opposed them could not win, Leo assured the Catholic activists, politicians, and priests. Their movement was growing, and the "renewal of our culture" would come from their continued work, he said. God, after all, was loyal to his people. "I have faith that together we will carry it forward and once again lift the eyes of America upward toward Christ," he promised. The audience leaped to its feet.

Leo's zeal was unwavering. But he also saw something about the fall of Roe that few others did.

THE DAY ROE was overturned, Leo woke up at his estate home on Mount Desert Island, an old-money enclave on the craggy coast of Maine. He had hosted a grand party the night before, where the former food-and-beverage director at Trump's defunct hotel in Washington picked the wines. The champagne, Pol Roger Reserve, was a Winston Churchill favorite. Two dozen federal and state judges mingled at his house with other conservative legal luminaries. The dinner coincided with a conference—a week in Maine, all expenses paid—put on by the Antonin Scalia Law School at George Mason University near Washington, which had become a growing nexus of conservative legal thought. The school bore Scalia's name thanks to Leo, who had coordinated $30 million in donations to honor his late friend. Security details stood guard around the perimeter of Leo's estate as the group feted their host and their victories.

The morning after the party ended, at 10:10 a.m., came the ultimate victory. The day was a triumph, a zenith of Leo's life's work, as it was for so many in the antiabortion movement. But unlike so many others, Leo stayed quiet.

Leo and his wife, Sally, went to Mass, lunch, and one of their late daughter Margaret's favorite places. The day was indeed an enormous celebration—but not just about Roe, he said. It was a celebration for Margaret Mary, their girl who shaped her father's view of how ending abortion and embracing suffering could redeem humanity. A girl whose casket Thomas carried and whose funeral Mass Roberts attended. A girl who, just maybe, their closest circle thought, inspired miracles and left divine signs of the Sacred Heart of Jesus behind.

The date of the decision—June 24, 2022—had not made sense to most people. But that particular Friday was not just a random Friday in June. The timing had a special significance.

On the Catholic calendar, it was a holy day, a feast day where Catholic believers across the world practiced a certain spiritual devotion. Of all the Catholic practices, this one began with a girl from France who, hundreds of years ago, was paralyzed as a child. A girl who had mystical visions of Jesus revealing his flaming heart to save humanity. A girl who followed what she, and then the church, saw as a divine call to propagate worship of that heart. A heart they believed beat for every human, from the moment of conception to the last breath.

Roe fell on the Feast of the Sacred Heart of Jesus.

One of the biggest legal decisions in American history fell not only on this specific sacred Catholic date but also on a holy day tied to the beloved daughter of Leo, the man who did more than perhaps anyone in America to help create a conservative Christian legal network that ended Roe and changed the nation.

Leo said he never spoke about the case—or timing of when it was released—with his friends on the court. The Supreme Court did not respond to requests for comment on the timing. The court probably didn't pick the day it was announced to coincide with his daughter's holy day, or the Catholic day at all, Leo said. The timing was most likely related to security concerns. Though he couldn't be totally certain. "It wouldn't have been Sam's, Clarence's decision anyway," he said, referencing Justices Alito and Thomas. "The chief would have decided the order of decisions that would come out that day. And I don't think he . . . well, I don't know. Maybe he knew it was the Feast of the Sacred Heart."

To many in the broader antiabortion movement who knew the Catholic significance of the date, if not the intimate meaning it had for Leo, the timing was more proof that the fall of Roe was, in fact, a miracle. The importance of that day, commemorating Jesus's love for the world, was to them a sort of divine code, yet another sign their God acted to save America and sounded the victory.

But in the pattern of the fall of Roe, the date they saw as providential might look to another part of America like a more earthly kind of coded message: a raw expression of political, legal, and Christian might.

35

After Dobbs

The reality was that Roe did not just fall once, on June 24, 2022. Roe collapsed over a transformational decade. Roe fell when Texas enacted its near-total abortion ban and turned neighbors into citizen law enforcers. It fell when Ruth Bader Ginsburg died during the Days of Awe and Amy Coney Barrett took her place. It fell when the Senate confirmed Brett Kavanaugh over Christine Blasey Ford's objections. When Jane Doe was initially denied an abortion. When Mike Pence worked to craft the Trump administration in his image. When Donald Trump survived "Grab 'em by the pussy" and was elected president. When Mississippi had just a single abortion clinic. When Wendy Davis's filibuster was interpreted as a victory, but was actually a defeat. Roe fell the day Marjorie Dannenfelser left that conference room, determined to fight back into the Republican Party that tried to kick her out.

Perhaps Roe was even falling the day it was decided, when John C. Willke and a small band of conservative Catholics decided to take it down. Nationally, the fall of Roe was the triumph of a minority view over a country that didn't fully understand the battle until it had all but lost.

It was a unique story but also, in some ways, a classically American one. Passionate minorities have changed the direction of the country since the founding. A small group of suffragists in white eventually gave women the right to vote. A coalition of Black pastors, students, and community leaders led the battle for civil rights protections. Gay activists cast equality as love and won the right to marry. Now an overwhelmingly Christian minority, who believed that a fetus should have the same fundamental rights as born humans, brought the end of Roe. They saw their win as a civil rights victory equal to those of the past.

But the essence of this battle was fundamentally different. The fetus was inextricably tied to the woman. Rights for one inherently meant fewer freedoms for another. Unlike those other fights—for gay rights, civil rights, and women's rights—the fall of Roe was a contraction of rights for women, not an expansion.

The antiabortion activists did not win by opening American hearts and minds to their cause, as those other activists did. Not a single state had a majority of adults that favored overturning Roe. Even in Mississippi, only 40 percent agreed with the court's decision. Nor did they convince large numbers of women to stop getting abortions: data suggested that legal abortions likely increased in the first six months of 2023, as tens of thousands of women crossed state lines to procure the procedure and access to medication abortion by telemedicine increased. Their victory was an undoing of what vast national majorities supported.

The antiabortion movement succeeded because most people did not believe it would. For all its efforts over the decades, it did not convert broad swaths of the country to its beliefs, even as Americans held complicated views about the details of abortion. Americans simply did not believe that a right that had become so integral to their understanding of women's lives, liberty, and their pursuit of happiness could disappear in the pages of a legal opinion. Widespread denial proved more powerful than the reality of a changing country, where conservative states were moving in great numbers to ban abortion. And then suddenly, the spell was broken.

With that one sentence in Dobbs, the Roe era in America ended. Roe had been decided at the end of its own transformational ten-year period, one in which the court expanded voting rights and instituted affirmative action. And it fell as those landmark laws and policies were being challenged, at the Supreme Court and by the rightward shift of Republican politics. Roe was decided when America was a majority white, Christian nation, in the early days of the sexual revolution transforming gender relations. It fell in a different America, one that was increasingly secular, religiously unaffiliated, and racially and sexually diverse.

For so many decades, the foundation of the discussion over women's rights and sexuality had been Roe. Now that was shattered. A new period began, and the nation was being remade in real time. From politics to medicine to law to the antiabortion movement itself, forces that had long been constant in American life were suddenly scrambled.

The fall of Roe marked the symbolic inauguration of a new generation of the religious right, a post-Roe movement that was more radical than the one that preceded it. Many of these activists saw their cause as intertwined with the broader swath of concerns animating Trump's Republican Party, issues like election denialism, eradicating transgender rights, and limiting what schools could teach about race and inequity. After Dobbs, the lawyers at ADF turned their attention to limiting rights for transgender people, using the legislation-to-court-to-culture pipeline that was the backbone of their anti-Roe strategy.

This new Christian legal movement had reached political maturity and gained power from statehouses to Congress. In late 2023 when Republicans failed over and over to successfully elect a Speaker of the US House of Representatives—a position second in line to the presidency—they finally agreed on a little-known congressman from Louisiana, Mike Johnson, who had worked as a lawyer for ADF. "I'm a Bible-believing Christian. I believe in the sanctity of every single human life," he said in an early interview with Fox News. "Until recently, actually, almost all of our nation's leaders openly acknowledged that they were also Bible-believing Christians."

Yet after Dobbs, ADF and its allies no longer benefited from the veil of denial that they would succeed. After the decision, views on abortion shifted rapidly. Nearly 70 percent of the country believed that abortion should be legal in the first three months of pregnancy, a record high. A majority said the procedure was "morally acceptable."

In a heartbeat, everything had changed. The laws that ADF helped usher in had been written as a litigation strategy, not as actual policy. Other bills had been crafted largely as political messaging, never expected to become actual law in a world without Roe. When they were instituted after Dobbs, they opened new questions over what dire circumstance qualified for a medical exception, and what procedures, exactly, remained legal.

What was once only theoretical to many Americans became startlingly real as stories of women and girls confronting difficult choices became public. The nation was plunged into the detailed reality of pregnancy, engaging in political and medical conversations that would have once seemed unimaginable. There were debates over ectopic pregnancies and miscarriage care, with frank descriptions of heavy bleeding and life-threatening complications. Graphic discussions happened in state legislatures over sexual assault and campaign ads featuring survivors of child rape. Hospitals in Republican states formed committees that debated whether providing each medically necessary abortion would trigger legal action under the new laws. And parents had quiet conversations about sending students—boys and girls—to college with packs of abortion pills in states where the procedure was prohibited. Even the term itself was reconsidered, as women realized the "termination" of their nonviable pregnancy had actually been something else entirely: an abortion.

Suddenly, it was Democrats who had political energy on their side. The abortion rights majority—a coalition of Democrats, independents, and moderate Republicans—was silent no longer. Alito had written in his decision that "women are not without electoral or political power." Now, they used that power to push back.

The 2022 midterm elections marked the best midterm result for a president's party in two decades. In Michigan, where an abortion-rights referendum was on the ballot, Democrats won full control of state government for the first time in forty years. In Arizona, Pennsylvania, Georgia, and Nevada, Democrats staved off an expected red wave in key races. Voters in five states voted to expand or protect abortion rights through ballot measures. And the Republican candidates who embodied the post-Roe religious right, even calling for the end of the separation of church and state, largely lost their races, some failing to survive even primaries within their own parties. The message Ilyse Hogue had pushed before the 2020 election—that abortion rights were a fundamental freedom—had become the dominant argument of her party, echoed from statehouses to the White House. NARAL, the organization she once led, even changed its name to Reproductive Freedom for All, an effort intended to reflect its expanded coalition and the stakes of the new fight.

Not every Democrat won in 2022. In Texas, Rochelle Garza, the attorney who had defended Jane Doe, lost her race to oust Texas attorney general Ken Paxton by nearly ten points, leaving Paxton in place to continue defending Texas's strict bans. Still, for the antiabortion movement, the overall results were a low point reminiscent of the one after 2012, when it felt like Republicans were trying to push them out of the party with the autopsy.

Abortion had transformed from a motivating issue for the conservative base to a political liability for Republicans with independent and moderate voters. Trump publicly distanced himself from the cause, blaming the antiabortion movement that helped boost him to the White House for the party's midterm defeats. And even SBA's donors began to waver. Most had supported the organization not because they were fervently against abortion but because they saw the group as an asset for Republican victories, which now it was seemingly not. SBA urged its allied lawmakers to move carefully: in a private strategy call just weeks before the midterm elections, the organization counseled lawmakers in Tennessee to wait several years before considering laws that would regulate IVF and contraception. But there were plenty of signs that their movement had moved beyond them. In Alabama, it only took twenty months for a state Supreme Court to rule that frozen embryos should legally be considered children, prompting some clinics in the state to halt IVF procedures and sparking a national panic over the possible widespread loss of fertility treatments.

Leonard Leo and the conservative justices also paid a political price for the decision, as they faced new scrutiny from the public, the media, and Congress. Senate Democrats and reporters dug into the justices' finances, discovering that Justices Alito and Thomas had accepted gifts and trips and gave paid speeches—the sum of which was worth hundreds of thousands of dollars. For the first time, the Supreme Court adopted an ethics code, but the policy did not have an enforcement mechanism. And as part of its investigation, the Senate Judiciary Committee authorized a subpoena of Leo. He refused to participate. "Senate Judiciary Committee Democrats have been destroying the Supreme Court; now they are destroying the Senate. I will not cooperate with this unlawful campaign of political retribution," he said in a statement.

To Clinton, it seemed like a good start. For years, Democrats failed to "invest in the kind of parallel institutions" to the conservative legal establishment, she believed. "We could have done a much better job exposing Leonard Leo, exposing the Federalist Society, exposing their mission, their movement to overturn *Roe v. Wade*," Clinton said. Democrats were still relatively powerless to stop the new antiabortion regime. The federal standard set by Dobbs was the law of the land. Even Julie Rikelman, the Center for Reproductive Rights' lawyer who argued Dobbs, whom Joe Biden picked as a federal circuit court judge in Boston, promised to "apply Dobbs faithfully" in her confirmation hearings, as she was required to follow new Supreme Court precedent.

Even with Democratic control of the Senate, Biden was limited in what he could do. In the months after Dobbs, Congress codified protections for same-sex marriage and interracial marriage into federal law, but Democrats could not get the votes to do the same for abortion rights. The White House determined it had reached the legal limits of its powers by the end of the summer, after issuing a series of executive orders. During the midterm campaign, Biden publicly vowed that the first bill he would send to Congress after the election would be one enshrining abortion rights in federal law. It was a promise Democrats would be unable to fulfill, given that Republicans kept their narrow majority in the House. In the first post-Roe State of the Union address in 2023, Biden spent roughly forty-two seconds of his seventy-two-minute address on the topic—a quiet admission of the limits of his power to restore federal abortion rights. And almost two years after Dobbs, as he headed into his reelection campaign, Biden still had not held a formal White House meeting with the heads of the abortion-rights organizations.

Indeed, even as the antiabortion movement seemed to lose the immediate political fight, there was little question that it had reshaped the country. A year after the decision, 17.5 million women of reproductive age lived in fourteen states where abortion was completely or mostly banned. In another seven states, abortion bans had been passed but were blocked by the courts. At the local level, the tactics that led to the Texas law spread across the country, as a growing constellation of conservative cities and counties passed local ordinances to effectively ban abortion within their borders.

For every step its opponents made, the antiabortion network pushed back in statehouses and the courts. Democrats celebrated the success of a ballot measure in Ohio that enshrined abortion rights in their state constitution in 2023, defeating an $18 million effort by a Leonard Leo–affiliated group. But as they did, antiabortion groups sued in Michigan, attempting to overturn the constitutional provisions that voters there passed in a similar measure the year before. "I think we're farther than anyone would have expected we would be," said Kristan Hawkins on the year anniversary of the ruling. "But am I complacent with that? Hell no."

The post-Roe world also scrambled the movement that ushered it in. Before the decision, some Republicans talked about embracing proposals like expanded child tax credits, expanded prenatal care and maternity leave, and even direct payments to families with young children. Those plans were a tacit acknowledgment of the future that would be arriving fast. With abortion soon to be illegal or tightly restricted in half the country, tens of thousands more babies would be born to parents struggling to afford housing, health care, food, and childcare.

When that future came, Republican leaders focused less on concrete help for the new babies that would now be born and more on the political crisis at hand. "Pro-life" had become synonymous with abortion bans, internal polling by Republican strategists found. In private memos and closed-door meetings, they urged Republican candidates to talk instead about "common-sense restrictions" and "compassionate exceptions" for rape, incest, and life of the mother. Dannenfelser tried to rally their party around a national fifteen-week ban, which she and her allies framed as "a reasonable fifteen-week limit." It was a way to cast a stricter restriction—five weeks earlier than the twenty-week ban their cause once pushed in Congress—as a compromise stance.

Just like Mississippi's fifteen-week law, their proposal did not grow first from health or science, though it argued that was the point in pregnancy when a fetus could feel pain—a claim that continued to be widely discredited by the mainstream medical establishment. Nor would it stop the vast majority of abortions, given that more than 93 percent happen before that stage in pregnancy. Rather, fifteen weeks was the point at which polling showed a majority of voters said they might consider limitations. But in this new post-Roe era, those kinds of tactics didn't work as well as they once did. Independent and Democratic voters now understood the ultimate goal to be banning all abortion.

The new, fifteen-week positioning was also a compromise that many in the antiabortion movement were no longer willing to accept. Hawkins pushed for the abolition of all abortion and still wanted Congress to ban abortion as early as possible, at around six weeks of pregnancy. She wasn't worried about what was politically possible or would help their allies win elections. At lunch with Dannenfelser before the midterm election, Hawkins compared their split views to divisions among leaders of the women's suffrage and civil rights movements, in the final years before those victories. In each case, she told Dannenfelser, there was a more established leader, plotting carefully and methodically toward the goal, but there was also the more extreme leader of an allied group who came in near the end and demanded uncompromising change. In this analogy, Hawkins was the radical. "They felt that these activists were messing things up for them, that they were speeding up the timeline too fast, or that they didn't have all the pieces in place," she said. "I'm like, oh my gosh, that is literally the argument."

The post-Roe activists were ready to take their birthright and control the movement. They had fought for this new world, one where they no longer had to accept incremental advancement. For years, allies had told Hawkins to stop saying they would overturn Roe, that the goal sounded "politically naive" and was "giving people false hope," she said. But history had proved them wrong, and with Roe gone, she wanted more. Not just banning surgical abortions after fifteen weeks but all of it—abortion pills, morning-after pills, birth control pills, and IUDs. She wanted a museum of abortion in Washington to accompany the Holocaust Museum.

Just as Dannenfelser had her supporters in the Republican Party establishment, Hawkins and the post-Roe generation had powerful allies too. The same lawyers who pushed the fall of Roe were at the vanguard of the next fight. Ten days after abortion cost Republicans in the midterm elections, ADF filed a lawsuit in the Northern District of Texas asking the Food and Drug Administration to revoke its 23-year-old approval of mifepristone, the first pill in the two-drug medication abortion regimen, which is also a standard drug used in miscarriage care. Leo's web of dark money groups helped fund the antiabortion organizations, which were the plaintiffs—and ADF's clients.

As part of the case, ADF lawyers resurrected the Comstock Act, a 150-year-old law that made it a federal crime to mail or deliver "obscene, lewd, or lascivious" material, specifically any item related to an abortion or birth control. It was the same law that ensnared Margaret Sanger, back in 1916 when she opened her first clinic in Brooklyn, selling instructions on using birth control for ten cents a pamphlet. Roe had largely turned the law into an unconstitutional relic, but now it was back—an old weapon made new. Over the months that followed, the Supreme Court announced it would take up the case. Trump allies began planning how they could enforce the old law, effectively instituting a national abortion ban, through the Department of Justice if he won a second term. It would be a version of the work through executive actions they did during his administration, just supercharged for this new era.

Whatever the court's decision and whoever won the 2024 presidential election, it was clear that the case would not mark the end of the post-Roe religious right's legal and political efforts to roll back America's cultural transformation. If its efforts with Roe showed America anything, it was that its success never depended on just one argument. Even with federal abortion rights gone, the new, post-Roe religious right was using the same tactics: an overwhelming, unrelenting march to banning all abortion and beyond. But in this new decade, they would face a far more potent opposition from a newly energized left, now fully aware of the new reality revealed by the fall of Roe.

What is less certain is how the court will assess these arguments in the decades to come. Or even if plaintiffs will be arguing before the same court. The tumultuous events of the past decade showed that for all the careful legal planning, even the Supreme Court was limited by another marker of human life: its end.

36

What Is a Woman?

A decision of the Supreme Court, once made, nearly always stands. Less than 1 percent of the court's more than twenty-five thousand decisions have ever been expressly reversed since the founding of America. When the court rules about the meaning of the Constitution, it has lasting power to define the country.

But words of a dissent are not always lost to history. There is a tradition in the United States, Ruth Bader Ginsburg had said, where eventually, over time, the greatest dissents become the law of the land. "That's the dissenter's hope: that they are writing not for today but for tomorrow," she said in 2002. Dissents can point the country toward a future age, hinting at a path for justices on future courts to change the country.

In a way, the dissent in Roe from 1973 became the majority opinion in Dobbs. Justice Byron White, the justice whom Ginsburg replaced in 1993, wrote the opinion disagreeing with the court's decision in Roe and expressing the yearnings of the then nascent abortion opposition to one day fight back.

"The Court apparently values the convenience of the pregnant mother more than the continued existence and development of the life or potential life that she carries," he wrote. "I cannot accept the Court's exercise of its clear power of choice by interposing a constitutional barrier to state efforts to protect human life and by investing mothers and doctors with the constitutionally protected right to exterminate it. This issue, for the most part, should be left with the people and to the political processes the people have devised to govern their affairs."

After forty-nine years, the antiabortion movement had made White's dissent America's new reality. Just as White argued in Roe that there was "nothing in the language or history of the Constitution" that supported a right to an abortion, so did Samuel Alito argue in Dobbs.

But now there was a new dissent. The three justices appointed by Democrats, two Jews and one Catholic—Stephen Breyer, Elena Kagan, and Sonia Sotomayor—had written an agonized opinion, warning that the court had done grave damage to women's equality and the court's own legitimacy. Their jointly authored dissent was unusual, a signal of how strongly they disagreed with the decision.

Their language was furious. "The Constitution will, today's majority holds, provide no shield, despite its guarantees of liberty and equality for all," they wrote. "And no one should be confident that this majority is done with its work."

Women's lives and the expectations they had for them would be fundamentally transformed by this decision, they argued, whether or not they became pregnant. In the stroke of a pen, Dobbs had remade the futures of 167.5 million American women.

"After today, young women will come of age with fewer rights than their mothers and grandmothers had," the dissenters wrote. "The majority accomplishes that result without so much as considering how women have relied on the right to choose or what it means to take that right away."

Yet the impact wasn't limited to women's lives. The decision, they wrote, threatened the very legitimacy of the court in American life by undercutting the legal doctrine that courts should honor previous decisions. The court appeared "not restrained but aggressive, not modest but grasping," they wrote.

"The majority has overruled Roe and Casey for one and only one reason: because it has always despised them, and now it has the votes to discard them," they said. "The majority thereby substitutes a rule by judges for the rule of law."

They concluded with overt words of sadness, a rare seeping of emotion into the legal language of the court. "With sorrow—for this Court, but more, for the many millions of American women who have today lost a fundamental constitutional protection—we dissent."

The three justices weren't the only dissenters. A year and a half after Dobbs, the Center for Reproductive Rights represented a Dallas mother of two, Kate Cox. She sued to be granted an abortion under the minimal medical exceptions in the Texas ban, after receiving a severe fetal diagnosis that threatened her health and future fertility. The Texas Supreme Court denied her appeal and she traveled to New Mexico for her procedure. "The state of Texas wanted me to continue a pregnancy where I would have to wait until a baby dies in my belly, or dies at birth, or lives for days, and put my own health at risk and a future pregnancy at risk," she told CBS News, a few weeks later.

Twenty-two other Texas women filed a separate lawsuit claiming the denials of their abortions violated their rights under the state constitution. Dr. Austin Dennard, an ob-gyn in Dallas who joined that lawsuit after leaving the state for her own abortion, said she never expected Roe to fall, even as she watched restrictions on abortion multiply in Texas over the past decade. She had been "blissfully naive," Dennard said. And then, suddenly, abortion laws were part of her daily life. A sixth-generation Texan, she considered moving to a state where abortion remained legal and she could practice obstetrics without the possibility of legal threats. Instead, she stayed and became engaged in politics, even agreeing to be featured in an early ad for Biden's reelection campaign. "Being so silenced and so gaslit in states like Texas, it's like a whole additional form of oppression," she said. "Almost more painful than having to go out of state is feeling like you had to be silent about it afterwards."

After Dobbs, Dennard, and so many other women, would no longer stay silent. There would be other women and other lawsuits. Their cases would move through the courts. It took nearly half a century for the antiabortion movement to take down Roe. But their fight showed that history was not stagnant. A victory once won could become a defeat in the future. A defeat could become a victory.

SIX DAYS INTO this new America, the first post-Roe justice took her oath of office for the Supreme Court. For the first time, there were four women on the court. And, for the first time, a Black woman. As she transformed the court, she also entered a court transformed, riven by polarization and mistrust, ruling over a divided nation.

Cameras flashed as Ketanji Brown Jackson took her seat at her Senate confirmation hearing, in the spring before the decision. She had clerked for Breyer, the man she replaced, two decades earlier. Now only Clarence Thomas remained as a justice from that time. Jackson, a Harvard graduate twice over, whose family descended from enslaved people, was a year older than Amy Coney Barrett and also a mother, with two daughters. She had been confirmed by the Senate three times for other positions, winning support even from a handful of Republicans. She looked like no one who had preceded her in the Supreme Court confirmation chair.

The hearing made clear the new questions that would define her era. As the questioning on the second day dragged into hour thirteen, Marsha Blackburn, the lone Republican woman on the committee, took the microphone. The senator, who famously preferred the title *congressman* during her earlier years in the House, had made her name through the antiabortion cause. She led one of the congressional committees that investigated Planned Parenthood in 2015, fanning the controversy with the audacious charge that the group was selling "baby body parts on demand."

"I'm a pro-life woman," Blackburn now explained, in her honeyed Tennessee twang, from the edge of a long U-shaped table. "I find it incredibly concerning that someone who is nominated to a position with life tenure on the Supreme Court holds such a hostile view toward a view that is held as a mainstream belief that every life is worth protecting."

The Dobbs decision was coming soon, Blackburn said. There would be a new precedent. Would Jackson commit to following the court's decision on Dobbs, should Roe no longer apply? It was the reverse of the standard question about Roe that Republicans had asked for decades. Now, Blackburn was asking whether Jackson would respect what her movement had spent so many decades working to achieve: the fall of federal abortion rights as a new precedent in American law.

The woman who would become the country's first Black female justice responded calmly and clearly, giving an upside-down—and yet the same—version of the answer used by Neil Gorsuch, Brett Kavanaugh, and Amy Coney Barrett. "Whatever the Supreme Court decides in Dobbs will be the precedent of the Supreme Court. It will be worthy of respect in the sense that it is the precedent."

Blackburn pivoted to another question, one that was far more unusual. It was one that no one could remember ever being asked of a Supreme Court nominee. "Can you provide a definition for the word *woman*?" she asked.

Jackson paused. "Can I provide a definition? No. I can't," she responded.

"You can't?" asked Blackburn, her voice rising.

"Not . . . not in this context," Jackson responded. "I'm not a biologist."

Blackburn pounced. She expressed concern about a transgender swimmer who won a collegiate swimming championship just days earlier. For conservatives, this was a gotcha moment, a way to stoke conservative outrage about transgender rights and show

how far the country had strayed from traditional values. "The fact that you can't give me a straight answer about something as fundamental as what a woman is, underscores the dangers of the kind of progressive education that we are hearing about," Blackburn said. "It tells our girls that their voices don't matter. . . . I think it tells them that they are second-class citizens."

Americans didn't have a clear answer either. Searches of the word *woman* spiked after the exchange, leading Dictionary.com to select it as the word of the year for 2022. The word *woman*, so simple and common, was "inseparable from the story of 2022," they wrote. Decades of political warfare happened over abortion and pregnancy, a nine-month period when women gave of their own bodies and blood to grow new beings. Yet the symbolism of Roe had been so much bigger than just the temporary phase of pregnancy. When the nation fought about abortion, it was debating the place of women in American life.

For nearly half a century, Roe was seen as a foundation of women's freedoms in America. A pregnant woman could legally choose whether she wanted to bear a child. It was a ruling ushered in by a rapidly changing understanding of women's place—economically, legally, and domestically—in the national project. When Roe was decided, women could not get a credit card in their own names, could not legally refuse sex to their husbands, lacked guarantees not to be fired if they became pregnant, and did not have legal protections against sexual harassment. There were no female senators, and the first female Supreme Court justice—Sandra Day O'Connor—would not be confirmed for another eight years.

The Dobbs decision effectively restored childbearing as an inescapable fate for pregnant women and girls in broad swaths of conservative America. Yet it could not turn back the clock. America was changing. And as Jackson's presence on the congressional dais underscored so vividly, the societal changes since Roe were now "deeply rooted"—if not in American history, then certainly in the reality of the American present.

Dobbs was now the guiding force for the country's laws. But the mass outrage that met the ruling showed that the country had not resolved the essential question intertwined with the long national battle over abortion: What rights is a woman owed?

In America, a nation that from its founding declared that all men were created equal, it was never in doubt that all white men had rights. But from the beginning, the place of women was always less certain, as Abigail Adams made clear to her husband in 1776 when he served in the Continental Congress to craft the foundation of this new nation: "I desire you would Remember the Ladies, and be more generous and favourable to them than your ancestors," she wrote. "Remember, all men would be tyrants if they could."

Generations later, even the most basic understanding of the role and rights of women in the American experiment, even the essence of what makes a woman herself, remained unresolved. The majority of justices in Dobbs, representing a minority of Americans, declared one answer.

A minority of justices in Dobbs, representing a majority of Americans, had their own reply.

And on the final day of Jackson's hearings, when the Republican senators returned to Blackburn's line of questioning about womanhood, the soon-to-be newest justice offered an answer of her own. It cut through political lines. It did not wrestle with faith or race or ideology or the law. Instead, it spoke both to a woman's sense of self-determination and the interdependent relationship that defined the abortion question for so many.

"I know I am a woman, I know Senator Blackburn is a woman," she said, her voice strong. "And the woman I admire most in the world is in the room today. My mother."

MARCH 2023

Las Cruces, New Mexico

The building on the corner of Fondren Place and North State Street in Jackson that once was the Pink House was now repainted a creamy white. There was a new green lawn, and a freshly paved parking lot. All the signs that supporters had posted on the big black fence in the clinic's final days—handwritten vows of resistance like "These people, this place has saved my life" and "Let this radicalize you rather than lead you to despair"—were gone. So was Diane Derzis, the owner of the bubble-gum-pink abortion clinic, and Shannon Brewer, the director. They had gone west to the desert of Las Cruces, New Mexico, 1,100 miles away, where Derzis had bought a former dentist's office with plans to make it the Pink House's new home, in a state where abortion seemed like it would remain legal.

The owner of a luxury consignment furniture shop up the street had snagged their old building when it went up for sale, and spent months renovating it. About a week after its grand opening, new women came. One waited under a blue awning for the shop to open at 10:00 a.m. so she could look at a lamp for her mother. Another came to find a dining room table.

They wandered inside, between manicured antique desks and porcelain dish sets, hutches with teacups behind the glass and Chinese calligraphy brushes hanging on the wall. On a console table rested a stack of Norman Rockwell books, and wood and iron statues of crosses and angels.

Asked what it felt like to own a piece of American history, the new owner did not seem to understand the question. David Carpenter instead focused on his customers, and had no comment on the Dobbs case. It had nothing to do with him, he said. This was just a building.

"It's an investment," he said, gesturing to the main street outside with a shrug.

In New Mexico, the new Pink House West—officially the Las Cruces Women's Health Organization, or LCWHO—would not be pink but beige, small, and with no sign. It was one medical building among many others, old territorial-style brick structures with red roofs—a dentist, a cardiologist, and a blood-draw site.

Derzis had started thinking about moving in 2021, after the Supreme Court had agreed to consider the Dobbs case. She knew that New Mexico would likely become the closest place for millions of women to get an abortion after it would be banned across so much of the South and Midwest.

The towns right on the Texas border would provide the closest access to the women who would be traveling across the country. But Derzis didn't see them as a real option. They were too "Trumpy," she reported after visiting. She'd been in the abortion business long enough to know her opponents. In those conservative areas, they would face constant threats from antiabortion activists pushing local ordinances to make the towns into sanctuary cities for the unborn—a way of putting them out of business. Derzis didn't want to deal with that if she could avoid it. But Las Cruces, a liberal city sandwiched between the Chihuahuan Desert and the angular spires of the Organ Mountains, about forty minutes from El Paso, could work. The sixteen-hour trek from Mississippi meant traveling across the northern reaches of Louisiana and the broad expanse of Texas, both states where abortion was banned.

For Brewer, the decision to uproot her life wasn't that difficult. She wanted to keep fighting. But the pain of leaving behind Mississippi women—her women, she thought—haunted her. "I can keep moving forward and helping women but there's something about Mississippi," she said on the day Roe fell. "I understand Mississippi women. I understand everything about their struggles and everything they go through because . . ." She paused to take a ragged breath, to hold back tears. The rest of her words came out in a rush. "Because those are the same struggles I've gone through in my life. . . . Nothing," she said, "about what went on today is going to tell me that this was right."

Brewer liked that the new building was surrounded on two sides by flash flood ditches, or arroyos, and that the entrance was behind the building, not right off the street. They were physical barriers, she thought, against the protesters she expected to soon see. It was nothing like the iconic old building in Jackson, with its unmissable exterior and corner lot. The only real identifying mark came inside on the brick floor: A black welcome mat with pink letters that read, "Welcome to LCWHO 'Pinkhouse West.'"

Derzis hated the austerity of the décor. The dentist had painted his offices in sterile medical tones of brown, green, and beige. She wanted some pop to create a place that felt warm and inviting. Color made her feel good. They painted the walls yellow, fuchsia, and orange.

She shipped art from her house up north in Pecos and installed her pieces in the new clinic. They were cheerful paintings of a blue dress shirt and a red tie, big blue hearts on a bright yellow background, and a woman in oversize white sunglasses—just like the ones Derzis wore to her last press conference at the old Pink House. When Derzis saw her art hanging on the walls, she cried.

As they prepared the clinic, Brewer called Derzis with surprising updates. People from the town were dropping off food. They were stopping by to welcome her. This felt nothing like Mississippi, she reported.

The Pink House West opened quickly—just weeks after the decision—and provided abortion pills along with surgical abortions until sixteen weeks, as it had in Mississippi. New Mexico, with its Democratic leadership, was touted as a haven for abortion access. But even there, it was limited. A year after Roe fell, New Mexico had only six surgical abortion clinics that provided abortions after about eleven weeks of pregnancy. The Pink House West was the only one outside of Albuquerque.

Inside the clinic, Derzis built a large fake-brick wall to block the nearly two-story-high windows. No one could see inside, where women would wait in a room with a cozy Southwestern-style area rug and a table offering tea and Folgers coffee. Behind the check-in counter, the staff took calls and filed papers. Other than Brewer, only one of the Mississippi staff made the long journey to a new home. It was quiet, except for a television in the corner of the small waiting room and a ceiling fan whirling slowly.

Derzis remembered reading about Roe in the paper when the decision was first announced in 1973. A year later, she got an abortion herself. She was married then but didn't feel ready for a baby. Her husband found a doctor in Birmingham, Alabama, who performed the procedure for $150. She'd never forget what he told her: "You didn't have any problem spreading your legs before, so spread them now." Her mother, back in the Shenandoah Valley, told her she would regret it. Derzis never did. When the first clinic later opened in Alabama, Derzis pestered the staff until they hired her as a counselor for $5 an hour. When a second clinic opened on Birmingham's south side, she was asked to run it.

Nearly a quarter century later, in 1998, the clinic she opened in Birmingham was bombed by Eric Rudolph, a domestic terrorist later convicted for a series of bombings across the South. The explosion, believed to be the first fatal bombing of an abortion clinic, would kill a security guard and severely injure a nurse. Derzis was back in the clinic days later, surveying the blown-out windows and doors.

Over the decade that followed, her opponents derided her as the "abortion queen." Derzis embraced the moniker. She opened clinics in Columbus, Georgia, and Richmond, Virginia, bought the Pink House, and kept ownership of her building in Birmingham as long as she could after losing an extended legal battle with the state health department.

Derzis's lifetime had encapsulated the Roe era. She gained the right as a young woman, and at sixty-nine, she couldn't imagine the federal right to abortion coming back in her remaining years or even within the lifetimes of these babies being born in Mississippi, Alabama, and the dozen other states where abortion was banned. Eradicating Roe, she thought, was only the beginning for the anti-abortion forces. "If anyone thinks they're going to stop there, they're crazy," she said. "They're predators, and we're the prey."

Building clinics was the only way to keep her sanity in this new reality, she thought. Along with Las Cruces, she opened a clinic in Illinois, another safe haven state. She moved a decades-old clinic over the border from Bristol, Tennessee, to Bristol, Virginia. The move was less than a mile, but it meant the difference between a near-total ban and abortion being legal until twenty-six weeks and six days.

Derzis intended to keep up the fight. But she knew that the newly motivated abortion-rights coalition was playing catch-up to an opponent that thought in terms of generations. Fundamentally, her movement—and the America it represented—had been outplayed. A right that had belonged to American women for half a century was gone. The country had been transformed, and the future was uncertain.

"We've given this right back," she said. "This was ours to keep, and we didn't do that."

If anyone understood just how strong faith and persistence made their opposition, it was Derzis. Wherever the Pink House went, its opposition would follow. Already antiabortion activists had leased space across the arroyo to open a pregnancy center that opposed abortion and contraception, and that offered free ultrasounds and assistance for mothers.

One day not long after the Supreme Court ruling, several hundred antiabortion activists fanned out over the parking lot to protest the new abortion clinic in the blazing early evening heat. They set up American flag lawn chairs and sold crosses in "MEMORY of the UNBORN." There was a Republican state senator, a Catholic priest, and the director of the new pregnancy center, Mark Cavaliere, another one of the movement's many foot soldiers.

He went to the microphone and looked beyond the crowd to the pink setting sun.

"If ever there was a place to respond to a challenge like we're facing, it's the City of the Crosses," he said. "We've seen what God can do."

ACKNOWLEDGMENTS

We are so grateful for the entire team that made this book possible. For Cameron Peters, our researcher extraordinaire. For Felice Belman, Rachel Dry, Michael Duffy, Reid Epstein, Ruth Graham, Dana Green, Seth Grossman, and Patricia Mazzei for their insights. For Hilary McClellen, our fact-checker, and Sheelagh McNeill for additional research.

For our wonderful and curious editor, Bryn Clark, and for Megan Lynch and everyone at Flatiron for unending support for two first-time authors, including Marlena Bittner, Malati Chavali, Bob Miller, Jeremy Pink, Mary Retta, Nancy Trypuc, and Emily Walters.

For our agents at CAA, Mollie Glick and David Larabell, who believed in our project long before Roe actually fell.

Special thanks to the leadership of *The New York Times*, for your commitment to independent journalism and to our work. To the dedicated reporters who have covered this challenging topic over the years. To our inspiring colleagues.

And especially to our families, for your unwavering love.

SOURCES

The reporting for this book comes from more than 350 interviews with people who had real-time knowledge of events, including elected officials, lawyers, activists, doctors, and everyday people whose lives were changed by the fall of Roe. Many interviews were conducted on the record, while in other cases sources spoke with the understanding that they would not be quoted but that their information would be used in our reporting. In those cases, we worked to verify their accounts with additional sources and through concrete records.

We combed through private documents, memoirs, video and audio recordings, family papers, thousands of pages of court records, and academic archives at Smith College, the Schlesinger Library at Harvard University, and Duke University. To guide our investigation, we compiled a 116,000-word timeline of abortion politics and policy spanning the last half century, based on thousands of contemporaneous news stories and dozens of books, and interwoven with the biographies, actions, and public words of the key decision-makers.

Our on-the-ground reporting included visits to sixteen states, as well as statehouses, the Supreme Court, the White House, Congress, abortion clinics, and antiabortion pregnancy centers. We drew on our own notes, interviews, and published work from over the course of our careers at *The New York Times*, the Associated Press, *Time*, *Bloomberg*, and *Politico*. Stories with our solo bylines are not listed here.

In particular, we relied on the following sources:

PREFACE

"Abortion, n." *Oxford English Dictionary*, December 2023.

Sanger-Katz, Margot, Claire Cain Miller, and Quoctrung Bui. "Who Gets Abortions in America?" *New York Times*, December 14, 2021.

JUNE 2022: CINCINNATI, OHIO

Garcia, Laura. "The Future of Roe: Women, Health and Law in the Obama Era." Americans United for Life, January 24, 2013.

New York Times. "Tracking Which States Banned Abortion Today." June 24, 2022.

1: THE AUTOPSY

Biskupic, Joan. "Clarence Thomas Calls Out John Roberts as Supreme Court Edges Closer to Overturning Roe v. Wade." CNN, May 20, 2022.

Bohlen, Celestine. "Pope Offers 'Gospel of Life' vs. 'Culture of Death.'" *New York Times*, March 31, 1995.

Byler, David. "Republicans Now Enjoy Unmatched Power in the States. It Was a 40-Year Effort." *Washington Post*, February 18, 2021.

Cassidy, John. "The Ringleader." *New Yorker*, July 24, 2005.

Cooper, Michael. "G.O.P. Factions Grapple over Meaning of Loss." *New York Times*, November 7, 2012.

Edsall, Thomas B. "GOP Right Prevails on Abortion Language." *Washington Post*, July 29, 2000.

Eligon, John, and Michael Schwirtz. "Senate Candidate Provokes Ire with 'Legitimate Rape' Comment." *New York Times*, August 19, 2012.

Goodstein, Laurie. "Christian Right Failed to Sway Voters on Issues." *New York Times*, November 9, 2012.

Guttmacher Institute. "States Enact Record Number of Abortion Restrictions in 2011." January 5, 2012.

Holland, Steve. "Romney Says Won't Pursue New Abortion Laws." Reuters, October 9, 2012.

Jaco, Charles. "Jaco Report: Full Interview with Todd Akin." KTVI-TV, August 19, 2012.

Langer, Emily. "John 'Jack' Willke, a Father of Antiabortion Movement, Dies at 89." *Washington Post*, February 23, 2015.

Lieb, David A. "Rape Remark Defined Akin's Campaign, McCaskill Win." Associated Press, November 7, 2012.

McDermott, Kevin. "Todd Akin Was Arrested at Least Three Times During '80s Abortion Protests." *St. Louis Post-Dispatch*, October 23, 2012.

New York Times. "Polling the Tea Party." April 14, 2010.

O'Keefe, Ed, and Rosalind S. Helderman. "Akin Comments Expose GOP Rift over Abortion." *Washington Post*, August 21, 2012.

Pew Research Center. "After Newtown, Modest Change in Opinion About Gun Control." December 20, 2012.

———. "Modeling the Future of Religion in America: How U.S. Religious Composition Has Changed in Recent Decades." September 13, 2022.

———. "The Complicated Politics of Abortion." August 22, 2012.

———. "The Tea Party and Religion." February 23, 2011.

Public Religion Research Institute. "The 2020 PRRI Census of American Religion." July 8, 2021.

Rappeport, Alan. "Grover Norquist, Anti-Tax Crusader, Says Carried Interest Tax 'Doesn't Matter.'" *New York Times*, September 29, 2015.

Saad, Lydia. "Majority of Americans Still Support Roe v. Wade Decision." Gallup, January 22, 2013.

Sheppard, Kate. "Susan B. Anthony List Founder: Republicans Hijacked My PAC!" *Mother Jones*, February 22, 2012.

Sullivan, Sean. "Todd Akin's Biggest Problem: GOP Critics." *Washington Post*, August 20, 2012.

Szegedy-Maszak, Marianne. "Calm, Cool and Beleaguered." *New York Times Magazine*, August 6, 1989.

Talbot, Margaret. "Justice Alito's Crusade Against a Secular America Isn't Over." *New Yorker*, August 28, 2022.

Tau, Byron. "SBA List Calls Obama an 'Abortion Radical' in New Ohio Ad." *Politico*, September 27, 2012.

Toner, Robin. "Conservatives Savor Their Role As Insiders at the White House." *New York Times*, March 19, 2001.

Toobin, Jeffrey. "How Scalia Changed the Supreme Court." *New Yorker*, February 13, 2016.

Weisman, Jonathan, and John Eligon. "G.O.P. Trying to Oust Akin from Race for Rape Remarks." *New York Times*, August 20, 2012.

Williams, Vanessa. "Romney: No Abortion Legislation on His Agenda." *Washington Post*, October 9, 2012.

Zernike, Kate. "How Did Roe Fall? Before a Decisive Ruling, a Powerful Red Wave." *New York Times*, June 25, 2022.

2: JOAN OF ARC

ABC News. "Texas State Sen. Wendy Davis Shared Abortion Stories During Filibuster." June 27, 2013.

Aguilar, Julián, Becca Aaronson, Jay Root, and Shefali Luthra. "Liveblog: Abortion Bill Fails amid Midnight Chaos After Filibuster." *Texas Tribune* and *KFF Health News*, June 26, 2013.

Batheja, Aman. "How Activists Yelled an Abortion Bill to Death." *Texas Tribune*, June 28, 2013.

Brown, Jennings. "Wendy Davis' Filibuster by the Numbers." *Esquire*, June 26, 2013.

Cohn, Nate. "Do Americans Support Abortion Rights? Depends on the State." *New York Times*, May 4, 2022.

Dallas Morning News. "49 Years Ago, the U.S. Supreme Court Struck Down Texas Abortion Law in Roe vs. Wade." January 22, 2020.

Davis, Wendy. *Forgetting to Be Afraid: A Memoir*. Blue Rider Press, 2014.

———. *Let Her Speak: Transcript of Texas State Senator Wendy Davis's June 25, 2013, Filibuster of the Texas State Senate*. Counterpath Press, 2013.

———. "Wendy Davis: 'My Stand on Abortion Showed Women What We Could Achieve.'" *The Guardian*, September 12, 2014.

Dewey, Caitlin. "Wendy Davis 'Tweetstorm' Was Planned in Advance." *Washington Post*, June 26, 2013.

Draper, Robert. "Can Wendy Davis Have It All?" *New York Times Magazine*, February 12, 2014.

Fernandez, Manny. "Abortion Restrictions Become Law in Texas, but Opponents Will Press Fight." *New York Times*, July 18, 2013.

Fleishman, Rachel. "I'm a Neonatologist. This Is What Happens When a Baby Is Born 5 Months Early." NBC News, May 7, 2022.

Glueck, Katie. "Wendy Davis' Daughters Defend Her." *Politico*, January 28, 2014.

Guttmacher Institute. "States Enact Record Number of Abortion Restrictions in 2011." January 5, 2012.

Johnson, M. Alex. "Texas Abortion Bill Fails to Pass After Epic Filibuster." NBC News, June 25, 2013.

Kliff, Sarah. "Anti-Abortion Push Gains Momentum." *Politico*, December 14, 2010.

———. "Wait, How Did Texas Republicans Pause Wendy Davis' Filibuster?" *Washington Post*, June 25, 2013.

Koppel, Nathan. "Texas Candidate's Misstatements Cloud Campaign." *Wall Street Journal*, January 30, 2014.

Lyman, Rick. "Ann Richards, Flamboyant Texas Governor, Dies at 73." *New York Times*, September 14, 2006.

Max, D. T. "Two-Hit Wonder." *New Yorker*, October 14, 2013.

Pew Research Center. "Section 2: Issues of the 2012 Campaign." April 17, 2012.

Ramshaw, Emily. "Required Delay Between Sonogram and Abortion Creates Logistical Issues." *Texas Tribune*, January 28, 2012.

Richards, Cecile, and Lauren Peterson. *Make Trouble: Stand Up, Speak Out, and Find the Courage to Lead*. Gallery Books, 2018.

Rocha, Alana, Justin Dehn, Todd Wiseman, and Tenoch Aztecatl. "Running Out the Clock: The Wendy Davis Abortion Filibuster, 5 Years Later." *Texas Tribune*, June 25, 2018.

Suro, Roberto. "The 1990 Elections: Texas: Richards Promises a New Direction." *New York Times*, November 8, 1990.

Toobin, Jeffrey. "Daughters of Texas." *New Yorker*, July 29, 2013.

3: A CONVERSION STORY

Balmer, Randall. "The Real Origins of the Religious Right." *Politico Magazine*, May 27, 2014.

Clines, Francis X. "Reagan Appeal on Abortion Is Made to Fundamentalists." *New York Times*, January 31, 1984.

Conohan, Sherry. "Hughes, Smith Spar over Pro-Life Caucus Staff Pay." *Asbury Park Press*, October 2, 1992.

Dannenfelser, Marjorie. *Life Is Winning: Inside the Fight for Unborn Children and Their Mothers*. Humanix Books, 2020.

Greenhouse, Linda, and Reva B. Siegel. *Before Roe v. Wade*. Yale Law Library, 2012.

Horowitz, Jason. "Woman Who Supported Abortion Rights Experienced Evolution That Changed Her Mind." *Washington Post*, May 14, 2010.

Houston, Paul. "'Silent Scream' Called 'Testament for Pro-Life': White House Showcases Abortion Film." *Los Angeles Times*, February 13, 1985.

Howley, Kerry. "The Woman Who Killed Roe." *New York Magazine*, May 9, 2022.

Langer, Emily. "Lennart Nilsson, Photographer Who Revealed Unborn Life, Dies at 94." *Washington Post*, February 2, 2017.

Marcus, Ruth. "'Silent Scream': Loud Impact." *Washington Post*, February 9, 1985.

McCombs, Phil. "The 'Scream' of Bernard Nathanson." *New York Times*, March 24, 1985.

Mullins, Brody. "Abortion Fight: Targeting a Former Boss." *Wall Street Journal*, March 21, 2010.

New York Times. "Editorial: A False 'Scream.'" March 11, 1985.

Nilsson, Lennart. "Drama of Life Before Birth." *Life*, April 30, 1965.

Peterson, Bill, and Herbert H. Denton. "President Backs Foes of Abortion." *New York Times*, September 9, 1982.

Reid, T. R. "Reagan Is Favored by Anti-Abortionists." *Washington Post*, April 12, 1980.

Sulzberger, A. O., Jr. "Reagan Says Ban on Abortion May Not Be Needed." *New York Times*, March 7, 1981.

Weber, Bruce. "Paul Weyrich, 66, a Conservative Strategist, Dies." *New York Times*, December 18, 2008.

Wilkerson, Isabel. "The Papal Visit; A Witamy for Wojtyla in Hamtramck." *New York Times*, September 19, 1987.

4: HER MOTHER'S TEXAS

Alexander, David. "Obama Says Abortion Rights Law Not a Top Priority." Reuters, April 29, 2009.

Belluck, Pam. "Cancer Group Halts Financing to Planned Parenthood." *New York Times*, January 31, 2012.

Belluck, Pam, Jennifer Preston, and Gardiner Harris. "Cancer Group Backs Down on Cutting Off Planned Parenthood." *New York Times*, February 3, 2012.

Brockell, Gillian. "How Jewish History and the Holocaust Fueled Ruth Bader Ginsburg's Quest for Justice." *Washington Post*, September 19, 2020.

Carmon, Irin. "It's a Wendy Davis Nation, Now." *Salon*, June 27, 2013.

Clymer, Adam. "Democrats Promise Quick Action on a Clinton Plan." *New York Times*, November 5, 1992.

Dallas Morning News. "Texas-Born Leader of Planned Parenthood Is Driven by Those Who Would Roll Back Abortion Rights." June 8, 2012.

Elving, Ron. "Abortion Vote Shows How Much Democrats' World Has Changed." NPR, January 26, 2015.

Finn, Robin. "Anti-Abortion Advocates? Bring 'Em On, Texan Says." *New York Times*, March 10, 2006.

Heilemann, John. "Cecile Richards." *Hell & High Water with John Heilemann*, February 28, 2023.

Hiltzik, Michael. "Susan G. Komen Foundation Discovers the Price of Playing Politics." *Los Angeles Times*, January 8, 2014.

Jackson, Nicholas. "Who Is Behind Susan G. Komen's Split from Planned Parenthood?" *The Atlantic*, February 1, 2012.

James, Frank. "Mississippi Voters Reject Personhood Amendment by Wide Margin." NPR, November 8, 2011.

Jennings, Diane. "Daughter of a Revolution: Planned Parenthood President Takes Helm amid Turbulent Waters." *Dallas Morning News*, March 13, 2006.

Kunhardt Film Foundation. "Cecile Richards Interview: Reproductive Rights, Family, and Women in Politics." Interview by Noah Remnick, June 17, 2022.

Luthra, Shefali. "Perry Signs Omnibus Abortion Bill into Law." *KFF Health News*, July 18, 2013.

Lyman, Rick. "Ann Richards, Flamboyant Texas Governor, Dies at 73." *New York Times*, September 14, 2006.

Maraniss, David. "Texas, Oklahoma and Louisiana Make Slow Comeback from '86 Oil Bust." *Washington Post*, November 18, 1990.

McGee, Kate. "Sarah Weddington, Lawyer in Roe v. Wade Case, Dies at 76." *Texas Tribune*, December 26, 2021.

Mitchell, Elizabeth. "The Genius of Cecile Richards." *The Nation*, March 7, 2012.

Morgan, Robin, ed. *Sisterhood Is Forever: Women's Anthology for a New Millennium*. Simon & Schuster, 2007.

Morris Bakken, Gordon, ed. *Icons of the American West*. Greenwood, 2008.

Mundy, Alice. "Women PACs See Surge in Giving." *Wall Street Journal*, October 25, 2012.

New York Times. "Liberals Aim to Win." March 19, 2008.

New York Times. "The 1992 Elections: Congress; New in the United States Senate." November 5, 1992.

New York Times. "Transcript of the Keynote Address by Ann Richards, the Texas Treasurer." July 19, 1988.

Pear, Robert. "Bishops Reject Birth Control Compromise." *New York Times*, February 7, 2013.

Preston, Jennifer, and Gardiner Harris. "Outcry Is Fierce to Cut in Funds by Cancer Group." *New York Times*, February 2, 2012.

Ramsey, Ross. "UT/TT Poll: Texans Split on Permissibility of Abortions in State." *Texas Tribune*, June 20, 2013.

Ratcliffe, R. G. "Midland Oilman Clayton Williams (1931–2020): Winner in Business, Not in Politics." *Texas Monthly*, April 2020.

Reid, Jan. *Let the People In: The Life and Times of Ann Richards*. University of Texas Press, 2012.

Richards, Ann, and Peter Knobler. *Straight from the Heart*. Simon & Schuster, 1989.

Richards, Cecile, and Lauren Peterson. *Make Trouble: Stand Up, Speak Out, and Find the Courage to Lead*. Gallery Books, 2018.

Richards, David. *Once Upon a Time in Texas: A Liberal in the Lone Star State*. University of Texas Press, 2002.

Sheehy, Gail. "What Hillary Wants." *Vanity Fair*, September 4, 2013.

Smith, Evan. "Texas Democrats Try to Keep Their Momentum Going." *New York Times*, July 1, 2013.

Smith, Morgan, Becca Aaronson, and Shefali Luthra. "Abortion Bill Finally Bound for Perry's Desk." *Texas Tribune* and *KFF Health News*, July 13, 2013.

Stevenson, Richard W. "Bush Signs Ban on a Procedure for Abortions." *New York Times*, November 6, 2003.

Strauss, Alix. "Key Moments Since 1992, 'The Year of the Woman.'" *New York Times*, April 2, 2017.

Sullivan, Sean. "Perry Calls for Special Session to Revisit Controversial Abortion Bill." *Washington Post*, June 26, 2013.

Sun, Lena H., and Sarah Kliff. "Komen Grants Flowing to Planned Parenthood." *Washington Post*, April 12, 2012.

Sun, Lena H., Sarah Kliff, and N. C. Aizenman. "Komen Gives New Explanation for Cutting Funds to Planned Parenthood." *Washington Post*, February 2, 2012.

Suro, Roberto, Isabel Wilkerson, and Felicity Barringer. "The Thomas Nomination: Woman in the News; A Private Person in a Storm: Anita Faye Hill." *New York Times*, October 11, 1991.

Toobin, Jeffrey. "Daughters of Texas." *New Yorker*, July 29, 2013.

Vicini, James. "U.S. Catholic Bishops Oppose Obama Birth-Control Plan." Reuters, February 12, 2012.

Zeleny, Jeff. "G.O.P. Captures House, but Not Senate." *New York Times*, November 2, 2010.

5: TEACHING THE MEN

Belluck, Pam. "Complex Science at Issue in Politics of Fetal Pain." *New York Times*, September 16, 2013.

Bennet, James. "Clinton Again Vetoes Measure to Ban a Method of Abortion." *New York Times*, October 11, 1997.

Burkett, Elinor. "In the Land of Conservative Women." *The Atlantic*, September 1996.

Center for American Women and Politics. "Election 2012: Record Number of Women Will Serve in Congress." November 7, 2012.

Conway, Kellyanne. *Here's the Deal: A Memoir*. Threshold Editions, 2022.

Fischer, Sara. "David Koch Is Pro-Choice, Supports Gay Rights; Just Not Democrats." CNN, August 23, 2019.

Gray, Jerry. "Abortion Foes Dealt Setback by the Senate." *New York Times*, November 9, 1995.

Greenhouse, Linda. "Justices Back Ban on Method of Abortion." *New York Times*, April 19, 2007.

Helderman, Rosalind S. "Congress Now Has More Women, Minorities than Ever." *Washington Post*, January 3, 2013.

Howley, Kerry. "The Woman Who Killed Roe." *New York Magazine*, May 9, 2022.

Hurdle, Jon, and Trip Gabriel. "Philadelphia Abortion Doctor Guilty of Murder in Late-Term Procedures." *New York Times*, May 13, 2013.

Jesserer Smith, Peter. "Kellyanne Conway: President Trump's Pro-Life Counselor." *National Catholic Register*, January 27, 2017.

Johnson, Brent. "Meet the N.J. Native Who's Running Donald Trump's Campaign." *NJ Advance Media*, September 26, 2016.

Jones, Jeffrey M. "Gender Gap in 2012 Vote Is Largest in Gallup's History." Gallup, November 9, 2012.

Kane, Paul. "House Republican Conference Holds More Somber Annual Retreat." *Washington Post*, January 20, 2012.

Konigsberg, Eric. "Washington's Sexual Awakening." *New York Magazine*, February 9, 1998.

Lizza, Ryan. "Kellyanne Conway's Political Machinations." *New Yorker*, October 8, 2016.

MacNair, Rachel. "My Personal Journey on the Abortion Issue." *Friends Journal*, February 1, 2010.

Marcotte, Amanda. "Why Are 'Free Market' Organizations Pouring Money Into Anti-abortion Activism? The Koch Brothers." *Slate*, November 6, 2013.

Mascia, Kristen. "Kellyanne Conway When the Cameras Aren't Rolling." *Cosmopolitan*, January 31, 2017.

New Yorker. "The Fifty-One Per Cent." With Kellyanne Conway, Margaret Hoover, Melissa Harris-Perry, and Cecile Richards. Interview by Dorothy Wickenden. The New Yorker Festival, October 6, 2012.

Nuzzi, Olivia. "Kellyanne Conway Is a Star." *New York Magazine*, March 18, 2017.

Parker, Ashley. "Ryan Returns to Spotlight at House Republican Retreat." *New York Times*, January 18, 2013.

Peters, Jeremy W. "Conservatives Hone Script to Light a Fire over Abortion." *New York Times*, July 24, 2014.

Pew Research Center. "Section 2: Issues of the 2012 Campaign." April 17, 2012.

Richardson, Valerie. "Feminist Launches PAC for Pro-Lifers; Sees Lopsided 'Year of the Woman.'" *Washington Times*, November 7, 1992.

Rovner, Julie. "'Partial-Birth Abortion': Separating Fact from Spin." NPR, February 21, 2006.

Sheppard, Kate. "Susan B. Anthony List Founder: Republicans Hijacked My PAC!" *Mother Jones*, February 22, 2012.

Sherman, Jake, and John Bresnahan. "GOP Pollster: Stop Talking About Rape." *Politico*, January 17, 2013.

Smith, Kathryn, and Ginger Gibson. "House OKs 20-Week Abortion Ban Bill." *Politico*, June 18, 2013.

Trinity Magazine. "Q&A with Kellyanne Conway '89." Interview by Trinity Washington University, February 5, 2013.

Weekly Standard. "Is There a Worldwide Conservative Crack-Up?" August 25, 1997.

6: THE PENDULUM

Balz, Dan, and Scott Clement. "Poll Shows Obama Approval Low, GOP Enthusiasm Higher Than Democrats'." *Washington Post*, October 15, 2014.

Barabak, Mark Z. "Wendy Davis Opens Texas Governor Bid with Slap at Republican Leaders." *Los Angeles Times*, October 3, 2013.

Bartels, Lynn. "Colorado's 'War on Women' and the U.S. Senate Race: The Sequel." *Denver Post*, September 24, 2014.

Berke, Richard L. "Clinton Names Ruth Ginsburg, Advocate for Women, to Court." *New York Times*, June 15, 1993.

Brown, Jennifer, and Lynn Bartels. "Cory Gardner Defeats Mark Udall for U.S. Senate in Colorado." *Denver Post*, November 4, 2014.

Davidson Sorkin, Amy. "A Very Bad Ruling on Hobby Lobby." *New Yorker*, June 30, 2014.

Dominus, Susan, and Charlie Savage. "The Quiet 2013 Lunch That Could Have Altered Supreme Court History." *New York Times*, September 25, 2020.

Frommer, Frederic J. "Justice Ginsburg Thought Roe Was the Wrong Case to Settle Abortion Issue." *Washington Post*, May 6, 2022.

Glenza, Jessica, and Alana Casanova-Burgess. "The US Air Force Gave Her a Choice: Your Baby or Your Job." *The Guardian*, December 13, 2019.

Heberlein, Martha, Tricia Brooks, Samantha Artiga, and Jessica Stephens. "Getting into Gear for 2014: Shifting New Medicaid Eligibility and Enrollment Policies into Drive." Kaiser Family Foundation, November 21, 2013.

Henderson, Nia-Malika. "Mark Udall Has Been Dubbed 'Mark Uterus' on the Campaign Trail. That's a Problem." *Washington Post*, October 13, 2014.

Jerman, Jenna, Rachel K. Jones, and Tsuyoshi Onda. "Characteristics of U.S. Abortion Patients in 2014 and Changes Since 2008." Guttmacher Institute, May 2016.

Kennedy, Lesley. "Why Was Joan of Arc Burned at the Stake?" *HISTORY*, April 16, 2019.

Kunhardt Film Foundation. "Cecile Richards Interview: Reproductive Rights, Family, and Women in Politics." Interview by Noah Remnick, June 17, 2022.

Lee, Jennifer 8. "Abortion Rights Group Plans a New Focus and a New Name." *New York Times*, January 5, 2003.

Lepore, Jill. "Ruth Bader Ginsburg's Unlikely Path to the Supreme Court." *New Yorker*, October 1, 2018.

Liasson, Mara. "Changing Tack, GOP Candidates Support Over-the-Counter Birth Control." NPR, September 12, 2014.

Liptak, Adam. "Court Is 'One of Most Activist,' Ginsburg Says, Vowing to Stay." *New York Times*, August 24, 2013.

———. "Supreme Court Rejects Contraceptives Mandate for Some Corporations." *New York Times*, June 30, 2014.

MacPherson, James. "Sole ND Abortion Clinic Halts Medication Abortions." Associated Press, October 29, 2014.

McCune, Greg, Mary Wisniewski, Edith Honan, and Jim Forsyth. "Planned Parenthood Sues Texas over Abortion Restrictions." Reuters, September 27, 2013.

Mitchell, Heidi. "Stand and Deliver: After Her 12-Hour Filibuster, How Far Will Texas Senator Wendy Davis Run?" *Vogue*, August 15, 2013.

Nash, Elizabeth, Rachel Benson Gold, Gwendolyn Rathbun, and Yana Vierboom. "Laws Affecting Reproductive Health and Rights: 2014 State Policy Review." Guttmacher Institute, January 1, 2015.

North, Anna. "Planned Parenthood Moving Away from 'Choice.'" *BuzzFeed News*, January 9, 2013.

Richards, Cecile. "Ending the Silence That Fuels Abortion Stigma." *Elle*, October 16, 2014.

———. "Inside the Brutal Fight to Include Women in the Affordable Care Act." *Cosmopolitan*, April 2, 2018.

———. "The Only Controversy About Birth Control Is That We're Still Fighting for It." *Time*, July 1, 2014.

Richards, Cecile, and Lauren Peterson. *Make Trouble: Stand Up, Speak Out, and Find the Courage to Lead*. Gallery Books, 2018.

Root, Jay. "Wendy Davis Lost Badly. Here's How It Happened." *Texas Tribune*, November 6, 2014.

Silverstein, Jake. "Daughter of the Republic." *Texas Monthly*, February 2014.

Stayton, Jennifer. "Former Ann Richards Campaign Manager Says Maintaining Hope Is Key to Surviving Texas Politics." Texas Public Radio, October 24, 2022.

Wall Street Journal. "Midterm Elections 2014 Exit Polls." November 5, 2014.

Weisberg, Jessica. "Supreme Court Justice Ruth Bader Ginsburg: 'I'm Not Going Anywhere.'" *Elle*, September 23, 2014.

Weisman, Jonathan, and Ashley Parker. "Riding Wave of Discontent, G.O.P. Takes Senate." *New York Times*, November 4, 2014.

7: THE RADICAL POST-ROE GENERATION

Abcarian, Robin. "Abortion Foe Goes Undercover." *Los Angeles Times*, April 26, 2009.

Beard Rau, Alia. "Alliance Defending Freedom: Fighting the Culture Wars from a Scottsdale Office Park." *Arizona Republic*, August 22, 2016.

Calmes, Jackie. "With Planned Parenthood Videos, Activist Ignites Abortion Issue." *New York Times*, July 21, 2015.

Charo, R. Alta. "Yes, Republicans Are Outraged About Planned Parenthood. But They Used to Support Fetal Tissue Research." *Washington Post*, August 4, 2015.

Condon, Stephanie. "Congressional Investigation Launched into Abortion Practices." CBS News, July 15, 2015.

Grady, Denise, and Nicholas St. Fleur. "Fetal Tissue from Abortions for Research Is Traded in a Gray Zone." *New York Times*, July 27, 2015.

Haberkorn, Jennifer. "Meet the 26-Year-Old Activist Who Could Close the Government." *Politico*, September 21, 2015.

Hawkins, Kristan. *Courageous: Students Abolishing Abortion in This Lifetime*, 2012.

Jesserer Smith, Peter. "Kellyanne Conway: President Trump's Pro-Life Counselor." *National Catholic Register*, January 27, 2017.

Khurshid, Samar. "Lawmakers Knew About Planned Parenthood Video Weeks Ago." *Roll Call*, July 16, 2015.

Kirkpatrick, David D. "The Next Targets for the Group That Overturned Roe." *New Yorker*, October 2, 2023.

Kliff, Sarah. "Abortion Sting Hits Planned Parenthood." *Politico*, February 1, 2011.

Richards, Cecile, and Lauren Peterson. *Make Trouble: Stand Up, Speak Out, and Find the Courage to Lead*. Gallery Books, 2018.

Rose, Lila. *Fighting for Life: Becoming a Force for Change in a Wounded World*. Thomas Nelson, 2021.

Schmidt, Michael S., David A. Fahrenthold, and Adam Goldman. "James O'Keefe Leaves His Post as the Leader of Project Veritas." *New York Times*, February 20, 2023.

Somashekhar, Sandhya. "Meet the Millennial Who Infiltrated the Guarded World of Abortion Providers." *Washington Post*, October 14, 2015.

Stolberg, Sheryl Gay. "The Next Battle in the War over Planned Parenthood." *New York Times*, March 31, 2017.

Swan, Jonathan, and Alayna Treene. "Leonard Leo to Shape New Conservative Network." *Axios*, January 7, 2020.

Wadman, Meredith. "The Truth About Fetal Tissue Research." *Scientific American*, December 9, 2015.

Ward, Paula Reed. "Rep. Tim Murphy, Popular with Pro-Life Movement, Urged Abortion in Affair, Texts Suggest." *Pittsburgh Post-Gazette*, October 3, 2017.

8: THE SYMBOL OF SANGER

Behrens, David. "Profile: Faye Wattleton of Planned Parenthood: Fundamentalist's Daughter Shapes Pro-Choice Strategy." *Los Angeles Times*, October 15, 1989.

Carroll, Lauren. "Jeb Bush: Planned Parenthood Isn't Involved in Women's Health." *PolitiFact*, August 26, 2015.

Gibbs, Nancy. "The Pill at 50: Sex, Freedom and Paradox." *Time*, April 22, 2010.

Gibson, Caitlin. "The Abortion Rights Movement Is Bolder Than It's Been in Years. That's Cecile Richards's Plan." *Washington Post*, August 16, 2016.

Gonzalez, Daniel. "Planned Parenthood of Arizona's Surprising Ties to Peggy Goldwater and Conservative Republicans." *Arizona Republic*, September 18, 2022.

Hirschberg, Lynn. "Former Planned Parenthood President Faye Wattleton on Why We're Still Fighting for Reproductive Healthcare." *W Magazine*, October 16, 2017.

Kleikesrud, Judy. "Planned Parenthood's New Head Takes a Fighting Stand." *New York Times*, February 3, 1978.

Kliff, Sarah. "Mike Pence Launched Republicans' War on Planned Parenthood." *Vox*, January 27, 2017.

———. "Pence's War on Planned Parenthood." *Politico*, February 16, 2011.

Latson, Jennifer. "What Margaret Sanger Really Said About Eugenics and Race." *Time*, October 14, 2016.

Lepore, Jill. "Birthright." *New Yorker*, November 6, 2011.

Levy, Pema. "How the Bush Family Aided Planned Parenthood's Rise." *Mother Jones*, August 11, 2015.

Nocera, Kate, and David Nather. "House Defunds Planned Parenthood." *Politico*, February 18, 2011.

Rovner, Julie. "Calls to Cut Off Planned Parenthood Are Nothing New." NPR, August 3, 2015.

Sanger, Margaret. *Margaret Sanger: An Autobiography*. W. W. Norton & Company, Inc., 1938.

Shepard, Charles E. "Operation Rescue's Mission to Save Itself." *Washington Post*, November 24, 1991.

Span, Paula. "The Faye Wattleton Counterattack." *Washington Post*, October 14, 1987.

Stack, Liam. "A Brief History of Deadly Attacks on Abortion Providers." *New York Times*, November 29, 2015.

Stone, Geoffrey. "'Sex and the Constitution': Margaret Sanger and the Birth of the Birth Control Movement." *Washington Post*, March 24, 2017.

Szegedy-Maszak, Marianne. "Calm, Cool and Beleaguered." *New York Times Magazine*, August 6, 1989.

Young, Neil J. "How George H.W. Bush Enabled the Rise of the Religious Right." *Washington Post*, December 5, 2018.

9: THE HEARING

ABC News. "Hillary Clinton Calls Planned Parenthood Videos 'Disturbing.'" July 29, 2015.

Altman, Alex. "Reigniting the Abortion Debate." *Time*, September 24, 2015.

Associated Press. "Indiana Clears Planned Parenthood of Wrongdoing After Videos." July 30, 2015.

Calmes, Jackie. "Planned Parenthood Videos Were Altered, Analysis Finds." *New York Times*, August 27, 2015.

———. "Reacting to Videos, Planned Parenthood Fights to Regain Initiative." *New York Times*, September 26, 2015.

Cohen, Rachel M. "Cecile Richards: Grace Under Fire at Planned Parenthood." *American Prospect*, December 17, 2015.

Crockett, Emily. "Congress Has Spent 15 Months 'Investigating' Planned Parenthood Using McCarthy-Like Tactics." *Vox*, December 7, 2016.

Dannenfelser, Marjorie. *Life Is Winning: Inside the Fight for Unborn Children and Their Mothers*. Humanix Books, 2020.

Flegenheimer, Matt. "Fusion GPS Founder Hauled from the Shadows for the Russia Election Investigation." *New York Times*, January 8, 2018.

Gibson, Caitlin. "The Abortion Rights Movement Is Bolder Than It's Been in Years. That's Cecile Richards's Plan." *Washington Post*, August 16, 2016.

Griffin, Drew, and David Fitzpatrick. "The Real Story Behind Those Planned Parenthood Videos." CNN, October 20, 2015.

Harris, Gardiner. "Obama Vetoes Bill to Repeal Health Law and End Planned Parenthood Funding." *New York Times*, January 8, 2016.

Hook, Janet. "Planned Parenthood Emerges Unscathed from GOP Attacks—WSJ/NBC Poll." *Wall Street Journal*, September 28, 2015.

Lizza, Ryan. "A House Divided." *New Yorker*, December 6, 2015.

Markay, Lachlan. "Planned Parenthood Sought Soros Cash to Protect Federal Subsidies." *Washington Free Beacon*, August 22, 2016.

Ollstein, Alice Miranda. "GOP Lawmakers' Reality: They Won't Cut Planned Parenthood." *Politico*, December 2, 2018.

Pierson, Brendan. "Abortion Foes Largely Lose $2.4 Mln Appeal over Planned Parenthood Videos." Reuters, October 21, 2022.

Richards, Cecile, and Lauren Peterson. *Make Trouble: Stand Up, Speak Out, and Find the Courage to Lead*. Gallery Books, 2018.

Riffkin, Rebecca. "In U.S., 59% View Planned Parenthood Favorably." Gallup, October 14, 2015.

Steinhauer, Jennifer. "John Boehner, House Speaker, Will Resign from Congress." *New York Times*, September 25, 2015.

———. "John Boehner, Strong Abortion Foe, Is Imperiled by the Like-Minded." *New York Times*, September 17, 2015.

St. John, Paige. "State Attorney General Seizes Videos behind Planned Parenthood Sting." *Los Angeles Times*, April 5, 2016.

Turkewitz, Julie, Richard Fausset, Alan Blinder, and Benjamin Mueller. "Robert Dear, Suspect in Colorado Killings, 'Preferred to Be Left Alone.'" *New York Times*, November 28, 2015.

10: TITANS AND SAINTS

Baker, Peter, and Gardiner Harris. "Washington Pauses for Justice Antonin Scalia's Funeral." *New York Times*, February 20, 2016.

Barnes, Robert. "Antonin Scalia's Funeral Reflects the Justice's Life of Faith." *Washington Post*, February 20, 2016.

Baum, Lawrence, and Neal Devins. "Federalist Court." *Slate*, January 31, 2017.

Bella, Timothy. "Who Is Conservative Activist Leonard Leo? A Friend of Clarence Thomas." *Washington Post*, May 5, 2023.

Berman, Mark, and Jerry Markon. "Why Justice Scalia Was Staying for Free at a Remote West Texas Resort." *Washington Post*, February 17, 2016.

Biskupic, Joan. *American Original: The Life and Constitution of Supreme Court Justice Antonin Scalia*. Farrar, Straus and Giroux, 2009.

Brittain, Amy, and Sari Horwitz. "Justice Scalia Spent His Last Hours with Members of This Secretive Society of Elite Hunters." *Washington Post*, February 24, 2016.

Carroll, James. "The Sins of the High Court's Supreme Catholics." *New Yorker*, August 19, 2022.

Elliott, Justin, Joshua Kaplan, and Alex Mierjeski. "Justice Samuel Alito Took Luxury Fishing Vacation with GOP Billionaire Who Later Had Cases Before the Court." *ProPublica*, June 20, 2023.

Hakim, Danny, and Jo Becker. "The Long Crusade of Clarence and Ginni Thomas." *New York Times Magazine*, February 22, 2022.

Hulse, Carl. *Confirmation Bias: Inside Washington's War over the Supreme Court, from Scalia's Death to Justice Kavanaugh*. HarperCollins, 2019.

Kamen, Al. "Federalist Society Quickly Comes of Age." *New York Times*, February 1, 1987.

Kaplan, Joshua, Justin Elliott, and Alex Mierjeski. "Clarence Thomas and the Billionaire." ProPublica, April 6, 2023.

Kennedy, Merritt. "Mourners Honor Antonin Scalia at Funeral Service in Washington." NPR, February 20, 2016.

Kirkpatrick, David D., and Laurie Goodstein. "Group of Bishops Using Influence to Oppose Kerry." *New York Times*, October 12, 2004.

Kroll, Andy, Andrea Bernstein, and Ilya Marritz. "We Don't Talk About Leonard: The Man Behind the Right's Supreme Court Supermajority." ProPublica, October 11, 2023.

Liptak, Adam. "Antonin Scalia, Justice on the Supreme Court, Dies at 79." *New York Times*, February 13, 2016.

———. "Stevens, the Only Protestant on the Supreme Court." *New York Times*, April 10, 2010.

Markels, Alex. "Why Miers Withdrew as Supreme Court Nominee." NPR, October 27, 2005.

Michaelson, Jay. "The Secrets of Leonard Leo, the Man Behind Trump's Supreme Court Pick." *Daily Beast*, July 9, 2018.

Moravec, Eva Ruth, Sari Horwitz, and Jerry Markon. "The Death of Antonin Scalia: Chaos, Confusion and Conflicting Reports." *Washington Post*, February 14, 2016.

Novak, Viveca, and Peter Stone. "The JCN Story: How to Build a Secretive, Right-Wing Judicial Machine." *Daily Beast*, April 14, 2017.

O'Harrow, Robert, Jr., and Shawn Boburg. "A Conservative Activist's Behind-the-Scenes Campaign to Remake the Nation's Courts." *Washington Post*, May 21, 2019.

Pew Research Center. "Religious Landscape Study: Views About Abortion." May 30, 2014.

Quinn, Melissa. "Inside the Mind of Leonard Leo, Trump's Supreme Court Right-Hand Man." *Washington Examiner*, January 28, 2018.

Roberts, Roxanne. "Who Showed Up at Scalia's Funeral—and Who Didn't." *Washington Post*, February 20, 2016.

Ruse, Austin. "I'll Be Doing Opus Dei No Matter What." *Crisis Magazine*, September 15, 2023.

———. *Littlest Suffering Souls: Children Whose Short Lives Point Us to Christ.* TAN Books, 2017.

Shear, Michael D., Julie Hirschfeld Davis, and Gardiner Harris. "Obama Chooses Merrick Garland for Supreme Court." *New York Times*, March 16, 2016.

Thomas, Evan. "Washington's Quiet Club." *Newsweek*, March 8, 2001.

Toobin, Jeffrey. "The Company Scalia Kept." *New Yorker*, March 2, 2016.

———. "The Conservative Pipeline to the Supreme Court." *New Yorker*, April 10, 2017.

Totenberg, Nina, and Michael Martin. "Originalism: A Primer on Scalia's Constitutional Philosophy." NPR, February 14, 2016.

Vogel, Kenneth P., and Shane Goldmacher. "An Unusual $1.6 Billion Donation Bolsters Conservatives." *New York Times*, August 22, 2022.

11: THE LIST

ABC News. "Inside the South Carolina Exit Poll: A Closer Look at Donald Trump's Win with Evangelical Voters." February 22, 2016.

Brody, David. "Brody File Exclusive: Donald Trump Explains Pro-Life Conversion." Christian Broadcasting Network, April 8, 2011.

DeSilver, Drew. "Turnout Was High in the 2016 Primary Season, but Just Short of 2008 Record." Pew Research Center, June 10, 2016.

Diamond, Jeremy. "Donald Trump Waffles on Totally Defunding Planned Parenthood." CNN, August 12, 2015.

Enrich, David. "How a Corporate Law Firm Led a Political Revolution." *New York Times Magazine*, August 25, 2022.

Haberman, Maggie. "Trump Says He Was Kidding in Suggesting His Sister for the Court." *New York Times*, February 14, 2016.

Healy, Patrick, and Michael Barbaro. "Donald Trump Calls for Barring Muslims from Entering U.S." *New York Times*, December 7, 2015.

Healy, Patrick, and Jonathan Martin. "Donald Trump and Bernie Sanders Win in New Hampshire Primary." *New York Times*, February 9, 2016.

Horowitz, Jason. "Familiar Talk on Women, from an Unfamiliar Trump." *New York Times*, August 18, 2015.

Johnson, Jenna. "Antiabortion Activists to Iowa Voters: 'Support Anyone but Donald Trump.'" *Washington Post*, January 26, 2016.

Kane, Paul. "Trump Courts Lawmakers at Capitol Hill Law Firm, Wins Lobbyist Backing." *Washington Post*, March 21, 2016.

Klein, Edward. "Trump Family Values." *Vanity Fair*, March 1994.

Lazarus, Edward. "Bush and the Court." *Washington Post*, October 24, 2000.

Lee, Michelle. "Fact Check: Trump's Views on Abortion Rights." *Washington Post*, October 19, 2016.

Lizza, Ryan. "Kellyanne Conway's Political Machinations." *New Yorker*, October 8, 2016.

Martin, Jonathan, and Alexander Burns. "Donald Trump Wins South Carolina Primary; Cruz and Rubio Vie for 2nd." *New York Times*, February 20, 2016.

McManus, Doyle. "McManus: Republican 'Autopsy' Reveals a Divide in the Party." *Los Angeles Times*, March 20, 2013.

New York Times. "Abortion Rights Leader Honored." April 13, 1989.

Pew Research Center. "Support for Same-Sex Marriage at Record High, but Key Segments Remain Opposed." June 8, 2015.

Rappeport, Alan, and Charlie Savage. "Donald Trump Releases List of Possible Supreme Court Picks." *New York Times*, May 18, 2016.

Shear, Michael D., Julie Hirschfeld Davis, and Gardiner Harris. "Obama Chooses Merrick Garland for Supreme Court." *New York Times*, March 16, 2016.

Shear, Michael D., and Jennifer Steinhauer. "More Republicans Say They'll Block Supreme Court Nominee." *New York Times*, February 15, 2016.

Totenberg, Nina. "Donald Trump Releases List of Possible Supreme Court Picks." NPR, September 23, 2016.

Zitner, Aaron. "Ted Cruz's Iowa Win Powered by Evangelicals, Conservatives." *Wall Street Journal*, February 2, 2016.

12: HILLARY

Biskupic, Joan. "Justice Ruth Bader Ginsburg Calls Trump a 'Faker,' He Says She Should Resign." CNN, July 13, 2016.

Caldwell, Leigh Ann. "Herstory Made: Hillary Clinton's Big Moment Caps a Long Journey." NBC News, July 24, 2016.

Clinton, Hillary Rodham. *What Happened*. Simon & Schuster, 2017.

Crockett, Emily. "It Could Take Years for Texas Abortion Clinics to Reopen, Even After a Supreme Court Victory." *Vox*, June 27, 2016.

Flanagan, Caitlin. "Losing the Rare in 'Safe, Legal, and Rare.'" *The Atlantic*, December 6, 2019.

Gibson, Caitlin. "The Abortion Rights Movement Is Bolder Than It's Been in Years. That's Cecile Richards's Plan." *Washington Post*, August 16, 2016.

Kliff, Sarah. "The Pro-Life Movement Is Winning. It'll Take More Than One Supreme Court Ruling to Change That." *Vox*, June 28, 2016.

Krieg, Gregory. "Hillary Clinton's Would-Be Campaign Slogans, Ranked." CNN, October 19, 2016.

Liptak, Adam. "Ruth Bader Ginsburg, No Fan of Donald Trump, Critiques Latest Term." *New York Times*, July 10, 2016.

Meltzer, Marisa. "A Feminist T-Shirt Resurfaces from the '70s." *New York Times*, November 18, 2015.

Mettler, Katie. "Hillary Clinton Just Said It, but 'the Future Is Female' Began as a 1970s Lesbian Separatist Slogan." *Washington Post*, February 8, 2017.

Palmieri, Jennifer. *Dear Madam President: An Open Letter to the Women Who Will Run the World*. Grand Central Publishing, 2018.

Paquette, Danielle. "Planned Parenthood Announces It Will Fight Abortion Laws in Eight States After Supreme Court Ruling." *Washington Post*, June 30, 2016.

Pender, Geoff. "Politics Aside, Nomination of a Woman Is Historic." *The Clarion-Ledger*, July 28, 2016.

Redden, Molly. "Clinton Leads Way on Abortion Rights as Democrats Seek End to Decades-Old Rule." *The Guardian*, July 26, 2016.

Richards, Cecile, and Lauren Peterson. *Make Trouble: Stand Up, Speak Out, and Find the Courage to Lead*. Gallery Books, 2018.

Ronayne, Kathleen. "Planned Parenthood Backing Clinton in Primary Race." Associated Press, January 10, 2016.

Schouten, Fredreka. "Hillary Clinton's Bid Draws Legions of Female Donors." *USA Today*, August 3, 2016.

Sherrill, Martha. "The Education of Hillary Clinton." *Washington Post*, January 11, 1993.

Sullivan, Peter. "Hillary Slams 20-Week Abortion Ban." *The Hill*, May 13, 2015.

Thomas, Ken. "Clinton: Supreme Court's Future Hangs in the Balance in 2016." Associated Press, March 28, 2016.

13: THE ODDEST COUPLE

Alberta, Tim. *American Carnage: On the Front Lines of the Republican Civil War and the Rise of President Trump*. Harper, 2019.

Barbaro, Michael, and Erik Eckholm. "Indiana Law Denounced as Invitation to Discriminate Against Gays." *New York Times*, March 27, 2015.

Boorstein, Michelle. "What It Means That Mike Pence Called Himself an 'Evangelical Catholic.'" *Washington Post*, July 18, 2016.

Cha, Ariana Eunjung. "Mike Pence Has Made No Secret About His Views on Abortion. Will This Help or Hurt Trump?" *Washington Post*, July 15, 2016.

Cook, Tony, and Chelsea Schneider. "What We Know About Gov. Mike Pence's Position on Gay Rights over the Years." *Indianapolis Star*, January 4, 2016.

Crockett, Emily. "Mike Pence Is One of the Most Anti-Abortion Republicans in Washington. Here's His Record." *Vox*, January 27, 2017.

Graham, Ruth. "Why It Matters That Karen Pence Pursued Medical Assistance When Trying to Get Pregnant." *Slate*, April 26, 2017.

Indianapolis Monthly. "Outtakes from the Bio of Mike Pence." November 2, 2016.

Kruse, Michael, Ekaterina Pechenkina, and Adam Wren. "55 Things You Need to Know About Mike Pence." *Politico Magazine*, June 7, 2023.

Langsam Braunstein, Melissa. "Second Lady Karen Pence Opens Up About Her Struggles with Infertility." *The Federalist*, April 25, 2017.

LoBianco, Tom. "How Pence's Camp Persuaded Trump to Pick Their Guy as VP." *Politico Magazine*, September 11, 2019.

———. *Piety & Power: Mike Pence and the Taking of the White House*. Dey Street Books, 2019.

Mahler, Jonathan, and Dirk Johnson. "Mike Pence's Journey: Catholic Democrat to Evangelical Republican." *New York Times*, July 20, 2016.

Mayer, Jane. "The Danger of President Pence." *New Yorker*, October 16, 2017.

Nussbaum, Matthew. "Pence Puts Conservative Credentials on Display." *Politico*, July 28, 2016.

Parker, Ashley. "Karen Pence Is the Vice President's 'Prayer Warrior,' Gut Check and Shield." *Washington Post*, March 28, 2017.

Parker, Ashley, Alexander Burns, and Maggie Haberman. "A Grounded Plane and Anti-Clinton Passion: How Mike Pence Swayed the Trumps." *New York Times*, July 16, 2016.

Parlapiano, Alicia. "Pence Ranks Low in Approval, but Not as Low as Trump and Clinton." *New York Times*, July 15, 2016.

Pence, Charlotte. *Where You Go: Life Lessons from My Father*. Center Street, 2018.

Pence, Mike. *So Help Me God*. Simon & Schuster, 2022.

Sanneh, Kelefa. "The Intensity Gap." *New Yorker*, October 20, 2014.

Smith, Mitch. "Indiana Governor Signs Abortion Bill with Added Restrictions." *New York Times*, March 24, 2016.

Smith, Mitch, and Erik Eckholm. "Federal Judge Blocks Indiana Abortion Law." *New York Times*, June 30, 2016.

Ward, Ken. "Flip-Flop Opinion: Abortion Issue Divides Pence, Sharp." *The Republic*, September 24, 1988.

14: "GRAB 'EM BY THE PUSSY"

Bump, Philip. "Donald Trump Will Be President Thanks to 80,000 People in Three States." *Washington Post*, December 1, 2016.

Conway, Kellyanne. *Here's the Deal: A Memoir*. Threshold Editions, 2022.

Dannenfelser, Marjorie. *Life Is Winning: Inside the Fight for Unborn Children and Their Mothers*. Humanix Books, 2020.

Fahrenthold, David A. "Trump Recorded Having Extremely Lewd Conversation About Women in 2005." *Washington Post*, October 8, 2016.

Inskeep, Steve. "Conservative Female Voters Disagree on Trump Tape Fallout." NPR, October 12, 2016.

Khalid, Asma, and Joel Rose. "Millennials Just Didn't Love Hillary Clinton the Way They Loved Barack Obama." NPR, November 14, 2016.

Kliff, Sarah. "No, Donald Trump, Abortions Do Not Happen at 9 Months Pregnant." *Vox*, October 19, 2016.

Martínez, Jessica, and Gregory A. Smith. "How the Faithful Voted: A Preliminary 2016 Analysis." Pew Research Center, November 9, 2016.

Pence, Mike. *So Help Me God*. Simon & Schuster, 2022.

Rappeport, Alan. "John McCain Withdraws Support for Donald Trump After Disclosure of Recording." *New York Times*, October 8, 2016.

Stahl, Lesley. "President-Elect Trump Speaks to a Divided Country." CBS News, November 13, 2016.

Tavernise, Sabrina, and Sheryl Gay Stolberg. "Abortion Foes, Emboldened by Trump, Promise 'Onslaught' of Tough Restrictions." *New York Times*, December 11, 2016.

15: THE NEW GIANTS

Associated Press. "Justice Alito Rallies Conservatives in Tribute to Scalia." November 17, 2016.

Chappell, Bill. "Supreme Court Rejects North Dakota's Bid to Save Strict Abortion Law." NPR, January 25, 2016.

Clinton, Hillary Rodham. *What Happened*. Simon & Schuster, 2017.

Eckholm, Erik. "Arkansas Adopts a Ban on Abortions After 12 Weeks." *New York Times*, March 6, 2013.

Hartocollis, Anemona, and Yamiche Alcindor. "Women's March Highlights as Huge Crowds Protest Trump: 'We're Not Going Away.'" *New York Times*, January 21, 2017.

Hellman, Jessie. "SBA List Seizing Its Moment." *The Hill*, June 20, 2017.

Nash, Elizabeth, Rachel Benson Gold, Zohra Ansari-Thomas, Olivia Cappello, and Lizamarie Mohammed. "Policy Trends in the States: 2016." Guttmacher Institute, January 3, 2017.

Pence, Mike. *So Help Me God*. Simon & Schuster, 2022.

Richards, Cecile, and Lauren Peterson. *Make Trouble: Stand Up, Speak Out, and Find the Courage to Lead*. Gallery Books, 2018.

Tucker, Neely. "Emails Show Outside Group's Influence on Mississippi's 'Religious Freedom' Bill." *Washington Post*, July 21, 2016.

Wolf, Richard. "Supreme Court Wannabes Audition in Scalia's Shadow." *USA Today*, November 20, 2016.

16: STACKING THE ADMINISTRATION

Alberta, Tim. "Social Conservatives Are 'Over the Moon' About Trump." *Politico Magazine*, April 26, 2017.

Armour, Stephanie. "Trump Appointee Harnesses Civil-Rights Law to Protect Anti-Abortion Health Workers." *Wall Street Journal*, April 13, 2018.

Bassett, Laura. "Trump Sends Anti-Birth Control Delegates to UN Commission on Women." *HuffPost*, March 17, 2017.

Cheney, Kyle, and Matthew Nussbaum. "Donald Trump's Man on the Hill." *Politico*, January 18, 2017.

Christie, Chris, and Ellis Henican. *Let Me Finish: Trump, the Kushners, Bannon, New Jersey, and the Power of In-Your-Face Politics*. Hachette Books, 2019.

Chuck, Elizabeth. "Trump Administration Abruptly Cuts Funding to Teen Pregnancy Prevention Programs." NBC News, August 25, 2017.

Cobler, Nicole. "Lawmaker Wants to Position Texas to Outlaw Abortion with 'Trigger Law.'" *Houston Chronicle*, February 6, 2017.

Conway, Kellyanne. *Here's the Deal: A Memoir*. Threshold Editions, 2022.

Dickerson, Caitlin. "Detention of Migrant Children Has Skyrocketed to Highest Levels Ever." *New York Times*, September 12, 2018.

Gambino, Lauren. "'Author of Controversy': How Andrew Puzder Made His Name Fighting Abortion." *The Guardian*, February 16, 2017.

Hirschfeld Davis, Julie. "Trump Signs Law Taking Aim at Planned Parenthood Funding." *New York Times*, April 13, 2017.

Johnson, Eliana. "New White House Counsel to Arrive as Democrats, Mueller Close In." *Politico*, December 4, 2018.

Karni, Annie, Eileen Sullivan, and Noam Scheiber. "Acosta to Resign as Labor Secretary over Jeffrey Epstein Plea Deal." *New York Times*, July 12, 2019.

Kelly, Meg. "A Year Later: Does Trump's Mexico City Policy Ban Funds to Groups That 'Even Mention' Abortion?" *Washington Post*, March 28, 2018.

Khan, Nisa. "We Found a New Batch of Trump Administration Appointees." ProPublica, July 31, 2018.

Kodjak, Alison. "Civil Rights Chief at HHS Defends the Right to Refuse Care on Religious Grounds." NPR, March 20, 2018.

LeVine, Marianne, and Timothy Noah. "Exclusive: Puzder's Ex-Wife Told Oprah He Threatened 'You Will Pay for This.'" *Politico*, February 15, 2017.

Levintova, Hannah. "The Trump Official Who Failed to Reunify Dozens of Separated Children Is Getting a New Role." *Mother Jones*, November 2018.

———. "Two Decades Ago, He Blocked Abortion Clinics and Dodged Police. Now He's Helping Wage Trump's War on Reproductive Rights." *Mother Jones*, February 22, 2019.

Liptak, Adam. "White House Announces Slate of 11 Judicial Nominees." *New York Times*, June 7, 2017.

Lithwick, Dahlia. *Lady Justice: Women, the Law, and the Battle to Save America*. Penguin Books, 2022.

Martin, Rachel. "Trump Hosts White House Dinner for Evangelical Supporters." NPR, August 29, 2018.

Mayer, Jane. "The Danger of President Pence." *New Yorker*, October 16, 2017.

Pear, Robert, and Jeremy W. Peters. "Trump Gives Health Workers New Religious Liberty Protections." *New York Times*, January 18, 2018.

"Pro-Life Weekly." EWTN, September 27, 2018.

Rinkunas, Susan. "Trump's New Health Secretary Could Be Disastrous for Women." *New York Magazine*, February 10, 2017.

Scheiber, Noam. "Eugene Scalia Confirmed by Senate as Labor Secretary." *New York Times*, July 12, 2019.

Shear, Michael D., and Helene Cooper. "Trump Bars Refugees and Citizens of 7 Muslim Countries." *New York Times*, January 27, 2017.

Shear, Michael D., Maggie Haberman, and Michael S. Schmidt. "Vice President-Elect Pence to Take Over Trump Transition Effort." *New York Times*, November 11, 2016.

Siegel, Rachel. "The Trump Official Who Tried to Stop a Detained Immigrant from Getting an Abortion." *Washington Post*, October 26, 2017.

Stolberg, Sheryl Gay. "The Next Battle in the War over Planned Parenthood." *New York Times*, March 31, 2017.

Thrush, Glenn, and Maggie Haberman. "Trump and Staff Rethink Tactics After Stumbles." *New York Times*, February 5, 2017.

Victor, Daniel. "Chris Christie Says Jared Kushner's Father Committed a 'Loathsome' Crime." *New York Times*, January 30, 2019.

Woellert, Lorraine. "Trump's Speech to March for Life Marks a U-Turn on Abortion." *Politico*, January 17, 2018.

17: THE LEFT'S DENIAL

Cobler, Nicole. "Lawmaker Wants to Position Texas to Outlaw Abortion with 'Trigger Law.'" *Houston Chronicle*, February 6, 2017.

Combe, Rachael. "Don't Cry. Organize." *Elle*, November 9, 2016.

DePaulo, Lisa. "Growing Up Trump: Ivanka Trump Tells All." *Harper's Bazaar*, August 8, 2016.

Dwyer, Colin. "Trump Signs Law Giving States Option to Deny Funding for Planned Parenthood." NPR, April 13, 2017.

Eckardt, Steph. "Planned Parenthood's Cecile Richards on the Problem of Ivanka Trump." *W Magazine*, April 16, 2018.

Goldberg, Michelle. "Why Did Planned Parenthood Supporters Vote Trump?" *Slate*, December 22, 2016.

Hulse, Carl. "McCain Provides a Dramatic Finale on Health Care: Thumb Down." *New York Times*, July 28, 2017.

Kantor, Jodi, Rachel Abrams, and Maggie Haberman. "Ivanka Trump Has the President's Ear. Here's Her Agenda." *New York Times*, May 2, 2017.

Kaplan, Thomas, and Robert Pear. "Senate Republicans Say They Will Not Vote on Health Bill." *New York Times*, September 26, 2017.

Petroski, William. "Planned Parenthood to Close Four Iowa Clinics After Legislative Defunding." *Des Moines Register*, May 18, 2017.

Pradhan, Rachana, and Dan Diamond. "Price Traveled by Private Plane at Least 24 Times." *Politico*, September 21, 2017.

Richards, Cecile, and Lauren Peterson. *Make Trouble: Stand Up, Speak Out, and Find the Courage to Lead*. Gallery Books, 2018.

Safronova, Valeriya. "Why You'll See Planned Parenthood Pins at New York Fashion Week." *New York Times*, February 6, 2017.

Shannon, Delisa, Richard Feloni, and Alana Kakoyiannis. "What Really Happened When Ivanka Trump Met with Cecile Richards." *Business Insider*, April 10, 2018.

Winfield Cunningham, Paige. "Planned Parenthood Defunded for One Year Under GOP Health Bill." *Washington Post*, May 4, 2017.

18: PURGING "PRO-LIFE" FROM THE PARTY

ABC News. "DNC Head: Dems Will Be a 'Big Tent Party,' Build Presence 'in Every Zip Code' in 2018." April 20, 2017.

Associated Press. "Trump Now Says Abortion Laws Should Be Left As Is." April 2, 2016.

Apgar, Blake. "Sanders, Perez Aim to Unify Democrats during Las Vegas Speech." *Las Vegas Review-Journal*, April 22, 2017.

Bassett, Laura. "Democratic Party Draws a Line in the Sand on Abortion Rights." *HuffPost*, April 21, 2017.

Benning, Tom. "Abortion Rights Activist Tells Texas Dems That Trump Wants to Keep 'Women in the Home.'" *Dallas Morning News*, July 25, 2016.

Bevan, Susan, and Susan Cullman. "Why We Are Leaving the G.O.P." *New York Times*, June 24, 2018.

Combe, Rachael. "The Head of NARAL on Why It's Not Strange That She's Pregnant." *Elle*, September 24, 2015.

Cooney, Samantha. "All of the 'Pro-Life' Democrats in Congress Are Men." *Time*, May 18, 2017.

Detrow, Scott. "Bernie Sanders Defends Campaigning for Anti-Abortion Rights Democrat." NPR, April 20, 2017.

Devins, Neal. "Rethinking Judicial Minimalism: Abortion Politics, Party Polarization, and the Consequences of Returning the Constitution to Elected Government." *Vanderbilt Law Review* 69, no. 4 (2019).

Epstein, Reid J., and Natalie Andrews. "Democrats Reload for Georgia Runoff, but Party Divisions Remain." *Wall Street Journal*, April 19, 2017.

Fingerhut, Hannah. "Women Drive Increase in Democratic Support for Legal Abortion." Pew Research Center, November 3, 2016.

Haberkorn, Jennifer, and Didi Martinez. "House GOP Closes Ranks on Abortion." *Politico*, June 28, 2018.

Hogue, Ilyse. "NARAL Pro-Choice America President Ilyse Hogue Shares Her Abortion Story." *Teen Vogue*, January 17, 2017.

Kamisar, Ben, and Reid Wilson. "Dem Campaign Chief Vows No Litmus Test on Abortion." *The Hill*, July 31, 2017.

Kilgore, Ed. "How the GOP Abandoned Pro-Choice Republicans." *New York Magazine*, May 19, 2022.

Lovelace, Berkeley, Jr. "Democratic Sen. Heitkamp Explains Why She Broke Ranks and Voted for Trump's Supreme Court Pick." CNBC, April 11, 2017.

Martin, Jonathan. "At a 'Unity' Stop in Nebraska, Democrats Find Anything But." *New York Times*, April 21, 2017.

Martin, Jonathan, and Alexander Burns. "As Primaries Begin, Divided Voters Weigh What It Means to Be a Democrat." *New York Times*, March 4, 2018.

McCarthy, Ellen. "Abortion Rights Leader's Pregnancy Surprises Opponents: 'Is That Real?'" *Washington Post*, June 7, 2015.

Pathé, Simone. "NARAL Goes on Air Against Democrat Dan Lipinski." *Roll Call*, November 30, 2017.

Riess, Jeanie. "The President of NARAL Gets Coiffed for Battle." *New Yorker*, November 12, 2018.

Silver, Nate. "Many Previously Pro-Choice Dems Voted for Stupak Amendment." *FiveThirtyEight*, November 9, 2009.

Tumulty, Karen. "Pelosi: Democratic Candidates Should Not Be Forced to Toe Party Line on Abortion." *Washington Post*, May 2, 2017.

Weigel, David. "Democrats Turn to Sanders and His Star Power to Rebuild the Party." *Washington Post*, April 19, 2017.

———. "Omaha Mayoral Race Reveals Tensions between NARAL, Democrats over Abortion." *Washington Post*, April 20, 2017.

19: JANE DOE

Diamond, Dan. "HHS Reviews Refugee Operations as Trump Calls for Border Crackdown." *Politico*, October 23, 2018.

Farias, Cristian. "Meet the Texas Lawyer Who Helped an Undocumented Teen Fight for an Abortion." *New York Magazine*, November 3, 2017.

Fernandez, Manny. "U.S. Must Let Undocumented Teenager Get an Abortion, Appeals Court Says." *New York Times*, October 24, 2017.

Garsd, Jasmine. "Meet the Women Who Escorted Jane Doe to Her Abortion." WGBH, October 26, 2017.

Hylton, Antonia. "Jane Doe Speaks About Her Abortion Battle with the Trump Administration." *VICE News*, October 25, 2017.

Lauter, David. "How Long Can the Trump Administration Prevent a 17-Year-Old Immigrant from Getting an Abortion? Case Tests Limit." *Los Angeles Times*, October 23, 2017.

Levintova, Hannah, and Pema Levy. "Internal Emails Reveal How the Trump Administration Blocks Abortions for Migrant Teens." *Mother Jones*, November 29, 2017.

Lithwick, Dahlia. *Lady Justice: Women, the Law, and the Battle to Save America*. Penguin Books, 2022.

Sacchetti, Maria, and Sandhya Somashekhar. "An Undocumented Teen Is Pregnant and in Custody. Can the U.S. Stop Her from Getting an Abortion?" *Washington Post*, October 17, 2017.

Stern, Mark Joseph. "SCOTUS Rejects the Trump Administration's Attempt to Punish the ACLU in Jane Doe Abortion Case." *Slate*, June 4, 2018.

JUNE 2022: SIOUX FALLS, SOUTH DAKOTA

Nieves, Evelyn. "S.D. Makes Abortion Rare Through Laws And Stigma." *Washington Post*, December 26, 2005.

Reuters. "South Dakota Law Requires 3-Day Abortion Wait." March 22, 2011.

Strubinger, Lee. "With Roe v. Wade Decision and Trigger Law, Most Abortions Now Illegal in South Dakota." South Dakota Public Broadcasting, June 24, 2022.

20: EXACTLY FIFTEEN WEEKS

Amy, Jeff, and Sarah Mearhoff. "Mississippi Imposes Toughest Abortion Ban in US; Clinic Sues, Hearing Set." Associated Press, March 19, 2018.

Associated Press. "GOP Gains Control of Miss. House for First Time Since Reconstruction." November 14, 2011.

Campbell, Larrison. "Mississippi's Only Abortion Clinic Sues State over New 15-Week Ban." *Mississippi Today*, March 19, 2018.

Cha, Ariana Eunjung, and Rachel Roubein. "Fetal Viability Is at the Center of Mississippi Abortion Case. Here's Why." *Washington Post*, December 1, 2021.

Farris, Michael. "I Helped Start the Moral Majority. Trump Is the Opposite of What We Wanted." *Washington Post*, June 23, 2016.

Federalist. "Here's The Speech Jeff Sessions Delivered To Christian First Amendment Lawyers." July 13, 2017.

Goldberg, Michael. "Abortion Ruling Means More and Riskier Births in Mississippi." Associated Press, October 24, 2022.

Kitchener, Caroline, and Casey Parks. "How Mississippi Ended up with One Abortion Clinic and Why It Matters." *Washington Post*, November 30, 2021.

Kyle, Keegan. "Brad Schimel Planned to Keep Secret Records of Trip, His Emails Show." *The Post-Crescent*, May 18, 2018.

Montgomery, Peter. "ADF Attorneys Boast of Plans for Further Restrictions, Then Bans on Abortion." *Right Wing Watch*, January 22, 2018.

Newport, Frank. "Mississippi Retains Standing as Most Religious State." Gallup, February 8, 2017.

Peters, Jeremy W. "Fighting Gay Rights and Abortion with the First Amendment." *New York Times*, November 22, 2017.

Pittman, Ashton. "Officials: Mississippi Unprepared for 5,000 More Babies Born Yearly After Dobbs Ruling." *Mississippi Free Press*, October 3, 2022.

Roberti, Amanda. "Pro-Life and Pro-Woman? Republican Women and Anti-abortion Legislation." *Gender Policy Report*, July 21, 2022.

Ura, Alexa. "Abortion Legal Fight Cost Texas More Than $1 Million." *Texas Tribune*, June 29, 2016.

Zelinski, Andrea. "Unconstitutional Anti-Abortion Law Costs Texas Another $2.5 Million." *Houston Chronicle*, September 23, 2019.

21: THE PICK

Baker, Peter, and Nicholas Fandos. "Show How You Feel, Kavanaugh Was Told, and a Nomination Was Saved." *New York Times*, October 6, 2018.

Bradley, Laura. "Under Their Eye: The Rise of Handmaid's Tale-Inspired Protesters." *Vanity Fair*, October 9, 2018.

Brown, Emma. "California Professor, Writer of Confidential Brett Kavanaugh Letter, Speaks Out About Her Allegation of Sexual Assault." *Washington Post*, September 16, 2018.

Brown, Emma, and Jon Swaine. "Amy Coney Barrett, Supreme Court Nominee, Spoke at Program Founded to Inspire a 'Distinctly Christian Worldview in Every Area of Law.'" *Washington Post*, September 27, 2020.

Carlsen, Audrey, Maya Salam, Claire Cain Miller, Denise Lu, Ash Ngu, Jugal K. Patel, and Zach Wichter. "#MeToo Brought Down 201 Powerful Men.

Nearly Half of Their Replacements Are Women." *New York Times*, October 29, 2018.

Dias, Elizabeth, Rebecca R. Ruiz, and Sharon LaFraniere. "Rooted in Faith, Amy Coney Barrett Represents a New Conservatism." *New York Times*, October 11, 2020.

Everett, Burgess. "Conservative Group Drops Another $1.4 Million to Confirm Kavanaugh." *Politico*, July 16, 2018.

Garvey, John. "I Taught and Worked with Amy Coney Barrett. Here's What People Get Wrong About Her Faith." *Washington Post*, September 25, 2020.

Hoover, Margaret. "Leonard Leo." *Firing Line with Margaret Hoover*, October 12, 2018.

Hulse, Carl. *Confirmation Bias: Inside Washington's War over the Supreme Court, from Scalia's Death to Justice Kavanaugh*. HarperCollins, 2019.

———. "Kavanaugh Gave Private Assurances. Collins Says He 'Misled' Her." *New York Times*, June 24, 2022.

Lang, Marissa J. "'Stop Kavanaugh': Week of Protests in D.C. Asks Senators to Oppose Trump's Pick for Supreme Court." *Washington Post*, August 23, 2018.

Liptak, Adam, and Maggie Haberman. "Inside the White House's Quiet Campaign to Create a Supreme Court Opening." *New York Times*, June 28, 2018.

Marcus, Ruth. *Supreme Ambition: Brett Kavanaugh and the Conservative Takeover*. Simon & Schuster, 2019.

Massie, Victoria M. "How Racism and Sexism Shaped the Clarence Thomas/Anita Hill Hearing." *Vox*, April 16, 2016.

O'Harrow, Robert Jr., and Shawn Boburg. "A Conservative Activist's Behind-the-Scenes Campaign to Remake the Nation's Courts." *Washington Post*, May 21, 2019.

Reinhold, Robert. "2 Women Win Nomination in California Senate Races." *New York Times*, June 3, 1992.

Schwartzman, Paul, and Michelle Boorstein. "The Elite World of Brett Kavanaugh." *Washington Post*, July 11, 2018.

Swan, Jonathan, and Sam Baker. "Scoop: Trump 'Saving' Judge Amy Barrett for Ruth Bader Ginsburg Seat." *Axios*, March 31, 2019.

Tillman, Zoe. "Republicans Confirmed a Lot of Judges While Everyone Was Focused On Brett Kavanaugh." *BuzzFeed News*, September 12, 2018.

Treene, Alayna. "Exclusive Excerpt: Justice Kennedy's Secret Meeting with Trump." *Axios*, July 8, 2019.

22: THE WAR OVER WEN

Adler, Kayla Webley. "Alexis McGill Johnson Is Making Her Mark on Planned Parenthood." *Elle*, July 7, 2021.

Belluck, Pam. "Trump Administration Blocks Funds for Planned Parenthood and Others over Abortion Referrals." *New York Times*, February 22, 2019.

Cha, Ariana Eunjung. "New Federally Funded Clinics Emphasize Abstinence, Natural Family Planning." *Washington Post*, July 29, 2019.

———. "Tough Questions—and Answers—on 'Late-Term' Abortions, the Law and the Women Who Get Them." *Washington Post*, February 6, 2019.

———. "U.S. Joins 19 Nations, Including Saudi Arabia and Russia: 'There Is No International Right to an Abortion.'" *Washington Post*, September 24, 2019.

Cha, Ariana Eunjung, and Lena H. Sun. "Christian Conservatives in Trump Administration Build Global Antiabortion Coalition." *Washington Post*, March 15, 2019.

Dannenfelser, Marjorie. *Life Is Winning: Inside the Fight for Unborn Children and Their Mothers*. Humanix Books, 2020.

Enten, Harry. "Brett Kavanaugh Is the Least Popular Supreme Court Nominee in 30 Years." CNN, September 22, 2018.

Goldmacher, Shane. "Planned Parenthood Ousts President, Seeking a More Political Approach." *New York Times*, July 16, 2019.

Helm, Angela. "Meet the New Head of Planned Parenthood: Alexis McGill Johnson Is a Seasoned Soldier in the War for Women's Reproductive Health." *The Root*, September 18, 2019.

Kaiser Family Foundation. "Abortions Later in Pregnancy." December 5, 2019.

Liptak, Adam. "Confirming Kavanaugh: A Triumph for Conservatives, but a Blow to the Court's Image." *New York Times*, June 10, 2018.

Lu, Denise, and Keith Collins. "'Year of the Woman' Indeed: Record Gains in the House." *New York Times*, November 16, 2018.

O'Connor, Ema. "Planned Parenthood's New President Wants to Focus on Nonabortion Health Care." *BuzzFeed News*, January 7, 2019.

O'Connor, Ema, and Ruby Cramer. "Planned Parenthood Has Ousted Its President, Leana Wen, amid a Dispute over the Organization's Direction." *BuzzFeed News*, July 16, 2019.

———. "Planned Parenthood Is Losing Top Political Aides as Its Staff Worries over Its Changing Direction." *BuzzFeed News*, February 8, 2019.

Ottesen, KK. "Planned Parenthood President: Saying Abortion Is a Small Part of What Group Does Is Stigmatizing." *Washington Post Magazine*, December 29, 2020.

Peters, Jeremy W. "Republicans' Messaging on Abortion Puts Democrats on the Defensive." *New York Times*, May 16, 2019.

Peters, Jeremy W., and Elizabeth Dias. "With Republican Gains in Senate, Social Conservatives Tighten Their Grip." *New York Times*, November 7, 2018.

Pew Research Center. "Americans Divided on Kavanaugh's Nomination to the Supreme Court." July 17, 2018.

Riess, Jeanie. "The President of NARAL Gets Coiffed for Battle." *New Yorker*, November 12, 2018.

Saul, Michael Howard. "Antiabortion Billboard in SoHo Draws Ire." *Wall Street Journal*, February 24, 2011.

Vogel, Kenneth P., and Robert Pear. "Trump Administration Gives Family Planning Grant to Anti-Abortion Group." *New York Times*, March 29, 2019.

Wen, Leana. *Lifelines: A Doctor's Journey in the Fight for Public Health*. Metropolitan Books, 2021.

Wen, Leana S. "Leana Wen: My Miscarriage Has Made My Commitment to Women's Health Even Stronger." *Washington Post*, July 6, 2019.

WTOP. "Ask the Governor with Virginia Gov. Ralph Northam." January 30, 2019.

23: GAMING THE COURTS

Associated Press. "Arkansas Governor Signs 18-Week Abortion Ban into Law." March 15, 2019.

Berenson, Tessa. "Inside Brett Kavanaugh's First Term on the Supreme Court." *Time*, June 28, 2019.

Cha, Ariana Eunjung. "At Least 20 Abortion Cases Are in the Pipeline to the Supreme Court. Any One Could Gut Roe v. Wade." *Washington Post*, February 15, 2019.

Hoover, Margaret. "Leonard Leo." *Firing Line with Margaret Hoover*, October 12, 2018.

Israelsen-Hartley, Sara. "The Power Broker: Can Conservative Icon Gayle Ruzicka Stay Relevant in Today's Republican Party?" *Deseret News*, March 7, 2019.

Liptak, Adam. "Supreme Court Blocks Louisiana Abortion Law." *New York Times*, February 7, 2019.

Nash, Elizabeth, Rachel Benson Gold, Zohra Ansari-Thomas, Olivia Cappello, Sophia Naide, and Lizamarie Mohammed. "State Policy Trends 2018: With Roe v. Wade in Jeopardy, States Continued to Add New Abortion Restrictions." Guttmacher Institute, December 11, 2018.

Patel, Ronak, and Michael Hibblen. "Arkansas Officials React to Abortion Ruling; 'Trigger Law' to Take Effect." Little Rock Public Radio, June 24, 2022.

Romboy, Dennis. "Utah Lawmaker Wants to Ban Abortions Based on Gender, Race." *Deseret News*, November 30, 2012.

Tavernise, Sabrina. "How Banning Abortion in the Early Weeks of Pregnancy Suddenly Became Mainstream." *New York Times*, April 18, 2019.

Vogue, Ariane de, and Ted Barrett. "Susan Collins Defends Her Brett Kavanaugh Vote After He Dissents in Abortion Access Case." CNN, February 12, 2019.

Whitehurst, Lindsay. "Utah Bans Abortions after 18 Weeks, Teeing up Legal Showdown." Associated Press, March 26, 2019.

24: THE THREAD

Associated Press. "Near-Total Abortion Ban Signed into Law in Alabama." May 16, 2019.

Astor, Maggie. "On Abortion Rights, 2020 Democrats Move Past 'Safe, Legal and Rare.'" *New York Times*, November 25, 2019.

Dovere, Edward-Isaac. *Battle for the Soul: Inside the Democrats' Campaigns to Defeat Trump*. Penguin Books, 2021.

Glueck, Katie. "Biden Still Backs Hyde Amendment, Which Bans Federal Funds for Abortions." *New York Times*, June 5, 2019.

———. "Joe Biden Denounces Hyde Amendment, Reversing His Position." *New York Times*, June 6, 2019.

Kelley, Kitty. "Death and the All-American Boy." *Washingtonian*, June 1, 1974.

Lerer, Lisa, and Katie Glueck. "In Abortion Fight, 2020 Female Candidates Lead Call to Arms." *New York Times*, May 15, 2019.

Lucey, Catherine. "Support for 15-Week Abortion Ban Outweighs Opposition, WSJ Poll Finds." *Wall Street Journal*, April 1, 2022.

Malone, Matt. "'Everyone's Entitled to Dignity': A Conversation with Joseph R. Biden Jr." *America Magazine*, September 29, 2015.

Morton, Jason. "West Alabama Women's Center Sold to New Owners." *Tuscaloosa News*, May 16, 2020.

Nelson, Amy. "NARAL President Ilyse Hogue Tells Us Everything We Need to Know About Abortion Rights." *The Riveter*, May 22, 2019.

North, Anna. "Planned Parenthood Moving Away from 'Choice.'" *BuzzFeed News*, January 9, 2013.

Pew Research Center. "America's Abortion Quandary." May 6, 2022.

Ward, Myah. "How One Abortion Clinic Is Surviving in a Post-Roe World." *Politico*, June 23, 2023.

Witt, Emily. "The Last Abortion Clinic in North Dakota Gets Ready to Leave." *New Yorker*, July 13, 2022.

25: MISSISSIPPI WOMANHOOD

Adler, Kayla Webley. "Alexis McGill Johnson Is Making Her Mark on Planned Parenthood." *Elle*, July 7, 2021.

Associated Press. "Mississippi to Drop Charge of White Ex-Cop in Man's Death." May 28, 2020.

Bogel-Burroughs, Nicholas. "Dobbs, Named in Abortion Case Ending Roe, Had Little to Do with It." *New York Times*, June 24, 2022.

Cineas, Fabiola. "Black Women Will Suffer the Most Without Roe." *Vox*, June 29, 2022.

Crary, David. "Supreme Court's Abortion Ruling Raises Stakes for Election." Associated Press, June 30, 2020.

Ellis, Nicquel Terry. "'Pushed to the Margins': Why Some Activists and Lawmakers Say Abortion Bans Are a Form of White Supremacy." CNN, May 18, 2022.

Fitch, Lynn, and Jennifer Ingram Johnson. "History Is Lunch: The Life and Career of Evelyn Gandy." March 9, 2022.

Fowler, Sarah. "Treasurer, Governor: End Gender Pay Gap in Mississippi." *The Clarion-Ledger*, January 10, 2017.

Harrison, Bobby. "State Treasurer Fitch Advocates for Equal Pay, Financial Literacy." *Northeast Mississippi Daily Journal*, February 21, 2017.

Hille, Austin. "Mississippi Delegates Weigh In on RNC, Trump's Campaign." *Daily Mississippian*, July 21, 2016.

Judin, Nick. "Historic Protests for Black Lives Sweep Mississippi over Weekend." *Jackson Free Press*, June 8, 2020.

Kantor, Jodi, and Adam Liptak. "Behind the Scenes at the Dismantling of Roe v. Wade." *New York Times*, December 15, 2023.

Kaplan, Joshua, Justin Elliott, and Alex Mierjeski. "Clarence Thomas and the Billionaire." ProPublica, April 6, 2023.

Kitchener, Caroline. "The Woman Who Could Bring Down Roe v. Wade." *Washington Post*, December 1, 2021.

Long, Robert Lee. "Fowl Play." *Click Magazine*, October 2015.

McGill Johnson, Alexis. "The End of Roe and What It Would Mean for the Black Community." *St. Louis American*, May 12, 2022.

Onion, Rebecca. "The Stories of 'Segregation Academies,' as Told by the White Students Who Attended Them." *Slate*, November 7, 2019.

Ottesen, KK. "Planned Parenthood President: Saying Abortion Is a Small Part of What Group Does Is Stigmatizing." *Washington Post Magazine*, December 29, 2020.

Pew Research Center. "U.S. Public Continues to Favor Legal Abortion, Oppose Overturning Roe v. Wade." August 29, 2019.

Reuters. "Planned Parenthood Founder Margaret Sanger's 1939 Quote on Exterminating Black Population Taken Out of Context." May 9, 2022.

Rosenberg, Eli. "Clarence Thomas Tried to Link Abortion to Eugenics. Seven Historians Told the Post He's Wrong." *Washington Post*, May 30, 2019.

Ross, Loretta. "Planned Parenthood's Next President Should Be a Woman of Color." *HuffPost*, January 30, 2018.

Sanger, Margaret. *Margaret Sanger: An Autobiography*. W. W. Norton & Company, Inc., 1938.

Seid, Dennis. "Fitch: Women Need to Empower Themselves." *Northeast Mississippi Daily Journal*, October 22, 2014.

Shirley, James L. "Preborn Black Lives Matter, Too." *Washington Times*, August 2, 2020.

Tavernise, Sabrina, and Elizabeth Dias. "The Supreme Court Stopped Anti-Abortion Momentum. For Now." *New York Times*, June 29, 2020.

Troutman, Michele, Saima Rafique, and Torie Comeaux Plowden. "Are Higher Unintended Pregnancy Rates among Minorities a Result of Disparate Access to Contraception?" *Contraception and Reproductive Medicine* 5, no. 16 (October 1, 2020).

Upholt, Boyce. "These Birds Can Fly: At Holly Spring's Fitch Farms, an Old Tradition of Quail Hunting Lives On." *Mississippi Magazine*, September 1, 2015.

Wilson, George Tipton. "Hunter's Heaven." *Mississippi Magazine*, September 1, 2004.

Zhu, Alissa, and Justin Vicory. "'No Justice, No Peace': Protesters Rally in Downtown Jackson against Police Brutality." *The Clarion-Ledger*, June 6, 2020.

26: THE DAYS OF AWE

Anti-Defamation League. "Pro-Trump Rallies in DC Attract Extremists & Erupt into Violence." December 13, 2020.

Buchanan, Larry, and Karen Yourish. "Ginsburg Supreme Court Vacancy Is the Second Closest to a U.S. Election Ever." *New York Times*, September 19, 2020.

Eisner, Jane. "Jane Eisner Interviews Ruth Bader Ginsburg: Transcript." *The Forward*, February 5, 2018.

Friedman, Vanessa. "Ruth Bader Ginsburg's Lace Collar Wasn't an Accessory, It Was a Gauntlet." *New York Times*, September 20, 2020.

Gerhart, Ann, and Lucio Villa. "Rose Garden Ceremony Attendees Who Tested Positive for Coronavirus." *Washington Post*, October 3, 2020.

Gramlich, John. "How Trump Compares with Other Recent Presidents in Appointing Federal Judges." Pew Research Center, January 13, 2021.

Kim, Seung Min. "Both Sides on Abortion Certain Barrett Would Restrict, If Not Overturn, Landmark Court Decision." *Washington Post*, October 8, 2020.

Kirchgaessner, Stephanie. "Barrett Was Member of Anti-Abortion Group That Promoted Clinic Criticized for Misleading Women." *The Guardian*, October 11, 2020.

Kroll, Andy, Andrea Bernstein, and Ilya Marritz. "We Don't Talk About Leonard: The Man Behind the Right's Supreme Court Supermajority." ProPublica, October 11, 2023.

LeVine, Marianne. "Judicial Crisis Network Launches $3 Million Ad Campaign for Barrett." *Politico*, September 26, 2020.
Mitchell, Andrea. "'She Made the World a Better Place': Justice Stephen Breyer Remembers Ruth Bader Ginsburg." MSNBC, September 25, 2020.
Naylor, Brian. "Ginsburg, Champion of Gender Equality, Becomes 1st Woman to Lie In State." NPR, September 25, 2020.
Pogrebin, Abigail. *Stars of David: Prominent Jews Talk About Being Jewish.* Broadway Books, 2005.
Shimron, Yonat. "Ruth Bader Ginsburg Was Passionate About Judaism's Concern for Justice." *Religion News Service*, September 18, 2020.
Smith, Kate. "These Are the Abortion Cases Amy Coney Barrett Might Hear on the Supreme Court." CBS News, October 15, 2020.
Sparks, Grace. "CNN Poll: Americans Are Divided over Amy Coney Barrett." CNN, October 7, 2020.
Swan, Jonathan, and Sam Baker. "Scoop: Trump 'Saving' Judge Amy Barrett for Ruth Bader Ginsburg Seat." *Axios*, March 31, 2019.
Observer. "Law Professor Reflects on Landmark Case." January 20, 2013.
Zornosa, Laura. "Ruth Bader Ginsburg's 'Dissent Collar' Donated to the Smithsonian." *New York Times*, March 30, 2022.

27: THE COUP

Associated Press. "Clinic Bomber Freed from Prison." February 17, 1995.
Block, Melissa. "Biden Establishes a Gender Policy Council Within the White House." NPR, March 8, 2021.
Dias, Elizabeth, and Ruth Graham. "How White Evangelical Christians Fused with Trump Extremism." *New York Times*, January 11, 2021.
Dias, Elizabeth, and Jack Healy. "For Many Who Marched, Jan. 6 Was Only the Beginning." *New York Times*, January 23, 2022.
Kantor, Jodi, and Adam Liptak. "Behind the Scenes at the Dismantling of Roe v. Wade." *New York Times*, December 15, 2023.
Kroll, Andy, Justin Elliott, and Andrew Perez. "How a Billionaire's 'Attack Philanthropy' Secretly Funded Climate Denialism and Right-Wing Causes." ProPublica and *The Lever*, September 6, 2022.
Linhorst, Michael. "Scott Stewart Wasn't Well Known in the Antiabortion World. Now He's Leading the Charge to Overturn Roe at the Supreme Court." *Washington Post Magazine*, November 9, 2021.
Lipton, Eric, and Mark Walker. "Christian Conservative Lawyer Had Secretive Role in Bid to Block Election Result." *New York Times*, October 7, 2021.
McCammon, Sarah. "Biden Administration Moves to Undo Trump Abortion Rules for Title X." NPR, April 14, 2021.
———. "Biden's Budget Proposal Reverses a Decades-Long Ban on Abortion Funding." NPR, May 31, 2021.

Nash, Elizabeth, Lizamarie Mohammed, Olivia Cappello, and Sophia Naide. "State Policy Trends 2019: A Wave of Abortion Bans, But Some States Are Fighting Back." Guttmacher Institute, December 10, 2019.

Peters, Jeremy W. "In Restricting Early Voting, the Right Sees a New 'Center of Gravity.'" *New York Times*, March 19, 2021.

Schmidt, Samantha, and Caroline Kitchener. "Before He Stormed the Capitol, Ex-W.Va. Lawmaker Harassed Women at an Abortion Clinic." *Washington Post*, January 16, 2021.

Sherman, Carter. "This Convicted Planned Parenthood Bomber Was at the Capitol 'Fighting' for Trump." *VICE News*, January 14, 2021.

———. "Why 'Baby Lives Matter' Messages Are Popping Up All Over the US." *VICE News*, September 17, 2020.

WUSA 9. "GRAPHIC: Video Shows Chaos after a 35-Year-Old Woman Was Fatally Shot during Capitol Riots." January 8, 2021.

JUNE 2022: JACKSON, MISSISSIPPI

Brewer, Shannon. "We're Mississippi's Last Abortion Clinic, and We're Braced for the Worst." *New York Times*, June 9, 2021.

Crary, David. "Mississippi's Last Abortion Clinic Persists." Associated Press, December 28, 2004.

Jackson. Directed by Maisie Crow. Girl Friday Films, 2016.

Kitchener, Caroline, and Casey Parks. "How Mississippi Ended up with One Abortion Clinic and Why It Matters." *Washington Post*, November 30, 2021.

Krueger, Hannah. "In Deep South, Mass. Doctors Staff Last Holdout of Abortion." *Boston Globe*, May 22, 2022.

McCann, Allison. "Seven States Have Only One Remaining Abortion Clinic. We Talked to the People Keeping Them Open." *VICE News*, May 23, 2017.

Regan, Michael D. "Court Blocks Mississippi Law That Would Have Shuttered State's Only Abortion Clinic." *PBS NewsHour*, March 18, 2017.

Rojas, Rick. "Inside the Last Abortion Clinic in Mississippi." *New York Times*, November 30, 2021.

Taft, Isabelle. "With Roe on the Line, an Abortion Provider Travels to Jackson for What May Be Her Final Shift." *Mississippi Today*, June 16, 2022.

28: THE BRIEF

Allen, Virginia. "Mississippi Attorney General Details Abortion Case That Could Undo Roe v. Wade." *Daily Signal*, September 22, 2021.

Armiak, David. "Group Run by Trump's 'Judge Whisperer' Leonard Leo Provides More Than a Third of RAGA's Revenue So Far in 2021." Center for Media and Democracy, August 3, 2021.

———. "More Staff Flee GOP Attorneys General Group After It Doubles Down on Insurrection." Center for Media and Democracy, May 4, 2021.

Bluestein, Greg. "GOP AGs Group Promotes Operative Behind Robocalls Urging March to Capitol." *Atlanta Journal-Constitution*, April 22, 2021.

Bogan, Jesse. "Mother, Wife, Lawyer: Erin Hawley Calls the Fight to Overturn Roe 'the Project of a Lifetime.'" *St. Louis Post-Dispatch*, May 7, 2022.

Cain Miller, Claire. "Mississippi Asks: If Women Can Have It All, Is Roe Necessary?" *New York Times*, December 1, 2021.

Cole, Devan. "Mississippi GOP Governor: State Abortion Law 'a Vehicle' for Supreme Court to Revisit Roe v. Wade." CNN, June 6, 2021.

Dinzeo, Maria. "Abortion Foes Will Face Criminal Charges in Undercover Video Case." *Courthouse News*, December 6, 2019.

Egelko, Bob. "S.F. Judge Upholds State Privacy Law Cited in Prosecution of Antiabortion Activists." *San Francisco Chronicle*, December 19, 2023.

Erskine, Ellena. "We Read All the Amicus Briefs in Dobbs so You Don't Have To." *SCOTUSblog*, November 30, 2021.

EWTN. "Mississippi Attorney General Lynn Fitch On Supreme Court Abortion Case." September 25, 2021.

Fitch, Lynn. "Mississippi Supports Protecting Life at 15 Weeks. Give Abortion Debate Back to the People." *USA Today*, July 23, 2021.

Kinnard, Meg. "Republican AGs Group Leader Quits over Call Pushing Protest." Associated Press, January 11, 2021.

Kitroeff, Natalie, and Jessica Silver-Greenberg. "Pregnancy Discrimination Is Rampant Inside America's Biggest Companies." *New York Times*, February 8, 2019.

Klein, Ezra. "Sex, Abortion and Feminism, as Seen from the Right." *Ezra Klein Show*, May 31, 2022.

Kroll, Andy, Andrew Perez, and Aditi Ramaswami. "Conservative Activist Poured Millions into Groups Seeking to Influence Supreme Court on Elections and Discrimination." ProPublica and *The Lever*, December 14, 2022.

Linhorst, Michael. "Scott Stewart Wasn't Well Known in the Antiabortion World. Now He's Leading the Charge to Overturn Roe at the Supreme Court." *Washington Post Magazine*, November 9, 2021.

Los Angeles Times. "Serve's Up at Malibu for Stewart." March 22, 2002.

Nash, Elizabeth, and Isabel Guarnieri. "13 States Have Abortion Trigger Bans—Here's What Happens When Roe Is Overturned." Guttmacher Institute, June 6, 2022.

Orr Larsen, Allison. "The Supreme Court Decisions on Guns and Abortion Relied Heavily on History. But Whose History?" *Politico Magazine*, July 26, 2022.

Pierson, Brendan. "Abortion Foes Largely Lose $2.4 Mln Appeal over Planned Parenthood Videos." Reuters, October 21, 2022.

Praxis Circle. "Erika Bachiochi—Are You a Catholic Feminist?" YouTube, April 5, 2023.

Przybyla, Heidi. "'Plain Historical Falsehoods': How Amicus Briefs Bolstered Supreme Court Conservatives." *Politico*, December 3, 2023.

Stone, Peter. "US Dark-Money Fund Spends Millions to Back Republican Attorneys General." *The Guardian*, June 23, 2023.

Tracy, Abigail. "Erin Morrow Hawley Is Leading the Charge to Ban Abortion Medication. She's Also Josh Hawley's Wife." *Vanity Fair*, March 23, 2023.

Vogel, Kenneth P., and Shane Goldmacher. "An Unusual $1.6 Billion Donation Bolsters Conservatives." *New York Times*, August 22, 2022.

29: TEXAN REVENGE

Chesler, Ellen. "Defending Margaret Sanger, Planned Parenthood's Founder." *New York Times*, April 20, 2021.

Collins, Jeffrey. "SC Governor Signs Abortion Ban; Planned Parenthood Sues." Associated Press, February 18, 2021.

Douglas, Erin, and Carla Astudillo. "We Annotated Texas' Near-Total Abortion Ban. Here's What the Law Says About Enforcement." *Texas Tribune*, September 10, 2021.

Groves, Stephen. "GOP-Led States See Texas Law as Model to Restrict Abortions." Associated Press, September 2, 2021.

Heilemann, John. "Cecile Richards." *Hell & High Water with John Heilemann*, February 28, 2023.

Jaradat, Mya. "These Christian Lawmakers Are on the Offensive Against Abortion." *Deseret News*, July 20, 2021.

Kantor, Jodi, and Adam Liptak. "Behind the Scenes at the Dismantling of Roe v. Wade." *New York Times*, December 15, 2023.

Kitchener, Caroline, Meagan Flynn, Lola Fadulu, Donovan J. Thomas, and Paul Schwartzman. "Thousands Gather at Women's March Rallies in D.C., Across U.S. to Protect Roe v. Wade." *Washington Post*, October 2, 2021.

Kitchener, Caroline, Beth Reinhard, and Alice Crites. "A Call, a Text, an Apology: How an Abortion Arrest Shook up a Texas Town." *Washington Post*, April 13, 2022.

Liptak, Adam. "Supreme Court Allows Challenge to Texas Abortion Law but Leaves It in Effect." *New York Times*, December 10, 2021.

McCullough, Jolie. "After Pursuing an Indictment, Starr County District Attorney Drops Murder Charge over Self-Induced Abortion." *Texas Tribune*, April 10, 2022.

McGill Johnson, Alexis. "I'm the Head of Planned Parenthood. We're Done Making Excuses for Our Founder." *New York Times*, April 17, 2021.

Nash, Elizabeth. "State Policy Trends 2021: The Worst Year for Abortion Rights in Almost Half a Century." Guttmacher Institute, December 16, 2021.

Oxner, Reese. "U.S. Supreme Court Refuses to Block Texas' Six-Week Abortion Ban." *Texas Tribune*, September 1, 2021.

Rogers, Katie. "Biden Vows to Protect Abortion Rights in Face of 'Extreme' Texas Law." *New York Times*, September 2, 2021.

Schmidt, Michael S. "Behind the Texas Abortion Law, a Persevering Conservative Lawyer." *New York Times*, September 12, 2021.

Schor, Elana. "Abortion Foes Vent Disappointment after Supreme Court Ruling." Associated Press, June 29, 2020.

Simmons-Duffin, Selena. "3 Abortion Bans in Texas Leave Doctors 'Talking in Code' to Pregnant Patients." NPR, March 1, 2023.

Tavernise, Sabrina. "With Abortion Largely Banned in Texas, an Oklahoma Clinic Is Inundated." *New York Times*, September 26, 2021.

Ziegler, Mary, and Rachel Rebouché. "The Federal Suit against Texas's Abortion Law May Fail. It's Still Worthwhile." *Washington Post*, September 11, 2021.

30: THE ARGUMENT

Heilemann, John. "Cecile Richards." *Hell & High Water with John Heilemann*, February 28, 2023.

Pew Research Center. "The Complicated Politics of Abortion." August 22, 2012.

Purifoy, Parker. "Outside Supreme Court, Crowd Amplifies Abortion Arguments." Associated Press, December 1, 2021.

Rovner, Julie. "Conservative Justices Seem Poised to Overturn Roe's Abortion Rights." *KFF Health News*, December 1, 2021.

VanSickle, Abbie, and Steve Eder. "Clarence Thomas's Clerks: An 'Extended Family' With Reach and Power." *New York Times*, December 24, 2023.

Walsh, Mark. "'Feelings Run High': Two Hours of Tense Debate on an Issue That Divides the Court and the Country." *SCOTUSblog*, December 1, 2021.

31: DISBELIEF

Edwards-Levy, Ariel. "CNN Poll: As Supreme Court Ruling on Roe Looms, Most Americans Oppose Overturning It." CNN, January 21, 2022.

Guskin, Emily, and Scott Clement. "Majority of Americans Say Supreme Court Should Uphold Roe, Post-ABC Poll Finds." *Washington Post*, May 3, 2022.

Kunhardt Film Foundation. "Cecile Richards Interview: Reproductive Rights, Family, and Women in Politics." Interview by Noah Remnick, June 17, 2022.

Richards, Cecile. "The One Regret from My Time Leading Planned Parenthood." *New York Times*, January 21, 2022.

Sanger-Katz, Margot, Claire Cain Miller, and Quoctrung Bui. "Most Women Denied Abortions by Texas Law Got Them Another Way." *New York Times*, March 6, 2022.

32: THE LEAK

Akin, Todd. *Firing Back: Taking on the Party Bosses and Media Elite to Protect Our Faith and Freedom*. WND Books, 2014.

Associated Press. "Reward Posted to Find Woman in Video of Abortion Clinic Fire." June 8, 2022.

Barnes, Robert. "Clarence Thomas Says Supreme Court Leak Has Eroded Trust in Institution." *Washington Post*, May 14, 2022.

Cramer, Maria, and Jesus Jiménez. "Armed Man Traveled to Justice Kavanaugh's Home to Kill Him, Officials Say." *New York Times*, June 8, 2022.

Dias, Elizabeth, and Ruth Graham. "Vatican Removes Anti-Abortion Activist From the Priesthood." *New York Times*, December 18, 2022.

Ellis, Blake, and Melanie Hicken. "These Male Politicians Are Pushing for Women Who Receive Abortions to Be Punished with Prison Time." CNN, September 21, 2022.

Evans, Rowland, and Robert Novak. "Justice Kennedy's Flip." *Washington Post*, September 3, 1992.

Flegenheimer, Matt, and Maggie Haberman. "Donald Trump, Abortion Foe, Eyes 'Punishment' for Women, Then Recants." *New York Times*, March 30, 2016.

Gerstein, Josh, and Alexander Ward. "Supreme Court Has Voted to Overturn Abortion Rights, Draft Opinion Shows." *Politico*, May 3, 2022.

González, Oriana. "Louisiana Abortion Bill Allowing Homicide Charges against Patients Stopped for Now." *Axios*, May 13, 2022.

Hoffman, Jan. "The New Abortion Bans: Almost No Exceptions for Rape, Incest or Health." *New York Times*, June 9, 2022.

Howley, Kerry. "The Woman Who Killed Roe." *New York Magazine*, May 9, 2022.

Kaplan, Joshua, Justin Elliott, and Alex Mierjeski. "Clarence Thomas and the Billionaire." ProPublica, April 6, 2023.

Kitchener, Caroline. "The Next Frontier for the Antiabortion Movement: A Nationwide Ban." *Washington Post*, May 2, 2022.

Marist College. "NPR/PBS NewsHour/Marist Poll of 941 National Adults." June 25, 2022.

Mayer, Jane. "Scooping the Supreme Court." *New Yorker*, May 6, 2022.

Meyer, Theodoric, Leigh Ann Caldwell, and Rachel Roubein. "Inside Chris Christie's Antiabortion Blitz." *Washington Post*, September 13, 2022.

Nelson, Ryan. "'If Abortions Aren't Safe, Neither Are You': Hialeah Pregnancy Clinic Vandalized." NBC 6 South Florida, July 5, 2022.

Palmer, Anna, and Tarini Parti. "Akin Un-Apologizes." *Politico*, July 10, 2014.

Pulliam Bailey, Sarah. "A Catholic Priest Put an Aborted Fetus on the Altar in an Appeal for Donald Trump." *Washington Post*, November 7, 2016.

Raza, Sarah. "Vandals Leave Threat, Break Windows at Dearborn Heights Pregnancy Center." *Detroit Free Press*, June 23, 2022.

Romano, Andrew. "Poll: Confidence in Supreme Court Has Collapsed Since Conservatives Took Control." Yahoo News, May 10, 2022.

Saad, Lydia. "'Pro-Choice' Identification Rises to Near Record High in U.S." Gallup, June 2, 2022.

Wall Street Journal Editorial Board. "Abortion and the Supreme Court." *Wall Street Journal*, April 26, 2022.

Washington Post. "Move by Burger May Shift Court's Stand on Abortion." July 4, 1972.

Watkins, Morgan. "Mitch McConnell Wants Whoever Leaked Supreme Court Roe v. Wade Draft Dealt with 'Severely.'" *Louisville Courier Journal*, May 3, 2022.

Welch, Monique. "Abortion Activists Strip Down to Underwear during Joel Osteen's Lakewood Church Service." *Houston Chronicle*, June 6, 2022.

33: THE OBITUARY

Ducharme, Jamie. "Alabama's Abortion Ban Isn't Only About Abortion. Opponents Are Afraid It May Drive Doctors Out of the State." *Time*, May 17, 2019.

Einbinder, Nicole, and Caroline Haskins. "Oklahoma Lawmakers Passed 5 Contradictory Abortion Bans. No One Knows Which Laws Will Be Enforced." *Business Insider*, June 24, 2022.

Ford, Matt. "What Samuel Alito Gets Wrong About English Common Law." *New Republic*, May 11, 2022.

Goldberg, Emma, and Lora Kelley. "Companies Are More Vocal Than Ever on Social Issues. Not on Abortion." *New York Times*, June 24, 2022.

Haberman, Maggie, and Michael C. Bender. "The Man Most Responsible for Ending Roe Worries That It Could Hurt His Party." *New York Times*, June 24, 2022.

Hawley, Erin. "Why Supreme Court Abortion Decision Empowers Women." Fox News, June 25, 2022.

HuffPost Video. "AOC: We Have To Fill The Streets." June 24, 2022.

Hulse, Carl. "Kavanaugh Gave Private Assurances. Collins Says He 'Misled' Her." *New York Times*, June 24, 2022.

Isaac, Mike, and Ryan Mac. "Meta Clamps Down on Internal Discussion of Roe v. Wade's Overturning." *New York Times*, June 24, 2022.

Kantor, Jodi, and Adam Liptak. "Behind the Scenes at the Dismantling of Roe v. Wade." *New York Times*, December 15, 2023.

Keefe, John, Shania Shelton, Kaanita Iyer, JiMin Lee, Ariella Phillips, Kenneth Uzquiano, and Christopher Hickey. "Track Changes between the Abortion Decision and the Leaked Draft." CNN, June 27, 2022.

Liptak, Adam. "In 6-to-3 Ruling, Supreme Court Ends Nearly 50 Years of Abortion Rights." *New York Times*, June 24, 2022.

Schneider, Gregory S., and Laura Vozzella. "Youngkin to Seek 15-Week Abortion Law in Virginia After Supreme Court Ruling," *Washington Post*, June 24, 2022.

Shepherd, Katie, Rachel Roubein, and Caroline Kitchener. "1 in 3 American Women Have Already Lost Abortion Access. More Restrictive Laws Are Coming." *Washington Post*, August 22, 2022.

Sneed, Tierney, and Veronica Stracqualursi. "Abortion Is Banned or Severely Limited in a Number of States. Here's Where Things Stand." CNN, September 23, 2022.

Sneve, Joe, Nicole Ki, Morgan Matzen, Jonathan Ellis, and Alfonzo Galvan. "Abortion Is Now Illegal in South Dakota. Here's What You Need to Know." *Sioux Falls Argus Leader*, June 24, 2022.

Stolberg, Sheryl Gay, and Emily Cochrane. "Becerra Was Visiting a Planned Parenthood in Missouri When Abortion Suddenly Became Illegal." *New York Times*, June 24, 2022.

Tingley, Anna. "What Moms Texted Their Daughters After the Supreme Court Ruling." *Washington Post*, June 27, 2022.

Vandell, Perry, and Stacey Barchenger. "Tear Gas Deployed as Protesters Bang on Senate Doors; GOP Likens Event to Insurrection." *Arizona Republic*, June 24, 2022.

34: THE HEART OF IT ALL

Astor, Maggie, and Nate Cohn. "Here's How Abortion Rights Supporters Won in Conservative Kansas." *New York Times*, August 3, 2022.

Borter, Gabriella. "Abortion Rights Wins in Michigan, Kentucky Give Fuel for Future Ballot Measures." Reuters, November 9, 2022.

Kroll, Andy, Andrea Bernstein, and Ilya Marritz. "We Don't Talk About Leonard: The Man Behind the Right's Supreme Court Supermajority." ProPublica, October 11, 2023.

Kroll, Andy, Andrea Bernstein, and Nick Surgey. "Inside the 'Private and Confidential' Conservative Group That Promises to 'Crush Liberal Dominance.'" ProPublica and *Documented*, March 9, 2023.

Merica, Dan. "'Kansas Will Not Be Our Last Fight': Abortion Rights Victory Gives Democrats New Hope for Midterms." CNN, August 4, 2022.

Shepherd, Katie, Rachel Roubein, and Caroline Kitchener. "1 in 3 American Women Have Already Lost Abortion Access. More Restrictive Laws Are Coming." *Washington Post*, August 22, 2022.

35: AFTER DOBBS

Barragán, James. "Ken Paxton Wins Third Term as Attorney General, Beating Democrat Rochelle Garza." *Texas Tribune*, November 8, 2022.

Becker, Amanda. "Dark Money Is Flowing to Groups Trying to Limit Medication Abortion. Leonard Leo Is Again at the Center." *19th News*, January 4, 2024.

Elliott, Justin, Joshua Kaplan, and Alex Mierjeski. "Justice Samuel Alito Took Luxury Fishing Vacation with GOP Billionaire Who Later Had Cases Before the Court." ProPublica, June 20, 2023.

Gorney, Cynthia. "The Dispassion of John C. Willke." *Washington Post*, April 21, 1990.

Hulse, Carl. "Senate Panel Approves Subpoenas in Supreme Court Ethics Inquiry." *New York Times*, November 30, 2023.

Johnson, Mike. *Fox News Sunday.* Interview by Shannon Bream, November 5, 2023.

Kaplan, Joshua, Justin Elliott, and Alex Mierjeski. "Clarence Thomas and the Billionaire." ProPublica, April 6, 2023.

Kaplan, Joshua, Justin Elliott, Brett Murphy, and Alex Mierjeski. "The Supreme Court Has Adopted a Conduct Code, but Who Will Enforce It?" ProPublica, November 13, 2023.

Kim, Seung Min. "Biden Vows Abortion Legislation as Top Priority next Year." Associated Press, October 18, 2022.

Kirkpatrick, David D. "The Next Targets for the Group That Overturned Roe." *New Yorker*, October 2, 2023.

Kitchener, Caroline, Rachel Roubein, Andrew Ba Tran, Caitlin Gilbert, and Hannah Dormido. "A Fragile New Phase of Abortion in America." *Washington Post*, June 22, 2023.

Marquez, Alexandra. "New Kentucky Governor Ad Features Rape Victim Criticizing GOP on Abortion Exceptions." NBC News, September 20, 2023.

Mauer, Craig. "Democrats Win Control of Michigan Legislature for 1st Time in Decades." *Detroit Free Press*, November 9, 2022.

Perez, Andrew. "Leonard Leo's Fight Against Abortion Access." *The Lever*, October 27, 2023.

Public Religion Research Institute. "Abortion Attitudes in a Post-Roe World: Findings from the 50-State 2022 American Values Atlas." February 23, 2023.

Rascoe, Ayesha. "In States with Abortion Bans, Hospital Ethics Boards Have the Power to Make Exceptions." NPR, March 12, 2023.

Saad, Lydia. "Broader Support for Abortion Rights Continues Post-Dobbs." Gallup, June 14, 2023.

Santhanam, Laura. "Support for Abortion Rights Has Grown in Spite of Bans and Restrictions, Poll Shows." *PBS NewsHour*, April 26, 2023.

Schoenfeld Walker, Amy, and Allison McCann. "Abortions Rose in Most States This Year, New Data Shows." *New York Times*, September 7, 2023.

Smith, Peter. "Evangelical Conservatives Cheer One of Their Own as Mike Johnson Assumes Congress' Most Powerful Seat." Associated Press, October 27, 2023.

Surana, Kavitha. "Their States Banned Abortion. Doctors Now Say They Can't Give Women Potential Lifesaving Care." ProPublica, February 26, 2024.

Surana, Kavitha. "'We Need to Defend This Law': Inside an Anti-Abortion Meeting With Tennessee's GOP Lawmakers." ProPublica and *WPLN*, November 15, 2022.

Wells, Kate. "Abortion Rights Opponents Sue to Overturn Prop 3." Michigan Public, November 8, 2023.

36: WHAT IS A WOMAN?

Andrews, Helena. "The Lady Prefers 'Congressman.'" *Politico*, April 15, 2008.

French, Lauren. "House Plans Special Committee to Probe Planned Parenthood." *Politico*, September 28, 2015.

Goodman, J. David. "Texas Supreme Court Rules Against Woman Who Sought Court-Approved Abortion." *New York Times*, December 11, 2023.

Klibanoff, Eleanor. "Kate Cox's Case Reveals How Far Texas Intends to Go to Enforce Abortion Laws." *Texas Tribune*, December 13, 2023.

Liptak, Adam. "Justice Jackson, a Former Law Clerk, Returns to a Transformed Supreme Court." *New York Times*, July 18, 2022.

Smith, Tracy. "Texas Mother Kate Cox on the Outcome of Her Legal Fight for an Abortion: 'It Was Crushing.'" CBS News, January 14, 2024.

Zornosa, Laura. "Ruth Bader Ginsburg's 'Dissent Collar' Donated to the Smithsonian." *New York Times*, March 30, 2022.

MARCH 2023: LAS CRUCES, NEW MEXICO

Boodman, Eric. "The 'Abortion Queen' Wants Patients to Have 'Skin in the Game.' Is That Restricting Access?" *Stat News*, October 11, 2023.

Bragg, Rick. "Bomb Kills Guard at an Alabama Abortion Clinic." *New York Times*, January 30, 1998.

McCann, Allison, and Amy Schoenfeld Walker. "One Year, 61 Clinics: How Dobbs Changed the Abortion Landscape." *New York Times*, June 22, 2023.

McCullough, Jolie. "After Losing Battle to Preserve Roe v. Wade, Mississippi's Last Abortion Clinic Is Moving to New Mexico." *Texas Tribune*, June 29, 2022.

McDevitt, Michael, and Leah Romero. "Mississippi Abortion Clinic at Center of Supreme Court Case Is Moving to New Mexico, Drawing Hundreds in Protest." *Las Cruces Sun-News*, July 20, 2022.

Nave, R. L. "Inside the Abortion Clinic Battle." *Jackson Free Press*, August 1, 2012.

Totiyapungprasert, Priscilla, and Victoria Rossi. "Las Cruces Becomes a Battleground in National Abortion Fight." *El Paso Matters*, July 21, 2022.

Wagster Pettus, Emily. "Abortion Clinic Owner Committed Despite Pressure." Associated Press, November 23, 2013.
Whitehead, Sam. "Abortion Is Just the Latest Dividing Line between the Twin Cities of Bristol and Bristol." *KFF Health News*, August 17, 2022.